Sociology and Health Care

For Laura and Ewan

For Churchill Livingstone:

Editorial Director: Mary Law
Project Development Manager: Ellen Green
Project Editor: Dinah Thom
Editor: Valerie Bain
Production Controller: Neil Dickson
Sales Promotion Executive: Hilary Brown

Sociology and Health Care

An Introduction for Nurses and other Health Care Professionals

John Bond BA

Reader in Social Gerontology, Centre for Health Services Research, The University of Newcastle upon Tyne, Newcastle, UK

Senga Bond PhD MSc BA RGN FRCN

Senior Lecturer in Nursing Research, Centre for Health Services Research, The University of Newcastle upon Tyne, Newcastle, UK

SECOND EDITION

CHURCHILL LIVINGSTONE
EDINBURGH LONDON MADRID MELBOURNE NEW YORK AND TOKYO 1994

CHURCHILL LIVINGSTONE
Medical Division of Longman Group UK Limited

Distributed in the United States of America by
Churchill Livingstone Inc., 650 Avenue of the Americas,
New York, N.Y. 10011, and by associated companies,
branches and representatives throughout the world.

First edition 1986
Reprinted 1988, 1989, 1990(twice), 1991, 1992
Second edition 1994

ISBN 0-443-04059-1

British Library Cataloguing in Publication Data
A catalogue record for this book is available from the British
Library.

Library of Congress Cataloging in Publication Data
A catalog record for this book is available from the Library of
Congress.

Produced by Longman Singapore Publishers Pte Ltd
Printed in Singapore

Contents

Contents

Preface to second edition

As the initial professional education of nurses and others allied to medicine increasingly becomes integrated into higher education there will be a tendency to increase the liberal arts and social science components of the curriculum and decrease the amount of clinical experience. Justification of this move rests on producing generations of practitioners who are able more effectively to apply knowledge drawn from diverse sources, both to understand their work and carry it out. Sociology is one such source of knowledge relevant to all of those who are engaged in the production of health and the alleviation of ill health.

In this second and long overdue edition of this introductory text on sociology written for health professionals, we have more or less kept to the same formula and structure as in the first edition, but have changed some of the emphases and updated the content where required. We have introduced the ideas of critical theorists and made more of feminist theory throughout. Since writing the first edition, the National Health Service and the delivery of health care has changed in a number of ways. While high-technology medicine continues to expand, community services have been transferred to Local Authority management and much long-term care has been transferred out of the public sector. There has been a cultural change from administration to management, with increased emphasis on value for money, a split between the purchasers of health services and their providers, and a nod towards consumerism. The profile of equal opportunities has been raised while changes remain to be demonstrated.

Despite these developments in an increasingly dynamic society, many of the issues, and certainly the underlying social structures, remain unchanged. Thus, we have again stressed issues like social class, unemployment and health inequalities, and gender and status effects in social life. We have also retained our stress on appreciating the implicit and explicit theoretical basis of sociological research and the knowledge which it generates. Without such an emphasis sociology would be reduced to an assortment of unconnected and insignificant facts.

In producing this second edition we owe a debt of gratitude to many of our colleagues at the Centre for Health Services Research: Freda Bolam, Debbie Buck, Wendy Clarke, Maureen Craig, Barbara Ingman, Jessie Rogers and Shirley Walworth who edited our work, produced diagrams and coped with the references. The tedious job of proof reading was cheerfully assisted by Sarah Grabham, Janet Storrie and Madeline Tyers, along with many cups of coffee. We sorely tried the patience of our publishers, and their goodwill is acknowledged here.

Finally, we have dedicated this book to our children, Laura and Ewan, in recognition not only of the parental deprivation they have endured during its production but also of their reminders of the things in life which matter most.

Hexham, Northumberland, 1994   J.B.
S.B.

Preface to first edition

We have written this book to provide an introduction to sociology, particularly sociology relevant to health and illness, for members of the health care professions. Its intention is to develop a sociological awareness which will assist health professionals to understand the social basis of much of their work and to use sociology to ask appropriate questions, consider relevant factors and provide workable solutions to some of their problems. Because a number of texts already exist which are devoted to medical sociology or written with a bias towards doctors we have written for a readership we regard as principally nurses, midwives, health visitors and remedial therapists, although some of the material has been used to teach doctors.

The approach we have taken differs from that of texts which already exist to serve this readership and we have tried to go beyond them to provide a grounding in the mainstream of sociological theory, albeit still at an introductory level.

Sociology is included in the curriculum of most health professionals. As long ago as 1968 the Royal Commission on Medical Education recommended that all medical students should pursue studies of sociology. Since then it has been included in the curriculum of other health professionals, though with varying degrees of explicitness. This has allowed sociology to be taught as just 'common sense'. One of the purposes of this book is to demonstrate that sociology is more than just 'common sense' and to provide some ideas about how the subject matter may be taught.

While meeting curriculum requirements is important, we feel that there are more fundamental reasons for health professionals acquiring some knowledge of sociology. Of particular importance is gaining an understanding of the social changes taking place – for example, in the age structure, marriage patterns, the types of illness being treated, patient expectations, the organisation and structure of professions – all of which have implications for the work of health professionals. We recognise the relevance of broad social changes and changes more directly relevant to health and illness, but it is also important to consider why other social features, such as the structure of British society, are relatively enduring, and to consider their implications for health. Because the delivery of health care is essentially a social activity, gaining an understanding of the social processes involved should prove useful in caring for patients and their families. This is equally relevant for social interaction with colleagues, supervisors and subordinates, and all of those with whom health professionals deal in the course of their work. A sociological understanding should help us to appreciate why people indulge in particular behaviour or take particular decisions, and why differences exist between individuals and groups in relation to health and illness. In writing this book we have tried to avoid an over-simplistic approach while recognising that some readers will be coming to sociology for the first time. We assume that readers will be critical, generally interested in society and examining it from a number of perspectives. We have therefore introduced a range of sociological perspectives which necessitate asking different questions about the social world and include some of the debates which exist between those favouring one approach or another. We have tried to be eclectic but inevitably personal biases are evident.

We have also attempted to take account of readers's likely knowledge and interests, using examples which will be familiar to some and giving them less explicit definition than would be required by a lay readership. British sources are drawn on heavily since this is the system of state health provision with which the majority of readers are likely to be familiar. Many issues, however, are of international significance; sometimes no British work is available to illustrate a point and, because American theorists are currently so influential in medical and mainstream sociology, we have referred to many of their studies.

We have selected issues which we consider are of concern to health professionals generally. Inevitably personal interests also influence selection and emphasis. The authors are: a sociologist working in health care research with a bias towards structuralist sociology (JB); and a nurse with a background in psychology but with leanings toward interactionist sociology (SB). This may help to explain the emphasis given to social structure and the heavy use of nursing sources, with a whole chapter devoted to death, dying and bereavement. We have taken account of comments from other sociologists and health professionals and we have attempted to provide a balanced set of chapters while introducing such topical issues as unemployment and health, and managerialism in nursing.

The book is divided into 13 chapters, the first of which constitutes an introduction to the subject and points out some of the distinctive features of sociology as an autonomous and vital discipline within the social sciences, and how it is relevant to health care. The idea of different perspectives in sociology is taken up in Chapter 2. We identify some major theories and concepts used in different interpretations of society. The idea that there exist a variety of sociological perspectives is carried forward throughout the book and we demonstrate how they have contributed in relevant ways to identifying problems in the health field, adding to

our understanding of them and offering solutions for them.

Chapter 3 focuses on a major aspect of social structure, namely social stratification and the concept of class, status and power. The chapter reviews briefly inequalities in the health status of different social groups and presents some of the competing explanations of inequalities in health.

Chapter 4 expands on some of the themes introduced in Chapter 3 by exploring social influences on health and the role of prevention. It examines broad structural influences in society on health and illness, using the example of the production and consumption of food, and describes a social model of the causes of illness. Chapter 5 introduces the concept of the life career and focuses on the nature of the family in different cultures and subcultures. It discusses the functions of the family in modern Britain. In Chapter 6, the role of the family in the maintenance of health and at times of illness is discussed. A review of family care and community care is provided.

Chapter 7 focuses on the concepts of institution and organisation by examining the stucture of and behaviour in health care organisations. It explores competing approaches to the study of organisations, highlighting the strengths and weaknesses of each for the study of health care organisations.

Chapter 8 is concerned with the patient career and introduces the concepts of deviance and labelling. The processes experienced by people when becoming patients are discussed. The medical model of disease and the social model of illness are described and two models of illness behaviour are explored.

Chapter 9 focuses on interaction between health professionals and their clients. It draws on some ideas introduced in Chapter 7 on role and negotiation and in Chapter 8 on the patient career. The important idea that professionals respond to patients as a limited number of types is developed and the chapter concludes by considering interaction in relation to the management of pain.

This is followed, in Chapter 10, by sociological aspects of death, dying and bereavement. This topic has only recently achieved prominence in the education of health professionals and the sociological literature remains relatively sparse. We give attention to definitions of dying and to social processes which surround death, particularly in institutions. As a case example, we focus on miscarriage, still birth, and perinatal death.

In Chapter 11, we turn our attention to the professional career, with an emphasis on how lay persons are socialised through their formal and informal education to become professionals. How different sociological perspectives deal with the theme of professional socialisation is discussed. We conclude the chapter with an examination of the relationship between gender and profession.

Our penultimate chapter revives the theme of sociological perspectives. Chapter 12 is devoted to an examination of methods of sociological research and presents this in relation to perspectives and the knowledge base of sociology. Research on suicide is used as a means of demonstrating that different perspectives raise different kinds of sociological questions and finding answers to these questions is done in different ways. We advocate a position of methodological pluralism.

Finally, we provide an overview of the contribution we think that sociology can make to health professionals as they go about their work and, more generally, to society. To this end we appeal to ways of using and producing sociological knowledge in the field of health care.

Every chapter stands on its own, but it is important to grasp the major ideas of different sociological perspectives outlined in Chapter 2 in order to appreciate fully subsequent chapters. Major concepts are introduced at the first most appropriate place throughout the book. It is logical therefore to read from the beginning. A glossary is provided to assist the understanding of unfamiliar sociological concepts.

We are aware of the offence caused to some people by the sexist nature of the English language. When the book was first drafted we attempted to use male and female pronouns in alternate chapters when the gender of the referent was not relevant. This proved too confusing and so we have had to revert to using, where possible, plurals and nongender words. We have, however, tended to refer to female health professonals since he/she, or worse (s)he is cumbersome.

The preparation of this book was greatly assisted by the help we received from a number of people, in particular the painstaking comments made on an early draft by Malcolm Colledge, Helen Evers, Eileen Fairhurst, Marion Ferguson, David O'Brien, Rex Taylor and Jean Walker. We have drawn extensively on the work of some authors; notably Berger and Berger whose approach to writing an introductory text influenced our style, Cuff and Payne whose work influenced Chapter 2, and Dingwall and Lewis whose reader on the sociology of the professions made a timely arrival when Chapter 11 was being rewritten. Rik Walton of Newcastle Polytechnic took many of the photographs for us and Margaret Derby, Malcolm Sellers and Graham Walton proved to be effective librarians. We would particularly like to thank Eva Brown who typed and retyped the manuscript and Joyce Crawley who assisted in preparing the references.

We have found writing this book an arduous task but we, and our students, have gained enormously from the labour. Its eventual appearance is in no small way due to the patience of our publishers.

Newcastle upon Tyne, 1986 J.B.,S.B.

Acknowledgements

We are grateful to the following for permission to reproduce copyright material: the author W. Wallace and Aldine Publishing Co for Figure 12.2; the authors E. C. Cuff and G. C. F. Payne and George Allen and Unwin Ltd for Figure 2.1; the authors S. V. Kasl and S. Cobb and *Archives of Environmental Health* for Figure 8.5; the author R. Dingwall and Basil Blackwell for Figure 8.6; the authors G. W. Brown, J. L. T. Birley and J. K. Wing and *The British Journal of Psychiatry* for Figure 6.1; the Economist for Table 11.1; the Controller of Her Majesty's Stationary Office for Figures 10.1, 12.3 and Tables 3.4–3.8, 12.2; the authors G. Marshall, H. Newby, D. Rose and C. Vogler and Hutchinson Books Ltd for Figure 3.3; the author A. Antonovsky and Jossey-Bass Ltd for Figure 4.4; the author A. Cartwright and the *Journal of Public Health Medicine* for Table 10.1; Laing and Buisson for Figure 13.1; the author J. M. Atkinson and Macmillan Ltd for Table 12.1; the author L. Prior and Macmillan Ltd for Table 10.5; *Nursing Standard* for Figure 10.2; the author P. Armitage and *Nursing Times* for Table 7.1; the author T. Griffin and the Office of Health Economics for Figure 10.2; the author W. Worsley and Penguin Books Ltd for Figure 5.2; the author C. Seale and *Social Science and Medicine* for Table 10.4; the authors E. J. Miller and G. V. Gwynne and Tavistock Publications for Figure 7.3; the author E. O. Wright and Verso Publications Ltd for Figure 3.2.

We are also grateful to the following for permission to reproduce photographic material: Derek Bayes and Dame Cicely Saunders; BBC Hulton Picture Library; Calderstones Hospital; City and Hackney Community Health Council; Department of Environmental and Occupational Medicine, University of Newcastle upon Tyne; Hexham Courant; Nursing Mirror; Nursing Standard; Nursing Times; University of Chicago Library.

1

Sociology and health care

Sociology is a relatively recent addition to the syllabuses of health care professionals; yet appreciation of the interrelationship between aspects of the society in which we live and the health of the population is not new. Indeed, the very early social surveys by Rowntree (1901) and Booth (1892, 1894) showed that ill health was related to poverty and one of the early classic works in sociology took death, in the form of suicide, as its subject (Durkheim 1952, first published in French in 1897). As our views about the nature of health and health care evolve, and the interconnectedness of features of our existence become apparent, so the range of knowledge relevant to the work of health professionals increases. This expansion means that more and more subjects jostle for inclusion in professional education, each competing for time in the curriculum. Sociology, itself a relatively recent discipline, is one such subject.

To some the inclusion of sociology is regarded as unnecessary because it is nothing more than 'common sense'. That some people view sociology in this way is not surprising given that sociology is the study of society and all of us know a great deal about the society in which we live and work. It is by virtue of our being social animals that we give particular meanings to everything and everyone we experience. Long before we understand the word 'sociology' we are already taking for granted much of what are the central concerns of sociology. It is this early introduction to some of the subject matter which makes sociology appear to be nothing more than 'common sense' by comparison with quantum physics or neurophysiology. In writing this book we believe, and will try to show, that sociology is more than common sense and may contradict common-sense views. For example, a common-sense belief is that since there will be unhappy people in all societies, suicide rates will be similar throughout the world. In fact, suicide rates vary enormously between even European societies, with the suicide rate in the United Kingdom being 4 times as high as in Spain but only a $\frac{1}{3}$ that of France (Charlton et al 1993). While common-sense ideas provide insights about our social world, sociologists must always be prepared to ask whether *this is really so*. While challenging common sense, sociology at the same time, like all disciplines, adds to what we regard as common sense. We know that both divorce rates and the number of married women with young children who are in employment have greatly increased since the Second World War. These facts, which are part of our common-sense knowledge, are based on the regular research of sociologists.

Learning to think sociologically, however, is not just about routine processes of acquiring knowledge: it is a particular way of interpreting the world. Developing an understanding of sociology is fundamental to a deeper understanding of the society in which we live and this is an important feature of professional knowledge. What, then, is sociology?

A SOCIOLOGICAL UNDERSTANDING

Often, introductory text books in sociology begin by posing the question 'What is sociology?'. This can be answered in a number of different ways. One is to say what sociology is not.

Sometimes it is confused with social work. But social work is not sociology although, like other caring professions, social workers may use the findings of sociological studies to help them understand aspects of their work. Social work offers a practical approach to the solution of social problems. This is not to say that social problems do not interest sociologists, for they

do. However, sociology is not only about what some regard as social problems but is about understanding what is ordinary and taken for granted in the wider universe of social activity in which we are all involved.

It is our view that sociology is about understanding the human social world, its social life, groups and societies, by examining it from particular perspectives. By focusing on the social world we distinguish it from the purely personal or private world of each of us; between what Mills (1970) calls society's public issues and individuals' private troubles. Private troubles occur within an individual's experience, resulting from personal characteristics or from relationships with others. Public issues, on the other hand, transcend the experiences of a single individual. They are concerned with the ways in which individuals' experiences overlap to form some wider fabric of social organisation (Mills 1970). Sociology does not deny or diminish the reality of individual experience but helps us understand and obtain a richer awareness of our own and others' individual characteristics, by developing a sensitivity towards the wider social activity in which we are all involved.

Let us consider a female student nurse in these terms. During her initial education she will experience a number of troubles. Examples of such troubles, which are sufficiently important to prompt individual nurses to leave nursing, may be poor staff relations, late notification of off-duty, absence of ward teaching, lack of someone to talk to, being physically tired out, or having to do night duty (Birch 1975, Mackay 1989). By attending to the problems of an individual nurse one may find some successful solution for her. However, in a school where 1- in-3 learners do not complete their training this represents a public issue, where solutions are found not so much in the characteristics of the individual student nurses but in the structure and functioning of the organisation, be it the educational or the clinical settings in which students receive their education. Effective actions to remedy the situation are likely to be oriented toward the institution and its organisation rather than individual student nurses or indeed individual teachers or ward sisters. It is to public issues or social issues that sociologists turn their attention. This involves a whole range of subject matter, from passing encounters between individuals in the street to global social processes.

Sociology and other social sciences

Sociology is one of a range of disciplines called the social sciences, which include psychology, anthropology, economics, politics and history. But can we really study social life in the same way as other sciences like chemistry or physics? The answer is both yes and no. All sciences use theory and systematic methods of investigation with logical assessment of argument to develop a body of knowledge. That knowledge, however, remains tentative and open to being revised or discarded in the light of new evidence or argument. The publication of findings and the criticism of these findings by other members of the scientific community is common to all sciences. To this extent sociology is the same as every other science.

But sociology differs from other sciences in the extent to which it can generate precise laws and predictions that have been developed by natural scientists about the physical world. This is because social science studies human beings in the social world and deals with activities which are meaningful to those involved. Unlike physical objects and chemical compounds, humans are self-aware and confer meaning, sense and purpose. Even engaging in describing social life accurately depends on grasping the meaning that people apply to their behaviour. For example, to describe a death as a suicide depends on learning the intention of the individual when he or she was killed, and ascertaining that the death was willed by the person involved. That we cannot study human beings in the same way as physical objects offers advantages as well as difficulties. On the one hand, sociologists can ask questions of those they study and gain their perspective on events. On the other hand, those who are the subjects of

sociological studies may react in different and atypical ways to being studied, both to assist the researcher or to obstruct or subvert the study. In this way, social sciences differ from natural sciences.

How then does a *sociological* understanding differ from that provided by the other social sciences? All social sciences, are concerned with human action or behaviour, but they differ in the particular attributes of behaviour they study. Consider the Stock Exchange as an example. In everyday life the Stock Exchange may not be particularly important to you. Yet, like events in Parliament and Prime Minister's Question Time, the daily financial report on Radio 4 is a British institution. Whereas journalists are interested in reporting the daily events of the Stock Exchange and quoting the Financial Times Index, our social science colleagues would have a broader perspective. Historians would be interested in the influences on its development and economists would study the process of economic transactions through share dealing. Psychologists might study risk-taking behaviour among brokers while sociologists would be concerned with the nature and variety of human relationships and interactions and may pay particular attention to the recent admission of women or the effects of new technology. They might want to describe the power and prestige of the different kinds of participants, and this can be done with only marginal reference to economics, history or psychology.

The above example illustrates the different interests of the social sciences, yet in one sense all social sciences are alike because they rely on providing knowledge about the world in a scientific way. That is, the statements they make about the world can be tested and verified empirically. While this basic scientific rationale provides a common grounding for asking essential questions about the validity of explanations, the social sciences differ in the concepts they use, the kinds of questions they pose about the world, the methods they use to answer the questions and the kinds of solutions or explanations they provide. They differ also in the kinds of assumptions they hold about the world and this influences the problems they select for study. For example, a major field of interest in psychology is individual differences – examining whether these are related to differences in genetic make-up, personality, intelligence or environment. Psychologists spend a great deal of effort in trying to tease out the genetic as compared with the environmental influences on human behaviour. Sociologists, on the other hand, generally assume that human action is culturally and socially shaped rather than genetically determined. While appreciating a genetic influence, they would be unlikely to explore individual differences from this perspective. Their interest lies in exploring how social life and the organisation of society influences and is influenced by individuals and groups, be it the society of which they are themselves members or a different one.

The kinds of questions social scientists ask about the world depend on the concepts and the theories they use. It is the way that concepts and theories are used that gives each social science, and indeed other sciences, their distinctive approach to the subject matter they study. As you read this book you will come across many of the major concepts and theories of sociology. Indeed, it is only through grasping and working with these concepts and theories as they are used in sociology that you will begin to develop a sociological understanding.

In order to achieve a sociological understanding we must suspend our taken-for-granted assumptions and take account of the variety of meanings of actions and events, which can be interpreted or explained in different ways by people who hold different perspectives. For example, one health education campaign was mounted on the assumption that the reason for women not attending for antenatal care was that they were unaware of the risks of postponing medical care. Yet studies which have asked women for their views report that women attend for antenatal care later than advised by obstetricians for a whole host of reasons. These reasons range from covering up the pregnancy because of the stigma of illegitimacy to the inconvenience of clinic appointments (Garcia

1982). However, the official explanation blames the ignorance of patients without considering women's understanding of and rational response to their pregnancy or the organisation of health services.

Consider also the issue of wearing cheap disposable paper face masks to carry out aseptic techniques. This practice continues in many hospitals. The official explanation is that it reduces the chance of hospital staff passing on potentially harmful microorganisms from their noses and mouths to patients and of inhaling microorganisms from patients. There is a mass of evidence, however, which shows that these particular masks provide a totally ineffective barrier; and when no such infection is present there is no point in wearing them anyway (Rogers 1981). Why then do some hospital workers, despite the evidence, continue to dress up in this ritualistic way? Many other rituals exist (Ford & Walsh 1990), such as nurses in the United Kingdom continuing to wear decorative caps and dresses while their North American counterparts often wear trousers as do physiotherapists in Britain. Why do they want to, and why do hospitals want to hold on to their own distinctive caps when mergers occur? Why do some groups continue to wear a specific uniform rather than the ubiquitous white coat worn by many other health workers?

Despite the recognition of the importance of parents staying overnight with young children who must be in hospital (Central Health Services Council 1959), why do some places still not readily offer accommodation? What makes some parents feel uncomfortable about staying with their child?

Posing questions like these to different kinds of people is likely to yield different answers and the official response as given by the organisation's officials is not necessarily the only or most helpful explanation of what is happening.

It is by addressing questions about social issues like those just mentioned that a sociological understanding of them emerges. An explanation of how this is done is given by Berger (1966) in his book *Invitation to Sociology*. He uses the analogy of the puppet theatre to represent

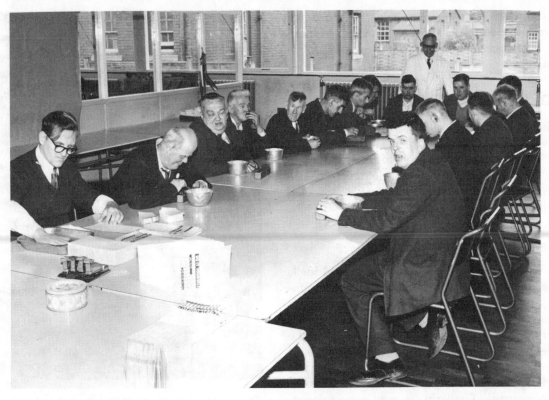

Fig. 1.1 Men with learning disabilities confined in an institution with their days filled doing repetitive activities (courtesy of Calderstone Hospital).

the actions of individuals in society (Berger 1966, p. 199). In a puppet theatre we can see the puppets dancing on their stage. We can see and know that they dance because the strings control their actions. In a similar way individuals in any society also obey a variety of rules. Some of these are practical, like driving on the left-hand side of the road, which has become law. Others have less obvious practical implications but have always existed, for example the fact that in Britain men and women marry only one spouse at a time. We know that this is not a universal form of social organisation for in some societies men may have more than one wife, while in others women may have more than one husband. Yet in our society we rarely challenge such a basic rule as 'one spouse at a time'. Those who do so create news. Even the increasing

numbers of cohabiting couples do not appear to challenge this rule. By responding to social rules, all of us are very much akin to the puppets. Unlike puppets, however, we have the possibility of stopping, standing outside our stage and becoming a member of the audience. In the audience we begin to see how our society works – how rules develop and are maintained or change. Of course, as with the puppet theatre, different members of the audience will perceive different explanations of why things are as they are. Yet to be able to ask questions and provide answers, about the forms of social organisations around us, such as the family, the political system or our working environment, we require a sociological understanding. It must be clear that such an understanding of our own society is not the monopoly of sociologists; we would recommend it to anyone who is concerned about the society of which they are a part. That, of course, includes all health care professionals.

SOCIOLOGY ON OFFER

What specifically does sociology have to offer the health professions? There are two kinds of sociological data which are relevant. First, there are data collected through sociology *in* health care and, second, there are data collected through a sociology *of* health care.

Sociology in health care

These data reflect the use of sociological ideas related to practice, client groups or professionals in ways that can be used by planners. For example, sociological concepts and methods were used in research commissioned by the Briggs Committee (Report of the Committee on Nursing 1972) and included a survey of the social characteristics of practising and nonpractising nurses. Similarly, it was a sociologist, Celia Davies, who drew together and interpreted the available evidence to produce the discussion papers which led to more recent developments in nurse education and the reforms of Project 2000 (UKCC 1986). We have recently studied the social and demographic characteristics of the providers of nursing care to frail elderly people in institutions as well as their views of their work and those they care for (Bond & Bond 1993). These studies, using sociological concepts and methods, reflect the concern of NHS management and policy makers with problems of the labour force and wastage as well as the quality of care and provide information as a basis for managing the service.

Health planners also make use of sociological knowledge in health care. Sociologists (Goffman 1961, Townsend 1962) carried out important studies of what happens to people who live in large groups in hospitals or asylums. For many years, people with mental illness and mental handicap, as well as frail elderly people, have been cared for in dehumanising institutions

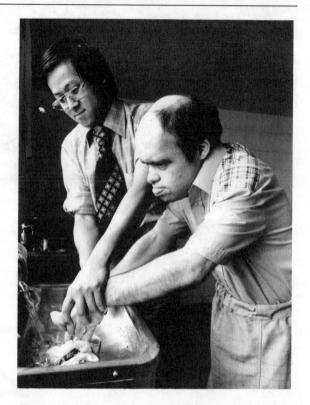

Fig. 1.2 Learning self-care skills to prepare for discharge from an institution (courtesy of Nursing Mirror).

(Fig. 1.1). Indeed, many continue to be housed in such environments. It was discovered that, in time, they learn particular ways of behaving, a process which has come to be known as institutionalisation. In our society most people do not live in large groups, nor are they confined to spending most of their days and nights within the institution (children at boarding schools, prisoners and closed religious orders being exceptions). We usually live in small groups – in families or with flatmates – and, as well as carrying out many activities with them, we go out to work and leisure in a range of different environments and meet different groups of people. While knowledge of the deleterious effects of institutional care has been around for a long time, it is only comparatively recently that health planners have used this knowledge in planning services. The move to community care for those groups which were formerly warehoused in institutions rests in part upon this knowledge and in part upon an economic analysis of the costs of different care environments. 'Normalising' the lives of those who have spent many years in institutions has resulted in them increasingly being cared for in small groups, living in ordinary housing in towns and villages and being encouraged to participate in local activities (Fig. 1.2). Yet an absence of employment opportunities means that many remain on the margins of society (Booth, Simons & Booth 1990).

Sociology of health care

In contrast, a sociology of health care has been concerned with analysis of providers of health care and what they have provided. A good example of this is Freidson's extended analysis of the medical profession (Freidson 1975). Towell (1976), Dingwall (1977) and Melia (1987) provide similar analyses of different nursing groups in the United Kingdom. Towell studied the way in which psychiatric nursing students became psychiatric nurses in a hospital which used different types of treatment in different wards. Dingwall studied the everyday world of health visiting, in order to provide insights into how nurses learn to do health visiting, while Melia examined students' accounts of their initial preparation for nursing. The insights which such studies provide frequently challenge the assumptions that health care professionals themselves hold about their own occupations.

The sociology of health care has also considered the practice of health care as social action. One of us (SB) undertook a study to examine communication processes in a radiotherapy department. This study examined the processes by which patients came to interpret their illness, going beyond what they were told or not told about it by hospital staff. The study also examined what nurses believed and assumed to be true about patients and how this influenced their communication practices (Bond 1978).

Kratz (1978), in her study of the care of the long-term sick in the community, also added to

our knowledge of the different ways that district nurses manage stroke patients by identifying how they implicitly categorise them. It is by using sociological theory and methods that a fresh perspective is obtained which aids our understanding of the way that health care is practised in a whole variety of settings.

Sociology in health care refers to those concerned with policy and planning using sociological concepts and methods to collect data to assist them in their work. It means applying sociological insights to policy and planning of the health services and the education of the workforce. *Sociology of health care* is about developing a sociological understanding of health providers and their practices. This is typically the work of professional sociologists and is embedded in sociological theory. It is the function of sociologists to yield this knowledge not only to fellow sociologists but to those who are the 'objects of study' – health professionals as well as lay carers and the recipients of health care.

Both types of study are used in developing this text with the objective of making links between sociologically derived knowledge and features of the social world that are encountered by health professionals.

A SOCIOLOGICAL ALTERNATIVE

As well as providing sociological data which has relevance for the organisation of the health professions and their practices, *sociology also offers other ways of viewing and explaining health care and health problems.*

The medical model

The traditional and generally accepted view of the health field is that improvements in health and the quality of health care are attributable to the art and science of medicine. This has become characterised as the medical or biomedical model of health. The link between health and the medical care system was created and is maintained by the powerful image of the role of medicine in the eradication of infections and parasitic diseases, advances in surgery, the application of technology and new drugs, and lowered infant mortality rates. The result of this orientation is an emphasis on the treatment of illness by medical means rather than on health or normality.

This emphasis is reflected in the education of health care workers, where curricula tend to be based on diseases according to medical specialties, and allocations for clinical experience similarly are organised around medical specialties. Such teaching often takes disease or ill health, rather than health or normality, as its starting point. Historically, it is easy to see why this is so. The history of medicine is full of examples of abnormality being presented to physicians, whose main endeavours have been in developing methods of treatment and in seeking causes within biological functioning. For this reason, preventing ill health has always run a very poor second to treating ill health, and medicine has dominated other groups, like sanitary workers and health visitors, whose primary task is prevention. Hospital-based medicine is similarly more prestigious than public health medicine which has a higher content linked to prevention.

The social model

The emphases of sociological perspectives of health and illness are on such aspects of health care as rehabilitation, prevention of illness and the social management of illness, rather than on biological and medical aspects of health care. This approach has become known as the social model of health. It contributes an understanding of illness and disease by pointing up the social rather than the biological contexts. A useful sociological model would illuminate how social processes work in defining illness, in understanding the causes of illness and promotion of health or in interpreting the organisational structures within the health care system. By 'model' we mean here a theoretical representation of reality.

An important distinction between medical and social models lies in the very definition of illness. The medical model defines patients as ill when they have certain biological and physiological signs. For example, when haemoglobin reaches a certain low level the patient is judged as anaemic and treatment advised. One very elderly women, who still managed and enjoyed going out for rides in her son's car, was thought very pale by her district nurse. A blood sample was taken and the resulting haemoglobin level was 6g/dl – less than half the desirable level. Her general practitioner urged her to have a blood transfusion. The old woman did not feel ill or incapacitated, and her lifestyle was not being interfered with by her poor blood chemistry. By her definition she was not ill and so she wanted nothing to do with blood transfusions. Her interpretation, unlike that of her doctor and nurse, was based not on medical criteria but on social criteria.

This description of medical and social models emphasises different aspects of health and illness. However, they provide complementary explanations, rather than alternative explanations. A good example of the value of both models is McKeown's historical analysis of improvements in health in England and Wales. McKeown (1979) concluded that the major contributions to improvements in health since the 18th century were, in order of importance, limitation in family size, an increase in food supplies, a healthier physical environment and specific preventive and therapeutic measures. He predicts that:

> Improvement in health is likely to come
> in the future, as in the past, from modification
> of the conditions which lead to
> disease, rather than from intervention in the
> mechanism of disease after it has occurred
> (McKeown 1979, p. 198).

The health field concept

Lalonde, as Canada's Minister of Health and Welfare, explicitly incorporated McKeown's ideas in his *health field concept*, which draws on medical and social models of health and illness. In this, health is attributed to four main elements: Human Biology, Environment, Lifestyle and Health Care Organisation (Lalonde 1974).

Human biology

The human biology element includes those aspects of mental and physical health which are a direct consequence of the basic biology of the individual. These include genetic inheritance, processes of maturation and ageing, and the complex biological systems of the human organism. The health implications of our complex biology are enormous and include malfunctions, chronic and degenerative diseases and genetic disorders.

Environment

In the environmental element Lalonde includes all those matters related to health which are external to the human body and over which the individual has little or no personal control. These include ensuring that food, drugs, cosmetics and the water supply are safe and uncontaminated, that the health hazards of all forms of pollution are controlled, that the spread of communicable diseases is prevented, that effective disposal of sewage is carried out and that the social environment, including rapid social change, does not have harmful effects on health.

Lifestyle

The lifestyle category in the health field concept includes those decisions made by individuals themselves, which have implications for their health. These include what we choose to eat, whether and how we exercise, our use of additive substances and how we get about. Many habits and decisions create self-imposed risks to health, and when illness or death results it is attributable to the victim's own lifestyle.

Health care organisation

Health care organisation consists of 'the quantity, quality, arrangement, nature and relation-

ships of people and resources in the provision of health care' (Lalonde 1974, p. 32). This is usually referred to as the health care system and includes medical practice, nursing, paramedical practice, hospitals, nursing homes, prescribed drugs, community health care, ambulance and dental services, as well as other health services such as chiropody, homoeopathy and osteopathy.

Lalonde contends that most of society's efforts to improve health, and the bulk of direct health expenditure, have been focused on this fourth element of the health field concept: health care organisation. Yet when the causes of ill health are examined they are rooted in the other three elements. In effect, we continue to promote an illness service rather than a health service. The health field concept, with its emphasis on four analytically separate yet complementary components, radically changes a perspective on health away from both health care organisation and the dominant medical model to one which is far more comprehensive as well as analytic. This is brought home by recent analysis which advocates that the way to improve the health problems and reduce the high fertility of developing countries is by increasing the education given to the women of these countries.

There is sometimes a tendency to regard the medical and social models as alternatives, presenting an either/or viewpoint regarding the appropriate way to conceptualise health concerns. By incorporating the social dimension into Lalonde's health field concept we can see more clearly that elements make differential contributions and will interact in different ways. The underlying causes of death from road-traffic accidents can be found in risks taken by individuals, with lesser importance given to the design and composition of cars and roads, and less again to the availability of emergency treatment. Human biology makes little contribution to causation in this area. When lifestyle factors are identified the risks taken by individuals can be considered under such headings as impaired driving, carelessness, failure to wear seat belts, or speeding. Impaired driving would include the effects of alcohol or drug abuse, sleepiness or distractions. In each of these there are social considerations.

Health professionals may find it helpful to consider illness and patients' responses to their predicament from viewpoints other than medical ones, by attending to the contributions of different disciplines and different perspectives. To some extent this is happening as concern with the effectiveness of health care turns to measuring outcomes for patients. Outcomes are measured not only in terms of physiological parameters but also in terms of functional and social response and quality of life. More refined analysis compares outcomes against patient expectations, thus individualising assessments and taking account of individual variation rather than assuming a norm.

That there are different ways of considering outcomes stems from the application of different perspectives in health. There are similarly different perspectives within sociology and sociologists themselves argue about how best to study human behaviour. It is to these different sociological perspectives and theories that we turn in Chapter 2.

FURTHER READING

Berger P 1966 Invitation to sociology. Penguin, Harmondsworth

Mills C W 1970 The sociological imagination. Penguin, Harmondsworth

2

Perspectives in sociology

INTRODUCTION

In Chapter 1 we spent some time identifying the distinctiveness of sociology. We argued that social phenomena could be studied from a sociological perspective, which would be different from but complement the perspectives of the other social sciences. It would be incorrect, however, to indicate that there is a single sociological perspective or that there is only one correct sociological approach. Indeed, sociology, like all other social sciences, is characterised by a variety of perspectives. In this chapter we introduce four major sociological perspectives – structuralism, interactionism, ethnomethodology and critical theory. We show that they make different assumptions, use different concepts in different ways, pose different questions and provide different explanations. We will argue that perspectives are not necessarily right or wrong: simply different and often complementary ways of considering society.

An appreciation of these different sociological approaches provides some organising principles for understanding why sociologists, interested in similar social issues, ask different questions about them and study them in a variety of ways. We shall highlight this difference briefly in relation to the medically defined phenomenon of mental illness. Furthermore, if sociological studies are not interpreted within the broad perspective in which they have their origins, their findings risk becoming nothing more than a series of disjointed facts which convey a sense of arbitrariness as to their scope and methods.

This chapter is intended to provide an understanding of the main features of the different perspectives from which sociological studies of health, illness and health care topics, and the social world more generally, are conceptualised, and hence assist in their interpretation throughout the remaining chapters. In order to grasp these differences it is important to appreciate the contribution theory makes to characterising sociological perspectives. We deal with this issue first.

THEORY IN SOCIOLOGY

The word 'theory' often gives rise to difficulties because it is used to describe everything which is not practical. When theory is used, as in economic, psychological or sociological theory, then it refers to a set of conjectures or tentative explanations of reality.

Each one of us uses theory constantly. We carry in our heads our personal theories or models which represent the world about us. To do this we use selected concepts and the relationships between them. It is because we do not all share the same theories that we see the world differently. In other words, facts do not speak for themselves; rather facts are interpreted in the light of some particular theory. It is because we have particular ideas about the nature of the 'family' and 'government' that we have difficulties in conceptualising kinship networks and political structures in cultures different from our own. Similarly, the views different people hold about the way that 'society' should care for sick old people are influenced by our personal theories of 'illness', 'old age' and 'the role of women'. We tend not to question these, but it is different perspectives of these issues which will influence both health policy about services for older people as well as family differences in how frail elderly people are cared for.

Some facts are more generally accepted than others and this may involve a process of accumulating particular knowledge which produces convergent theory. For example, we now take

for granted the fact that the world is spherical. Yet at the time of Columbus' famous voyage it was certainly not taken for granted and the world was believed to be flat by many people. We now find this almost inconceivable. It is by testing our hypothetical explanations that we accumulate knowledge and what may begin as facts at a scientific level gradually become accepted into common-sense knowledge. A medical example is our current 'common sense' knowledge of the microbiological origin of many current diseases and the process of infection. We still, however, do not have a common-sense knowledge of newer diseases like HIV infection where the generation of new knowledge is progressing quickly. Similarly we are in a position of uncertainty with some of the theories which are evolving about the origins and antecedents of child abuse and mental illness. But it is on the basis of accepted theory that interventions will be produced. Those holding different theories will produce different ideas about what is appropriate.

It is not only the facts which are disputed but also their explanations. If we return to the use of antenatal care services, a fact observed by many midwives and obstetricians is that more women from the lower social classes are 'late bookers' for maternity care. The facts are that a higher proportion of women with husbands in Social Class V occupations booked for maternity care 20 weeks after conception than did those in Social Class I. Competing theoretical explanations of why this should be the case are that it is due to the different amounts of knowledge about the benefit of antenatal care available to women in different Social Class categories, or that women regard antenatal care as of variable significance, and their individual viewpoints influence their attendance. It happens that a higher percentage of pregnant women in Social Class V are less informed about antenatal care and that a higher percentage do not regard antenatal care as sufficiently worthwhile to attend (Garcia 1981). These variable theoretical explanations of the nature of social behaviour, one emphasising class-based divisions and the other taking a perspective which emphasises the relevance of how individuals view their world, are typical of different sociological perspectives.

Sociological perspectives are made explicit or can be inferred from the research question asked, the facts collected and the methods used to carry out an investigation. In everyday life and in our professional lives we tend not to make our theories explicit. When a patient is admitted to care some form of assessment is generally carried out. Depending on who does the assessment, be it members of different professional groups or different individuals within a profession, given complete freedom they are likely to assess different patient features. That is, different facts will be collected about the patient. In some cases facts will also be collected about the family. The information collected will depend on the theory being used by the professionals concerned, which determines their interpretations of the nature of patients, their rights, the recovery process and so on. The theory-driven nature of what we assess may become explicit when, for example, care is said to be organised according to some particular theory. What we assess, however, may be constrained by a standard assessment procedure or a standard list of questions as is typically used in settings where there is a rapid throughput of patients such as in antenatal clinics. The contents of both paper- and computer-based assessments are theory derived, however, just as our individually designed ones would be if we were left to our own devices. In the last few years we have become aware of the value of supportive relationships to enhance social and psychological functioning and coping ability among those facing particular kinds of stress, such as childbirth, bereavement, amputation, mastectomy or myocardial infarction. Whether information about such relationships is collected and used will depend on whether professionals either individually or collectively incorporate this fact into their theoretical ideas about their responsibilities for patient well-being, recovery and the nature of rehabilitation itself. Patient assessment, as one example of social behaviour, is guided by theory and accumulated knowledge

of the kind mentioned above, operates within the confines of theory. The same rationale functions more explicitly in sociological theory.

We cannot ignore theory, we can only choose from the options available. Theory is not static, however, but dynamic and constantly changing. It is itself *socially constructed* according to the time at which it is developed and the prevalent belief system operating in society. Theory development, therefore, is best understood in a historical context, and fashions in the acceptability of different theories can be interpreted equally within a broader political or social context. That there are competing explanations of the connection between race and intelligence is a recent example of the fit between theories and the acceptability of broader ideas about the nature of people and society. Later in the chapter it will become obvious that sociological theories, and more generally perspectives, have evolved as products of their time.

The role of theory

It would be a mistake to regard theories as right or wrong. There are, rather, theories which are more or less useful or helpful to our understanding. No one theory is a completely accurate representation of reality but some provide better insight into a particular phenomenon than do others. The usefulness of any theory depends on how it functions to:

- explain past events
- predict future events
- generate new theory.

One function of theory is to provide explanations of the connections between what facts already exist about some phenomena. Often, facts appear trivial and disjointed yet they may be linked by some theoretical explanation. One example of this is the similar responses observed (facts) to bereavement, to retirement and to amputation. In all cases they may be explained by response to the loss of something valued. This kind of theorising is possible because of an existing system of relationships connecting different facts. When they are linked theoretically this adds to our understanding of otherwise disparate phenomena. By using theory we are able to summarise specific features which are generalisable beyond the immediate field of study. By the same token theory should be able to *predict* future outcomes. Using the above example, if a valued object is lost then similar responses would be anticipated to those already observed. In many areas of sociological concern theory is too embryonic for accurate prediction, and awaits refinement and empirical testing.

Finally, good theory should lend itself to generating new theory capable of more parsimonious explanation and prediction. One aspect of this is that good theory should generate testable hypotheses which give rise to empirical testing. Theory therefore should point to areas yet to be explored and indicate which facts to observe while defining them clearly. In this way, new findings and empirical generalisations emerge which are then used to amend and refine existing theory, if this is warranted. We will return to theory testing and development again in Chapter 12 when we deal with sociological methods.

PERSPECTIVES ON MENTAL ILLNESS

Let us begin to consider some different sociological perspectives by examining approaches to the sociological analysis of mental illness (after Cuff & Payne 1979, Cuff, Sharrock & Francis 1990). This topic has been of interest to scientists for a considerable period of time. Religious and supernatural explanations have also been available which suggest that mental illness means possession by spirits. Scientific explanations of what constitutes odd or abnormal behaviour may be biological, psychological and sociological (among others). Even definitions of what constitutes mental illness differ. Durkheim (1952, originally published 1897) was one of the earliest sociologists to study mental illness. Ever since he attributed suicide to social causes other aspects of health and illness have been regarded as the appropriate subject matter of sociology.

According to Durkheim, the behaviour of individuals depends on their social environment and what their society influences them into doing. For some sociologists, while there is acceptance that *individuals* can be mentally ill, they look for reasons not in these afflicted individuals themselves but in particular aspects of the structure of the society in which they live.

STRUCTURALISM

One such approach was demonstrated by Hollingshead and Redlich (1958), who sought to show that the incidence and type of mental illness varied as a consequence of position in the social class structure. Thus, while the highest social class contained 3.1% of the population, only 1% of mentally ill people came from this class. Conversely, they showed that the lowest social class included 17.8% of the population but contributed 36.8% of people with a mental illness. Illness designated as 'neurotic' was concentrated in the higher levels of social class while 'psychotic' types of illness predominated in the lower social classes. Without going into further detail, this analysis reveals a particular sociological perspective which makes certain assumptions about the nature of society and the causes of mental illness.

This perspective can be broadly labelled *structuralist* because it views society as being structured in certain ways, *social class* being one of them. People belonging to the same social class are assumed to be similar in certain ways – have similar roles in the economic order of society, similar lifestyles, attitudes and educational backgrounds. It is therefore considered appropriate to examine whether variations in the prevalence/or incidence of mental illness coincide with these socially constructed divisions. In Hollingshead and Redlich's study, mental illness does appear to differ by incidence and type in different social classes.

Another example of a structuralist approach to mental illness would be to relate it to different areas of residence, for example, between urban and rural areas. In this example the structuralist position postulates that there is an association between different areas of residence (and, arguably, different lifestyles and organisation) and rates and types of mental illness. Indeed, Dunham and Faris (1965) showed that in Chicago the incidence of schizophrenia varied in different parts of the city, with the highest rates in areas close to the city centre with many lodging houses, foreign-born communities and 'down and outs'. They suggest that it is the social disorganisation of these areas which predisposes to schizophrenia. The recent move toward 'community care' for former mental hospital patients in Britain may contribute to the concentration of people with schizophrenia who are attracted to such deprived inner-city areas. The researchers identify a link between the spatial pattern of the city and each area's distinctive ecology with different kinds and levels of social organisation. This in turn results in 'producing' schizophrenic illness at specific levels of incidence. In other words, the *structural* organisation of urban, social and economic life influences the condition of individuals who live there. An alternative explanation is that people who have mental illness are attracted to living or are forced to live in particular city areas.

INTERACTIONISM

In contrast with structuralists, sociologists who take an *interactionist* perspective provide a rather different view of mental illness. They begin with no taken-for-granted definitions of what mental illness is; they do not see it as something within the individual. Rather, it is a *social status* conferred on an individual by other members of society. For interactionists, mental illness is not like some disease within the person which can universally be observed and defined, like smallpox. Being regarded as mentally ill depends on individuals making that definition of others, labelling them and acting towards them as if they were mentally ill. The definition of mental illness occurs in the process of social interaction.

This contrasts with an understanding of mental illness founded on assumptions about society with a structure which exerts strong influences on individual members and how they behave. Interactionists stress the fundamental importance of individual actions and perceptions, each person taking account of the actions of others on the basis of the meanings and interpretations they give to them. It is not a case of individuals being governed by and reflecting back the structure of their society. Rather individuals, through social action, are also in the process of *creating* their society. Individuals have to interpret their social world, make sense of it and give meaning to it. Thus 'mental illness' and 'mental patient' are not absolute conditions or objects which exist 'out there'. Interactionists concern themselves with studying the processes by which people go about classifying others as 'mentally ill'.

In social life, some people who occupy particular roles have more power than others when it comes to assigning labels to people as mentally ill. Szasz (1971) has taken this approach in examining the process of a person's becoming so labelled. While most of us would say that we could recognise someone who was mentally ill, it is psychiatrists who are generally accepted as experts in doing so. Psychiatrists have considerable power to declare that someone is mentally sick, requires treatment and may be forcibly placed in an institution. Such is that power that others are likely to accept their categorisations of people as mentally ill and act towards those individuals accordingly. In this way, individuals become 'mentally ill' not simply on the basis of their behaviour but because of the particular label attached to them. If others apply the label it is less likely to stick if it is not also supported by a psychiatrist's opinion. What psychiatrists label as mental illness may change over time. For example, in 1974 the American Psychiatric Association voted to decide whether homosexuality was a mental illness. Only since 1974 has it not been considered to be an illness. In the former Soviet Union, dissidents from the prevailing political line were categorised as mentally ill and incarcerated in psychiatric hospitals. Within living memory in the United Kingdom, people who had illegitimate children were categorised as 'moral deviants' and incarcerated for the rest of their lives in hospitals for people with a mental handicap.

Not everyone agrees with the categorisations made. Studies based on interactionist assumptions have shown that disagreements occur over the interpretation and meanings given to the behaviour observed. The differentiation of 'mentally ill' from 'normal' members of society can be contingent upon the particular circumstances of the social situation in which people find themselves. Scheff (1964) examined the psychiatric screening procedures used to decide whether patients should be released from hospital. Scheff found that this decision is influenced more by the financial, ideological and political position of the examining psychiatrist than patient factors. The study demonstrated that court-appointed psychiatrists with particular ideological and political views were predisposed to assume that the person was *ill* from the outset. Within this frame of reference which pre-classifies the patient, psychiatrists then go on to interpret the patient's behaviour and records. Scheff argues that without this prior definition of the person as mentally ill, the patient's records, behaviour and responses to the psychiatrist's tests are interpreted differently.

On the other side of the coin, interactionists are also concerned with individuals' perceptions of themselves. This follows from the assumption that individuals have to interpret and give meaning to their own actions as well as make sense of those of others with whom they interact. How individuals act depends on their own self-image and this is constructed largely from our interpretation of how other people react to what we say and do. This has led to studies of the effects of labelling people as mentally ill and how these individuals subsequently see themselves. Conferring the label itself produces abnormal behaviour because of the way others start to act towards the people so labelled. This in turn produces actions by them which they recognise others expect of them. This is an example of a general phenomenon. Another example is that of trainees or learners becoming qualified and gaining new titles; people react to

them differently and, in turn, they behave differently.

These examples demonstrate the very different kinds of sociological analyses which are produced by sociologists who rely on the assumptions of the interactionist perspective, and the structuralists who take as their starting point a very different conception of the social world. As a result they use different conceptual frameworks, carry out different kinds of studies and use different methods to collect and analyse the data which provides the basis of their explanations. Neither is necessarily more correct than the other; they simply represent different ways of viewing the social world.

ETHNOMETHODOLOGY

A third and comparatively recent perspective in sociology is represented by an approach known as *ethnomethodology*, again choosing questions and investigating the social world on the basis of a different set of assumptions and choosing a different conceptual framework from the two perspectives described above.

The ethnomethodological approach assumes that the social world is constantly being created by members of society which for them is unproblematic because it is regarded as the result of society's members using their own common sense. Society is created by its members using their taken-for-granted commonsense knowledge about how the world works and how they can deal with it in acceptable ways. The concern of ethnomethodologists is to study and explain how it is that society's members actually go about accomplishing the social world which they create through commonly accepted, albeit sophisticated, methods. Of major importance is language; we accomplish social encounters largely through conversation as well as other forms of interaction. Individuals have learned methods for doing this and ethnomethodologists are interested in how they have achieved such methods.

Ethnomethodologists would be unlikely to study mental illness as a topic in its own right;

they would be more likely to have as their concern the society-building methods that people use which happen to have relevance to mental illness. Turner (1968) has shown that former mental patients can be faced with particular problems when renewing contact and taking up conversations with acquaintances after being discharged from a mental hospital. Cuff et al (1990) write:

His focus of study is in the way persons 'resume contact' after having been discharged from the mental institution. Turner suggests that in any subsequent encounter between any two persons, it may be the case that the parties to the conversation do some work of recognition. He argues that when persons engage in this 'resuming' work they offer identifications of themselves and the persons they are talking to, and in so doing they are suggesting a relationship between them. These identifications can be, and usually are, offered without explicitly announcing that one is a friend, or a long-lost acquaintance. For example, by saying, 'Hi Chuck, how did it go last night? I sure wish I could've made it,' as the opening utterance in an encounter the speaker is, without spelling it out word for word, probably identifying himself and the person he is talking to as 'friends'. Turner adds that part of this resuming work may involve bringing the parties to the conversation up to date, that is, filling each other in on newsworthy items which have happened to them individually since they last met. In the case of an encounter involving a 'former mental patient', however, Turner illustrates how troubles in everyday resuming work can be generated. For example, it may require the 'former mental patient' to accept unwanted identification. After all, it is likely that such an individual wants to forget that he has been mentally ill; he may consider his 'former state' is as irrelevant to his current life as a broken leg. But when resuming involves bringing the parties up to date, it is often difficult to avoid the topic of his recent experiences. Turner appeals to his materials and to our common-sense knowledge of the social world to suggest that the identity 'former mental patient' is one which persons who have not been mentally ill are most likely to use, in preference to any other, when they are doing resuming work with someone they know to have been mentally ill. Thus, the ethnomethodologists, by analysing conversational materials, can show us how interactional troubles can be generated and managed in everyday encounters. In particular, Turner's work illustrates how such analysis can illuminate some interactional problems involving persons who have been 'mentally ill'.
(pp. 21–22)

Critical theory

It is to critical theory, poststructuralism and postmodernism which we can turn to for a fourth sociological perspective. Poststructuralists and postmodernists hold a very different view of contemporary society to other theorists. Like ethnomethodologists, they would not be specifically interested in the study of mental illness. Their purpose in considering mental illness would be to use it as a general example of the processes whereby our society is being made ever more repressive. Although we might believe that different institutions in society, for example education and health care, are helpful, poststructuralists and postmodernists would argue that we are really being repressed by them. That we may feel perfectly happy with our society and do not feel imprisoned does not negate this view but supports it. It demonstrates how trapped we are within the structure of our ways of thinking.

In everyday life we take most things for granted. This applies equally to the way we structure knowledge as it does to everyday customs. We forget that we did not construct them but inherited them – we acquired them through learning language. Language is one of our most stable institutions (Berger & Berger 1976) but was created and developed in particular times and places. In order to understand language and the social categories it describes, and which we take for granted, poststructuralists and postmodernists would argue that we must take a historical perspective. This allows examination of the conditions under which our taken-for-granted ideas were created and developed.

Both poststructuralists and postmodernists approach mental illness in a similar way to that of the interactionists. Rather than explain mental illness in terms of labelling theory, however, which we have seen requires the legitimation of a label by others who act as agents of social control, postmodernists and poststructuralists charge that mental illness is nothing more than a response to a situation that contravenes typical symbolism. They argue that because a person fails or refuses to be limited by a particular portrayal of reality, he or she is identified as mad and sequestered from the rest of society. Madness, by this definition, simply pertains to someone who refuses to accept symbolic repression (Murphy 1988).

By taking a historical perspective we can explain this response to social reality. The practice of calling people 'witches' has been replaced by calling them 'mad'. It performs the same functions, namely stigmatising and controlling people who are a problem for others. The historical perspective also helps us understand why we incarcerate people who are 'mentally ill' in isolated institutions. Foucault (1973, first published in French in 1963) has suggested that this practice owes much to the fact that there were places available in which to contain people following the eradication of leprosy from Europe in the middle ages. This kind of practice continues today using surplus isolation hospitals and, more recently, wards surplus to requirement in hospitals for people with a mental handicap, for the warehousing of frail elderly people. These current practices may be of equal historical significance in understanding the portrayal of the social reality of old age.

The example of mental illness, which will be elaborated in Chapter 4, serves as a means of introducing and illustrating that within sociology there are different ways of conceptualising and studying any topic. As we will show in subsequent chapters, there is no one sociological approach to health and illness, the family, professional careers or indeed any subject of interest to sociologists. Particular sociologists themselves recognise and are recognised by others as adhering to a particular perspective. It is reflected in the way that they select and carry out sociological studies. Let us now begin to elaborate further some of the basic features of these sociological approaches.

STRUCTURALISM AS A PERSPECTIVE

Structuralism as a broad perspective is based on the assumption that all our social behaviour, our attitudes and values, are the result of the organisation and structure of society in which we live.

A major refinement of this, however, is to regard the components of the social structure as in consensus with each other or, alternatively, to consider them as in conflict.

Structural-functionalism – a consensus perspective

All sociological perspectives have in common a focus on the ordered nature of society, that is, a belief that in most situations the range of possible actions is fairly limited. We have a fair idea of how we would behave as well as being able to predict, within limits, the behaviour of others. The notion of order in how we behave is relevant to situations as diverse as a couple out on their first date to the stability of whole societies. It is at the societal extreme that the consensus perspective is situated, based on the assumption that, in the main, societies can be regarded as stable and generally integrated wholes. They differ according to their cultural and social structural arrangements.

This perspective in sociology owes a great deal to an analogy with natural and biological sciences. At the time sociology was emerging as a new discipline, there was also a thrust towards seeing the world according to the 'scientific methods' adopted in the natural sciences. Comte (1798–1857), a French philosopher who coined the word 'sociology', believed that sociology was about adapting and applying the methods of the physical sciences to social life. Its ultimate aim is the production of 'law-like' statements about the determinants of human behaviour so as to be able to reshape society by predicting and hence controlling its workings. Sociology, which attempts to adhere to the canons of physical science, is sometimes referred to as 'scientistic'. Comte's emphasis was on the structures of whole societies and the change of whole societies.

A second step in the notion of societies as integrated wholes was based in part upon a crude analogy between society and biological organisms. The analogy arises from the fact that both societies and biological organisms have, on the one hand, a propensity to survive against all odds and, on the other hand, a propensity to decay. Higher order biological organisms comprise systems made up of a number of distinguishable interrelated parts. Each of these parts affects and responds to changes in other parts of the organism. This analogy does not mean that the social system mirrors the biological system in terms of actual structure but that the different parts of the social system are similarly affected by and respond to changes in its other parts. Different parts of the biological system fulfil different functions; hence the sociological analogy of functionalism. Some functions are more essential to the organism's survival than others; so, too, individuals and institutions fulfil a variety of functions and roles. When the human organism loses an eye it adapts to changes in circumstances; in the event of heart failure the body eventually dies. The human organism is therefore an open and adaptive system which, however, is not immortal. Likewise, in its simplest form, structural functionalism describes society as an adaptive and open system whose different parts function to keep it unified and relatively unchanging.

Durkheim and functionalism

A major and long-lasting contribution to functionalism was made by Emile Durkheim (1858–1917). One feature of this was to regard the interrelated components of society as being *moral* entities. Furthermore, through their associations with each other, members of society develop what Durkheim (1964a, originally published 1893) called a 'collective consciousness' which constrains how they behave and which also gives rise to expectations and restraints in how others behave. The nature of these social constraints on our behaviour was what Durkheim meant by 'the moral reality' of society – that society, over and above individuals, had its own moral order which also included the collective values of its members. In order that individuals can operate in a society there has to be some framework of order which is rooted in members holding certain values in common. Consensus in society is achieved through this

sharing and cohesiveness. For Durkheim, this basic agreement is synonymous with an understanding of the concept of society itself.

Durkheim's emphasis on the moral nature of social relationships permeates his work. His analysis of the division of labour in society (the growth of ever more complex distinctions between different occupations) is a moral rather than an economic one. It is based on common values and expectations about what is appropriate for society at that time. Durkheim assumes a high degree of cohesiveness, with different components of the social structure adapting to maintain society in equilibrium. Stability does not mean that societies are static but that the systems within society are able to adjust and adapt in an orderly and evolutionary way to achieve a new state of equilibrium.

One repercussion of the functionalism of Durkheim is a tendency to regard society as an independently existing entity, existing in its own right over and above its constituent members. This is reflected in Durkheim's views of the appropriate subject matter for sociological research, that is, to study 'social facts' and to do so in a scientific way (Durkheim 1964b, originally published in 1895). 'Social facts' are different from other kinds of facts because they are the very fabric of society, evolving out of human relationships and association. An example of a social fact can be taken from Durkheim's study of suicide (Durkheim 1952, originally published in 1897). The *rate* of suicide, which cannot be reduced to single cases of suicide without losing sight of the *rate*, is an example of a social fact. Similarly, other collective phenomena like 'crime', 'fashion' and 'mental illness' which transcend the behaviour of individual people are social facts. Durkheim regarded some social facts as 'normal' in that they are appropriate to and necessary for the operation of a 'healthy' and well-ordered society. Social facts which were harmful to society were categorised as 'pathological', thus reinforcing the organic analogy.

The importance of Durkheim's contribution to sociology lies not only in his theory of society but also in his major work on methods to be used to study society. In sociology, as in all disciplines, it can be said that theory guides methods. We will demonstrate in Chapter 12 Durkheim's enduring influence on research methods from a functionalist perspective.

Developments in structural-functionalism

It would be misleading to characterise a universal functionalist approach but there is a limited number of variants. We can only touch on two of these here – the contributions of Talcott Parsons (1902–1979) and Robert Merton (b. 1910).

Parsons – the social system

Talcott Parsons' most significant contribution has been his attempt to construct a model of the working of all parts of the social system (Parsons 1951). In a vast output of work certain central and recurrent features emerge.

In explaining the concept of function, Parsons' view of the social system is of a network of interlocking systems and subsystems functioning together in order to meet the needs of each other. Order is achieved by integrating disparate motivations into a coherent and ordered society or, to use Parsons' own terminology, by integrating the *personality system* and the *cultural system* with the *social system*. These systems are linked by and share a *central value system* which Parsons, like Durkheim, claims as the basis of society. Stable expectations and behaviours are developed through the *role* relationships which arise; in turn these expectations enable others to meet them and to carry out role obligations in return for the rights which adhere to their respective roles. Thus behaviour is made predictable and society persists even though its members change. We will encounter the importance of this when we deal with socialisation in Chapter 5 and with the sick role in Chapter 8.

Before functions can be attributed to parts of systems, their value systems must first be defined. Value systems legitimise the *norms* upon which social processes are based, and so, in order to understand the components of social systems, a first concern is to define their prevail-

ing goals and values. Parsons devotes attention to four major subsystems which are themselves structural features of society. These are:

1. The economy, which provides and distributes the material resources needed by members of society.
2. The political subsystem, which serves the function of selecting the collective goals of society and motivating society's members to achieve them.
3. Kinship institutions, whose functions are to maintain accepted and expected forms of social interaction and control interpersonal tensions through the process of socialising individuals into competent role players.
4. Community and cultural institutions, such as religion, education and mass communication, which function to integrate the various elements of the social system. They may be reinforced by formal agencies of social control like the judiciary, police and the military.

From this approach we can identify the problem of explaining how these subsystems maintain their integration, and that of the whole social system, given the necessary diversity of roles and norms in modern societies.

The key for Parsons is the continual striving towards an ideal state of equilibrium. This is attained through the processes of *socialisation* and *social control* so that individuals are motivated towards the fulfilment of role expectations. In so doing, the *personality system* is related to the social structure in which the individual is situated. Socialisation and the internalisation of norms are key processes but they are related to the functions of the social structure. Individuals must be adequately socialised into roles appropriate to attain the goals of the particular institutions or subsystems, and goals are related to the functions of the institution. We shall show how this analysis applies to the family in Chapter 5.

Individual components of society are tied to the larger society by shared value systems and by their specific functional requirements, which they can only meet through the society and which must be met for them to 'survive'. Thus the continued existence of a system depends on its ability to *adapt*, to attain goals, to integrate constituent parts and to permit maintenance of the dominant value system and the pattern of interaction it lays down.

While there is an emphasis on integration and the persistence of social systems, Parsons does attend to social change. Change can arise in two ways: from pressures exerted by environmental transitions or from within the institution itself. Institutional pressures derive from *strain* within one of the subsystems, creating disequilibrium. Ultimately, however, the crucial change is the cultural value system of society which expresses its moral sentiments and normative expectations. Any change in society, according to Parsonian theory, must be to adjust and adapt towards a new type of stability or towards meeting more effectively the goals and functions of the system. This is expressed as the 'dynamic equilibrium' of social systems, with an emphasis on the functional consequences of change or conflict rather than on the sources or causes of conflict. In this sense it is emphatically a consensus perspective.

Merton's functionalism

Not all functionalists use the organic analogy, nor do they all attempt to consider the interrelatedness of the component parts of social systems. This has been the position of Merton (1967) who regards the Parsonian scheme as altogether too grand in its attempt to include all of society, at all levels, within its social structure. He argues that the tendency to dwell on the functions of social systems, as Parsons does, should be limited to the observed consequences of social events. He also considers that the functionalist view that particular social beliefs or practices are functional in the same way for the *entire* social or cultural system is too simplistic. His view is that a particular arrangement, activity or belief may be functional for only part of the total society. This has led Merton to develop a theory which can be said to be *middle-range*. Rather than try to consider total societal functions, he focuses on the consequences of one institutional area for another.

To help develop middle-range theories, Merton introduced three new concepts to functionalism:

1. Functions may be *latent*, i.e. unintended or unrecognised, as well as *manifest*, i.e. intended and recognised.
2. Because not all items necessarily fulfil positive functions, or not for the whole society, they can be *dysfunctional* – leading to instability and disruption rather than to stable maintenance of the system.
3. Rather than the conservative assumption that there are recognisable activities which are indispensable to a society because they fulfil functional prerequisites, for example the production and distribution of scarce resources in particular ways, Merton argues that there are *functional alternatives*, i.e. different and equally successful ways of providing for functions. This gets away from the functionalist conservative tendency to argue that something is indispensable for the well-being of society – that society could not survive without marriage, for example, to produce families and progeny.

Merton's brand of functionalism yields more for empirical sociologists than do the more grandiose theoretical schema of Parsons. It offers insights which suggest that behaviour is not always what it seems, that the consequences of actions are not always what they are intended to be, and that what may be regarded as 'bad' for a community could, in fact, turn out to perform vital functions. A structure which has existed unquestioned for generations could turn out to have *dysfunctional* consequences and *functional alternatives* may be available which could do the job more effectively.

Merton also deals with conflict, but his analysis points out that conflict can be functional as well as dysfunctional for social systems, in a number of ways. However, like other structuralists, Merton's analysis does not apply to individuals or to groups; like them he operates at the level of the needs of systems – whether of societies or their subsystems. Like the other structural-functionalists, Merton does not deal with consequences but with functions, i.e. whether or not actions meet needs which are held to prevail within a system. As such there is no satisfactory explanation of social change or the causes, as distinct from the consequences, of action.

Functionalism continues to be an important influence on sociological thought. In recent years, however, its influence has waned, although it still has its articulate defenders (Alexander 1985).

Structuralism – a conflict approach

Conflict theorists tend to regard themselves as radical critics of the consensus theorists, with their emphasis on maintaining the status quo. As such they are sometimes regarded as having political motives, most strongly exemplified in the writings of Karl Marx (1818–1883).

Marx as a sociological theorist

The sociologist who attempts to understand social phenomena within a Marxist perspective is not necessarily supportive of Marxist political theory or ideology, or only in as much as these provide meaningful explanations of society.

Marxism is essentially a historical interpretation of the evolution of societies or social systems. It explains social change historically by examining the evolution of modern industrial society, from ancient economies based on slavery, through the medieval economy based on serfdom, to the capitalist economy based on wage labour. Marxism is also deterministic in that it predicts the evolution of capitalist society into a socialist society. Like some other forms of structuralism it is synthetic in its approach to social change, being concerned with the whole of society rather than its component parts (Lefebvre 1968).

Some aspects of Marx's social philosophy are central to his sociological theory (Bottomore & Rubel 1965). For Marx, all societies are *stratified* into distinct *groups* or *classes*. In Chapter 3 we focus on the concept of *social stratification* and indicate how Marxism has influenced sociological thinking, and in Chapter 4 we demonstrate

through an understanding of the political economy of health approach, its relevance to studying the social causes of illness. Underlying Marxist theory is the notion that power and authority are linked closely to the economic organisation of society. In capitalist societies the owners of capital (*the bourgeoisie*) have power over the labour class (*the proletariat*). The relationship between these two social groups is characterised by exploitation and conflict. In modern industrial societies this power is vested in the State which determines laws favouring the bourgeoisie.

Marxism sees society as a product of the *conflict* between the bourgeoisie and the proletariat, and predicts that the struggle will be resolved through revolutionary rather than evolutionary social change. Societies pass through definite stages of development, with each stage containing contradictions and conflicts that lead to social change. But society and history are not seen as solely external to men and women. It is through our own activity as members of a social class having a distinctive class consciousness that the social and historical world is created and changed.

Like most structuralist theories, Marxism perceives society as a totality, a structure of interrelated levels. This is depicted in Figure 2.1. The economic substructure is closely bound up with the *superstructure* – that is, those institutions in society such as the mass media, the church, the family and the educational system, which produces knowledge – and with the relationship between the social classes.

Social change must begin with the forces of production. When they develop in such a way that they cease to fit with the relations of production, that is, the relations between the owners and the nonowners of the means of production, they create contradictions within the substructure of society. These contradictions occur between the new forces of production and the old relations of production. For example, a contradiction occurs between the social relationships in feudal societies, where serfs were tied to the landowners, and the demands for labour in capitalist societies, which required freedom of labour movement. In this instance, social change only occurred when the proletariat perceived that their freedom to move employers was threatened by the relationships of feudal society.

This notion was central to Marx's theory of social change in relation to capitalism and socialism. A socialist society would only come about when the bulk of the population, the free labourers, developed a consciousness of what was happening in their society and acted together as a social group, i.e. as a social class. Only through involvement in various forms of action could members of the proletariat develop their own ideology and begin to create a society which meets their own interest. Marx identified this process as developing a class consciousness.

Marxism is, of course, much wider-ranging than presented here, but all of it draws on the basic conflict between different classes based on different economic groups.

Max Weber

Max Weber (1864–1920) criticised Marx's position that only changes in the economic base can change society, arguing that many factors must

come together to produce social change. His major thesis *The Protestant Ethic* and the *Spirit of Capitalism* (1948, first published in German in 1904–5) argued that it was the religious ideals of Calvinism which transformed people's behaviour and produced capitalism, by turning their religious zeal into economic production through hard work rather than by detaching themselves from work to pursue their religious interests. Work on earth to gain God's favour of a place in heaven created the impetus for maximisation of efficiency and for finding the best means of doing the work. In his analysis of world religions Weber attempted to show that religious ideas – a component in Marx's superstructure – could affect economic behaviour.

Weber's other challenge to Marx was over the derivation of the power available to social groups. He did not agree that power derived solely from economic relations, the relations to private property and the means of production. For Weber there are different dimensions to power relationships. We take up these dimensions in Chapter 3 when we deal with social stratification and consider competing interests of class and status groups to establish the right to wield power. This is further discussed in relation to bureaucracy in health care organisations in Chapter 7. The conflict between different class groups is a core assumption of Weberian sociology which, despite its challenge to Marxism, owes its central ideas and concepts to Marxist theory.

Since Marx and Weber, other sociologists have continued to examine the structure of society along class lines as well as expanding ideas about the basis of class and class consciousness. Furthermore, as capitalist societies have been superseded by other forms of economic organisation, there is a continued analysis and refinement of Marx's concepts to accommodate these new types of social structure.

The structuralist contribution

We have compared some major ideas in consensus and conflict styles of structuralism, and have pointed out their basic difference in the way

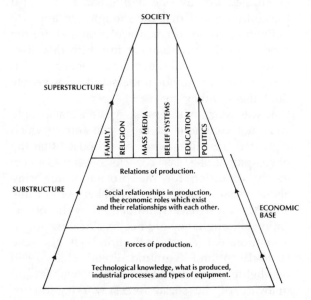

Fig. 2.1 Relationship between different levels in Marx's social structure (after Cuff & Payne 1979).

they view groups in society. On the one hand, consensus theory views the social system as essentially cohesive, with individuals and groups reciprocating and cooperating with each other by adhering to an integrating system of norms and values. Social life is therefore characterised by its continuity and stability rather than by change. On the other hand, conflict theorists point up divisiveness, conflict and hostility that is inevitably generated by social structures, creating groups with different and antagonistic interests. Social change comes about by groups attempting to preserve, extend or realise their own interests at the cost of other groups.

Despite these divergent views, both groups of structuralists are concerned with finding out how the whole of society works, identifying the interrelationships between its key parts and discovering how the social structure influences individuals. Inevitably, this leads to assumptions being made that social structures are systems of some sort, comprising some kind of parts which are related in some way, and when there is sufficient change in the nature of these parts, then this will bring about a change in the social structure as a whole. How the theorists differ in how they approach an understanding of the social world is in their respective views of the nature of the system, the parts, the relationships between parts and therefore the differential importance of certain parts. Nevertheless, the emphasis on the social world as a structured system allows them to be classified as structuralists.

CRITICAL THEORY: POSTMARXIST PERSPECTIVES

Contemporary structuralist theories have refined both the Marxian and Weberian perspectives of society. A number of their ideas, however, also have their origins in the theory of other 19th century writers. 'Critical theory' is a term coined to describe the Frankfurt School of sociologists. We use it here to encompass not only the different theories of the Frankfurt School but also to describe the work of other 20th century Marxists, the structuralists, the poststructuralists

and the postmodernists. The unifying theme of the critical theorists is their criticism of industrial and postindustrial society.

Since the Enlightenment period in the 17th and 18th centuries Western thought and culture has been dominated by the idea that through science and technology human life in general will be improved. This is clearly evident in modern capitalism, which argues that through economic growth and technological change society will increase wealth to the benefit of everyone. In 17th century philosophy (after Descartes 1596–1650), the study of human thought was dominated by the belief that knowledge emerged from the working of the mind through the power of reason. By studying the workings of the human mind philosophers at the time believed that we would be able to understand how we obtain knowledge and therefore identify the process by which we acquire new knowledge. The assumption that knowledge is the product of isolated individual minds was challenged toward the end of the 19th century and throughout the 20th century. The idea that people are guided by reason was questioned. The irrational behaviour observed in all individuals was explained by the existence of an unconscious mind which cannot be studied by any one individual. It was also forcefully argued that the thoughts of any one individual do not occur in isolation and are the product of the environment in which they live. Without reference to the environments in which people live we cannot understand why people think the way they do.

It was Marx who first suggested that people were not conscious of the social forces which regulated their lives when he proposed that the development of a class consciousness was a necessary condition for the proletariat to bring about social change. Those thinkers who came after Marx were clearly influenced by this observation although they did not specifically apply it to notions of class. Both Friedrich Nietzche (1844–1900) and Sigmund Freud (1856–1939) highlighted the extent to which we are all unaware of the social forces working on us. They stressed the extent to which people could be 'unconscious' of their motives for everyday actions. Following their lead we should all be sceptical of the ideals and motives that people declare in every day life.

Classical Marxism identifies the essentially repressive nature of the State which is designed to control opposition to the capitalist system. The State not only exerts economic and political control but also controls social knowledge. Gramsci (1891–1937) argued that it was the power of bourgeois ideas which controlled capitalist societies, not simply the economic and political power of the bourgeoisie. Western culture is dominated by the culture of the bourgeoisie. A number of 20th century Marxist thinkers followed this line of thought and rejected the idea that the economic base could determine the way societies evolved. Capitalist culture as a whole, rather than the specific economic system, became the focus of their criticism.

The Frankfurt School

The critical theory of the Frankfurt School has had an important influence on European social thought since the School first emerged in the 1920s. The School involved a number of people and they did not always agree. They did concur, however, like the 20th century Marxists, in giving priority to the criticism of bourgeois culture. The School was also critical of the way that reason and social knowledge is subordinated to the needs of capitalism. They developed the concept of instrumental reason to highlight their criticism. Social knowledge is seen to have developed in response to the needs of capitalism by focusing on the problems of capitalism, problems which are generally of an instrumental kind. The dominance of these instrumental processes within capitalism is reflected in the unstoppable movement in science and technology which has resulted in greater control over the people. The process of rationalisation, first identified by Weber as a key feature of capitalism, has triumphed over all social groups. Control has become an end in itself rather than suppression and control of one social group by another.

Members of the School were critical of the Marxist perspective which emphasised the influence of the economic base on the superstructure (see Figure 2.1). Their almost humanistic vision interpreted Marx as saying that human beings mould history and what actually happens is ultimately up to people themselves. Thus, control and oppression should be thought of not as overt processes forcing people to do things they do not want to do but covert processes encouraging people to think they want to do things that they would otherwise not do.

After Frankfurt

The Frankfurt School ceased to exist following the deaths of two of its postwar members Theodor Adorno (1903–1969) and Max Horkheimer (1895–1973). In some senses, however, the school continued to exist in the writings of Jurgen Habermas (b.1929) who developed and expounded many of the ideas of critical theory as the architect of neocritical theory. Like Marx, the writings of the young Habermas have developed in different directions in more recent writing. Any attempt to summarise his major ideas is fraught with difficulty not least because his thought is complex, opaque and poorly expressed.

Habermas has drawn on ideas from a variety of social science traditions including linguistics, philosophy and psychology. A central idea shared with the Frankfurt School is a critique of the scientific method of natural science and the positivism of many social scientists. We will leave further discussion of the critique of positivism until Chapter 12 when discussing sociological methods. It is sufficient to say, however, that the philosophical tradition of positivism is one example by which capitalism has attempted to suppress social thought by denying the legitimacy of other philosophical traditions.

Habermas (1972) distinguishes three forms of knowledge: instrumental, communicative and emancipatory. These relate to some fundamental interests of the human species, namely the development of science and technology, the need for understanding and communication between individuals and social groups, and emancipatory interests of individuals resulting from power relations in social life. Habermas emphasises the role of communication by construing rationality and truth as phenomena of communication. Truth is seen to be a matter of agreement arrived at through free discussions between individuals. In advanced capitalist societies, where communication is systematically distorted, not least by the mass media, Habermas argues that this process of arriving at the truth cannot occur. Participants in social discourse are not equal in advanced capitalist societies in which marked inequalities are endemic (see Ch. 3) and in which much social discourse does not proceed without interference and control. This oppression of free social discourse remains central to many recent critical theories and highlights the significance of spoken and written language in our social interactions.

Structuralism and poststructuralism

After Cuff and Payne (1979) we have used the term structuralism to categorise those sociological perspectives which focus on the way society shapes individual behaviour. Confusingly, the term has also been used to describe a specific theory which links sociological analysis to the study of language.

Structuralism and language

Structuralism was originally pioneered in linguistics by the Swiss linguist Ferdinand de Saussure (1857–1913) who distinguished between parole (speech) and langur (the language system). Saussure (1974, first published in 1915) argued that the meaning of words derives from the structures of language, not the objects to which the words refer. There are many words which have meaning but do not refer to specific things. If the meaning of words does not relate to objects, from where does the meaning originate? Saussure argues that meaning is created by the differences between related concepts which the rules of language recognise. In Eskimo language the meaning of the word

'snow' comes from the fact that the Eskimo language distinguishes 'snow' from 'sleet' (and many other words) which have similar, but distinct meanings.

'Structuralism' was used by the anthropologist Levi-Strauss in studying myths, religion and kinship. By applying the system of differences to myths he was able to show that stories which made no sense to us, appear intelligible when analysed in this way, just as they are intelligible in the society to which they belong. This approach also has an important bearing on a dominant view in Western culture, that it is in some way superior to traditional cultures. Levi-Strauss argues that the human mind is everywhere the same because the human brain operates through differences using binary oppositions like the modern computer. Thus human thought from other cultures is as intellectual as human thought in Western culture but expresses itself in different ways.

Poststructuralism and Foucault

Michel Foucault's (1926–1984) contribution to critical theory continues the theme of this section that all aspects of society are rooted in oppression. The 'structuralists' focused their analysis of society on language and systems of communication in an attempt to highlight order and unity in the social system. By conceiving social organisation as a system of signs, the 'structuralists' ignored the social context in which communication occurs and made no attempt to understand the role of communication in the system. Foucault remedied the limitation of the 'structuralist' approach by exploring the institutional context of language and systems of communication. He highlighted the central relationship between knowledge and power, an area we explore in greater detail in Chapter 9 when discussing interactions with patients and in Chapter 11 in relation to professional power. The 'structuralist' suggestion that social organisation originates in the system of meanings is countered by Foucault, who suggests that the organisation of meaning, or what he calls 'discourse', originates in historically quite specific social and organisational contexts. Thus it is the medical setting or 'clinic' which makes medical ways of talking possible, not the other way round (Foucault 1973, first published in French in 1963).

Foucault's analysis of knowledge and power contrasts markedly with that of the Marxists and other writers within the broader structuralist perspective. Whereas power is generally characterised as repressive, Foucault argues that power is 'productive' and an autonomous force. It is therefore wrong to conceive power as the means by which one social group controls others in its own interest. It is not the power of individuals or social groups which are repressive, although we can all have power, but the system itself which is repressive. Foucault argues that our search for truth, the reliance of science and technology to release us from the imprisonment of the poverty of historical lifestyles is self-deluding. Far from making us more capable of controlling our destiny, science and knowledge has only changed the nature of our imprisonment, which is characterised by an even more subtle system of control.

Postmodernism

The writings of Foucault, and more recently Jacques Derrida and Jean-Francois Lyotard, have led to the emergence of the era of postmodernism. Language as a system of communication remains central to postmodernist analysis. Postmodernism embraces the social sciences and the arts in the wholesale rejection of the Enlightenment perspective of industrial and postindustrial society which has dominated Western culture for the last 300 years. The central tenet of postmodernism is a resistance to theory. They do not, however, abandon truth and order. Likewise they do not believe that any interpretation of reality is true. To some commentators postmodernism is a continuity of critical theory but to others, notably Lyotard (1984), postmodernism represents the beginning of an era of unprecedented change which will affect the whole nature of the way we think and the nature of our knowledge. Much of this change is

seen as a product of the postindustrial information society and the way we are beginning to use computers and other new technology to reorganise social relations. Postmodernism is a major challenge to the way we think and process knowledge. Only time will tell whether this is a transient period in our understanding of social knowledge or whether there will be a long-lasting and critical reappraisal of Western culture and our way of life within capitalist society.

A note on feminism

Before we leave our discussion of the structuralist perspective there is one approach that we have not included so far, namely the feminist perspective. As Stacey (1988) makes eloquently clear, feminist issues are central to understanding health and illness in all societies. Yet feminism and the feminine viewpoint provide only one way of gaining insights. Women are never just women – they are also young or old, mothers or daughters, black or white, partnered or unpartnered, employed in public life or at home – and so a feminist viewpoint is contextualised among others (Gelsthorpe 1992). Feminist theory is not a homogeneous set of ideas and different feminist writers draw on pieces of theory included in both the structuralist and action perspectives. Feminism, however, has a unifying theme in the critique of the gender order in modern capitalist societies and recognises the basis of knowledge through dominant masculine viewpoints. Oakley (1972) has documented the way different societies allocate roles and responsibilities differentially between the sexes, noting that the ways in which this is done is variable. Gender order is not only about the division of labour between the sexes but the presence of authority relations and social stratification on the basis of gender. This social order is one of gender, and not of sex, for it is socially constructed and may be constructed in a number of ways. In most societies men, not women, are accorded the superior status and this is the case in modern capitalist societies. Because it explicitly recognises the political, i.e. power struggles underlying the production of all forms of knowledge, feminist sociology also tends to adopt methods which negate power hierarchies and include emancipation among its goals (Ramazanogulu 1992).

We will return to the issue of gender order in the next chapter when discussing social stratification, and in subsequent chapters since feminist issues cut across those of health and illness as well as family and professionals.

SYMBOLIC INTERACTIONISM AS A PERSPECTIVE

In some ways symbolic interactionism is an embracing term given to a number of sociological approaches in which an action perspective, rather than a structuralist perspective, is taken. The core ideas of the action perspective, known as *action theory* have evolved from Max Weber's simple idea that sociologists should proceed to *understand* those they study. This is achieved by attempting to look upon the world as they do — by appreciating how the world looks to them. To this is added learning the ideas, motives and goals which make people act. By learning these things about individuals, the sociologist should gain an understanding of why they act in certain ways in order to achieve particular ends in the face of their individual circumstances as they see them.

This approach, emphasising understanding the individual, is very different from that of the structuralist perspective with its emphasis on social structures and facts which exist independently of individual members of society. Though Parsons (1951) sought to build his structural functionalist theories from the elements of individuals' social action, he set them within the broader social systems which governed individual action. His emphasis therefore was on the understanding of social action by reference to social systems rather than of social action as generated through individuals in their particular circumstances. Thus, *social action* is attractive to a broad range of social theories but is difficult to study empirically while linked to broad social structures rather than small groups. It has been left to those with an action perspective to translate their theoretical position into empirical studies.

The bases of symbolic interactionism

The main ideas of symbolic interactionism were provided by George Herbert Mead (1863–1931, Fig. 2.2) in Chicago earlier this century, and the major contributions to this perspective have continued to be North American. At the heart of Mead's approach is the assumption that there is a difference between animal *reaction* and human *conduct*. Conduct requires the possession of *mind* which is distinctive to the human species. To this is added the concept of *self*. Individuals both undergo experiences and are aware of doing so.

Mead (1934) regards human action as very different from human behaviour. Behaviour is limited to a stimulus-response relationship. The concept of action depends on individuals' ability to plan their actions, reflect on past experience and reflect on themselves in the same way as they look upon other kinds of objects in the environment. It is the capacity for self-consciousness which makes human beings different from animals, and central to this is the ability of individuals to take the same attitude towards themselves as others take toward them. In this sense we become objects like any other objects; to look upon oneself as an object is to see oneself as others do.

For different individuals the same object, be it a pine tree or antenatal care, will have very different meanings which will depend on such factors as previous experiences and current purposes. The social significance of the pine tree will differ as a result of individuals' experiences. Post office engineers, through social interaction with fellow workers, may find themselves classifying pine trees as suitable or not suitable for telegraph poles. They will have learnt from other colleagues that elms and oaks are not suitable for the job. Country children learn from their peers that pine wood burns well but too quickly and is therefore not as suitable for fuel as oak or beech. When out on expeditions naturalists will refer to different pine trees by their various Latin names since this will have more significance for colleagues. Similarly, for a pregnant woman the value of antenatal care is determined by the individual's knowledge of her pregnancy, her experience of pregnancy and the experience of her peers. To health professionals the value of antenatal care will be determined by the kinds of information they receive during their professional training.

As individuals we all also experience the many different meanings we hold of ourselves for others, reflected back to ourselves. To handle this complexity, we construct pictures of ourselves according to the general, typical and predominant view of ourselves as shown by others. This is carried out largely through the medium of language – 'only human beings share language' – which Mead refers to as the *significant symbol*. Through such exchanges we learn the ways of acting which others expect of us and the self-consciousness necessary to engage in social life. The meanings of all objects are similarly derived from our social interaction with other members of society. Such meanings are handled in and modified through an interpretation process used by all of us in dealing with things we encounter.

It is explaining such processes that is the hallmark of symbolic interactionist approaches – providing an understanding of how and why things are as they are, by finding out about the circumstances of people's lives. Blumer (1969) contends these circumstances do not exist *in themselves* as stimuli to which the individual reacts. Rather, what constitutes circumstances depends on the purposes, plans and knowledge that the individual has *in mind*. Social action therefore has to be interpreted as the mindful action of individuals initiated to bring about certain purposes.

Blumer provides a major critique of those sociological approaches which attempt to ape the natural sciences by linking dependent and independent variables without any real understanding of either the variables themselves or what processes actually link them. This is because sociological abstractions used as variables, such as *authority* or *group morale*, have different indicators depending on the circumstances in which they are being studied. It would be inappropriate to use the same indicators, for example, of social integration, when applied to whole cities or a ward in a hospital. What Blumer is saying is that social life is extremely complex because of the elaborate and various processes which exist and about which we have only the most limited findings, and because the *inner* workings of social life which give rise to them are equally complex.

Blumer, therefore, advocates an approach to sociological enquiry which is distinctly sociological in that it examines in detail particular instances of social life as they occur in their natural settings. In advocating a *naturalistic* approach symbolic interactionists aim to put themselves in the position of seeing the world in the same way as the people they are studying. In carrying out studies which have been intensively concerned with topics limited to particular occasions or a narrow set of circumstances, symbolic interactionists have made a distinctive con-

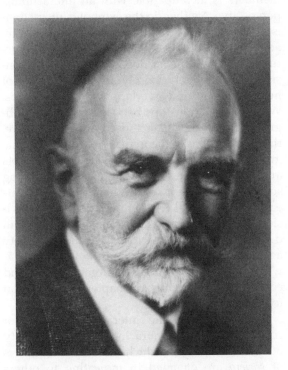

Fig. 2.2 The father of symbolic interactionism: George Herbert Mead (1863-1931) (courtesy of University of Chicago Library).

tribution to knowledge based on 'micro' sociological processes rather than the 'macro' analysis of the structuralists. One such contribution attempts to show how variable settings, which may differ by way of the content of their subject matter, display similar characteristics in terms of formal properties or structural arrangements. For example, much work has been done by symbolic interactionists on the concept of *career*. This is not only linked to occupational life; the career concept, as one of progression with differentiated stages, can also be applied to prisoners, patients and indeed the life cycle itself. Career can be said to have *formal* properties in that there is a chronological ordering of steps which are relatively predictable, each one bringing its typical experiences, tasks and problems. *Career* is therefore a formal generalisation, typical of the kind of formal approach used by symbolic interactionists; we pick it up in Chapter 5 in relation to the life career, Chapter 8 when we discuss the patient career and again in Chapter 11 for the professional career.

A similar idea is that social contexts influence interaction and, in Chapter 9, we discuss how *uncertainty* influences communication with patients and again in Chapter 10 in relation to the care of dying patients. Uncertainty, as a social context, would be equally relevant to playing bridge, arms and wage negotiations, managing information about a diagnosis or buying a house.

Symbolic interactionists have also shown how behaviour which from one perspective would be interpreted as totally irrational, from another perspective is a rational response to circumstances. We take up this idea in Chapter 8 when we discuss some ideas about illness behaviour and particularly the work of Goffman. This is associated with an interest in the processes by which members of society define their own circumstances and respective identities. This is encapsulated in a dictum attributed to W.I. Thomas: 'If men define situations as real, they are real in their consequences' (Merton 1968, p. 475). This definitional approach has had particular applications in what has come to be known as the *labelling theory of deviance*, that is,

how members of the community come to define and label some of its members as deviant in certain respects and interact with them in such a way that the person takes on the characteristics related to the label. We shall deal with labelling in Chapter 8, as it applies to patients.

The individual and society

For symbolic interactionists the organisation of social life arises from within society itself and out of the processes of interaction between its members. They do not accept that external factors, such as economic ones, determine the form that society takes, although such factors do exert influence. Such influences will vary, however, depending on how they are perceived and dealt with. While the organisation of social life arises from within, it does not take on any autonomous features like those attributed by structuralist sociologists. To assume that society imposes or determines the action of society's members is incompatible with an interactionist perspective. Neither do the symbolic interactionists regard the structure of society as rigidly adhering to some *basic*, almost universal structure, as Marxist theory does. Rather, society consists of a relatively loosely articulated array of heterogeneous and overlapping social groups. While the relationships between groups or subgroups may be characterised as competitive, there is no basic theoretical reason why one group should predominate. Relevant concepts and the processes of gaining or maintaining social dominance or control have been articulated by Strauss et al (1963) in relation to the division of labour in psychiatric hospitals. We will develop this idea of the *negotiated order* of society as groups continuously organising in Chapter 7, when we look at health care organisations, and consider its limitations in Chapter 11, in relation to professional power.

Typically, symbolic interactionists are not concerned with an embracing concept of society but with the way in which individual members of *society* are engaged in indicating to others who and what they take themselves to be. This draws heavily on Mead's view of the self as something created in and through social interaction. This self is portrayed in the conventional ways in which people communicate their social status, social role or sense of self. Goffman (1971) sought to understand how people come to decide, through social interaction, who they are. He also employs the metaphor of life being just like life on the stage. We develop this idea in Chapter 3, when we discuss how individuals engage in *impression management* in order to portray a particular identity and have this identity reaffirmed by others.

How do we achieve our sense of self? Particularly, what role does adult life play in modifying the sense of self achieved in childhood? Interactionists emphasise the continuous nature of socialisation extending throughout adulthood. This we shall elaborate when we discuss ageing in Chapter 5 and professional socialisation in Chapter 11.

Some criticisms of symbolic interactionism

Just as symbolic interactionists criticise sociological theory which conforms to natural science, which attempts an excessively deterministic view of the relationship between the individual and society, and which takes the macrostructure of society as its base, so reciprocal criticisms are levelled at symbolic interactionism. These include an indifference to problems of evidence, proof and systematic theory; an avoidance of regard for the structural constraints which foreclose available choices open to individuals; and an absence of any attempt to gain an overview of social organisation, with an accompanying neglect of the various sources of social stratification. Much of this criticism is directed not only at the basic theoretical assumptions of symbolic interactionism but also the *naturalistic* qualitative methods which it employs, with emphasis on lived experience as data, and which are at odds with the second order data and *quantitative methods* usually employed by sociologists using a structuralist perspective. Perhaps the most important criticism of symbolic interactionism is that offered by Cuff et al (1990) who highlight

the marginalisation of symbolic interactionism which has failed to produce a new idea for more than a decade. Symbolic interactionism, however, provides innumerable insights into our understanding of health and illness and for this reason we give the perspective more space than other introductory texts do. Moreover, a number of the ideas, which were spawned by symbolic interactionists, have been absorbed into mainstream sociology as everyday sociological knowledge.

ETHNOMETHODOLOGY AS A PERSPECTIVE

To some extent, ethnomethodology has taken over the role of symbolic interactionism as the minority critique of what was the dominant structuralist perspective in mainstream sociology. Here, we give far less attention to ethnomethodology as a perspective than its critique of other perspectives merits. This is because, to date, ethnomethodology has contributed relatively little to our sociological knowledge about health and illness. Its basic assumptions, deriving largely from the phenomenological philosophy of Edmund Husserl (1859–1938) are very different from those of other sociological theories and are often found to be confusing to those encountering these ideas for the first time.

Husserl attempts to describe the ultimate foundations which humans experience by 'seeing beyond' the particulars of everyday experiences to describe the 'essences' which underpin them. Only by grasping such essences do we have a foundation for all experience which enables us to recognise and classify it in an intelligible form. In order to grasp these essences it is necessary for the philosopher to disengage from our usual ideas about the world, to examine the stream of experiences available to us – past, present and future. Phenomenology is about perceiving phenomena in the world as objects or events which are, in essential respects, *common* – the same for others as they are for ourselves. Therefore, the foundations of social life are not within the mind and experience of the individual but in a commonly lived world of experience. This is a social world known in common with others.

It was Alfred Schutz (1899–1959) who developed this phenomenological approach into a sociological study of social life which has subsequently come to be known as ethnomethodology (ethno = people, hence ethnomethodology = the study of people's methods). Ethnomethodology especially, though not solely, is concerned with the language used in and to describe everyday life. The approach is concerned with the basis of the assumptions we all make in order to render comprehensible the routines and activities of everyday life. Such order is achieved through what Schutz (1972) has termed our *taken-for-granted assumptions*, in other words, our expectations of what should happen in a normal day and how we expect others to act. For example, we used to expect shops to close on Sunday but no longer, we expect the accident and emergency department to be busy on Saturday evenings, we know how to behave in the presence of our peers, teachers and parents. The social fabric is maintained by what Schutz (1972) has called *typifications*, that is, common ways of classifying particular objects (like tree or woman), events (like visits to the doctor or getting breakfast) and experiences (like pain or love) but in ways which are capable of being redesigned or adapted. One taken-for-granted assumption is that others, by and large, see the world as we do, something which is clearly not always borne out. This is nowhere more sharply focused as the disparity between adolescents and their parents! These elements of everyday life are not only learned through the process of socialisation but are also identified as 'mental tools' which we carry around with us in order that we can adapt our own actions according to the situations in which we find ourselves. Thus, like the interactionists, ethnomethodologists are concerned with how members of a social group perceive, define and classify the ways in which they actually perform their activities, and what meanings they assign to acts occurring in the context of their everyday lives.

We shall examine some ideas on professionals' typifications of patients, and their

effects, in Chapter 9 when we deal with social interaction.

The conceptual framework of ethnomethodology

In order to grasp the distinctiveness of ethnomethodology it is important to understand some rather basic though complex concepts. Their difficulty is partly due to the radical differences in perspective of ethnomethodologists, as well as to the language used by writers like Harold Garfinkel.

Rather than use the term actors or participants, ethnomethodologists follow the convention of Garfinkel (1967a) and talk about *members*. This term is preferred because it covers belief of a shared social life with others. Members recognise and produce social activities using methods which make them unproblematically available to other members. In order to produce routine unproblematic features of our everyday lives we engage in sense-making work. In other words, it is by *members' methods* of engaging in sense-making work that we actually accomplish the social world – be it telling a joke, carrying out a clinic or giving a lecture. Not only do we make it clear to others that this is what we are doing, but others also engage in sense-making work to comprehend and let us know that they comprehend what is going on – or that, in fact, they do not understand and would like us to make things clearer. This means that the social world is not something imposed from 'out there' or inherited by virtue of an assigned role. Rather, Garfinkel proposes that we must accomplish our social world and that we do so in ways which we ordinarily take for granted and do not stop to analyse. Ethnomethodologists regard it as their task to provide such an analysis in order to explain how we achieve the social world we inhabit.

Members' actions, and again their speech, are features of the organised social settings in which they are used and which they in turn produce. In this sense they are *indexical* to social settings. Garfinkel uses the term *indexicality* to stress the occasioned nature of everyday happenings –

the particulars of social occasions and events. For instance, there is no standardised use of words. How phrases like 'he's had it' are interpreted will depend on the particular occasion and the taken-for-granted analytic work of members. Similarly, the nature of the occasion, what it is, and what it means – be it a social chat or a disciplinary hearing – is not unambiguous. But making what it is has to be achieved by the members involved in it – there is no external reality.

This work is what ethnomethodologists refer to as 'repairing indexical particulars' – how members go about arriving at a limited definition of what they are engaged in. Not only members, but also ethnomethodologists studying members, must go through the same process to review and document what is of significance and arrive at a shorthand description of particular occasions. In every new situation the same processes have to be engaged in to produce the members' sense of it.

Garfinkel's analysis of the repair of indexical expression emphasises this as members' practical problems *and* the means whereby they manage to accomplish the social world. This whole enterprise is characterised by *reflexivity*. Reflexivity refers to the essential interdependence of the circumstances members attribute to social events and their descriptions or accounts of what the events themselves are. In other words, circumstances are embedded in descriptions or accounts of events and accounts or descriptions of events are embedded in their particular circumstances. Thus, members who are taking part in some social occasion use its features both to make visible to others what is happening and to make the features themselves come about. They do so by using members' common-sense methods to make this world describable to themselves and to others. Ethnomethodologists, in attempting to explicate these methods, are themselves confronted with making sense of what is happening and must examine their own reflexivity, something members take for granted.

In some respects, ethnomethodology is like symbolic interactionism in that it is concerned with studying social interaction as a process of meaningful communicative activity. There the similarity ends, however. Douglas (1976) has argued that while interactionists focus their attention on ongoing social interactions between individuals, they interpret these actions in a *scientistic fashion*. They, like the functionalists, are concerned with hypothesis testing and identifying cause and effect. To arrive at this level of explanation requires the translation of observations and statements about everyday happenings into more abstract theoretical statements. The ethnomethodological position is that this level of theorising and the methods used to achieve it are basically inappropriate for achieving a real understanding of everyday life:

There is no way of getting at the social meanings from which one implicitly or explicitly infers the larger patterns except through some form of communication with the members of that society or group; and, to be valid and reliable, any such communication with the members presupposes an understanding of their language, their use of language, their own understanding of what the people doing the observations are up to, and so on almost endlessly. (Douglas 1976, p. 9)

Thus the phenomena to be studied must be the phenomena as *experienced* in everyday life and not the phenomena observed and interpreted by the scientist with her or his own particular taken-for-granted assumptions, which will differ from those of the subject being studied. Similarly, the methods used for such empirical studies must be those which facilitate gaining this kind of understanding. Of course, this position is open to the criticism that while ethnomethodologists study members' methods they simultaneously employ these methods themselves. Ethnomethodologists would reply that it is necessary to construct methods of data collection and analysis appropriate to the empirical settings in which the search is conducted rather than producing a set of generalised methodological directives appropriate to particular settings. They will be judged, therefore, on the basis of the detailed arguments in reported empirical studies.

SOCIOLOGICAL PERSPECTIVES

At the beginning of this chapter we identified five broad sociological perspectives: consensus structuralist perspectives, conflict structuralist perspectives, critical theory, interactionism and ethnomethodology. As we unravelled the basic idea of each, it becomes apparent that each broad perspective comprises a number of different ideas and concepts. These have been labelled in different ways by sociologists, in different countries and over time. For example, we have included in the consensus perspective functionalism, structural functionalism and neofunctionalism. In an attempt to distinguish between the five broad perspectives we have drawn a sociological family tree of the different perspectives indicating links between different writers, their ideas and theories (see Fig. 2.3). The unbroken lines in the diagram show where there is a direct influence between writers, the dotted lines an indirect connection.

Our aim in writing this chapter has been to emphasise not only the central position of theory in sociology but also its relevance to our everyday lives. Our actions and how we interpret the world are guided by personal and often implicit theories. By contrast, the interpretations of the social world and the studies carried out by sociologists depend on theories which have been made explicit and are open to public scrutiny. One aspect of becoming familiar with sociology is to recognise these different major theories before making a decision about which to subscribe to as most useful, in what situation, for explaining particular social phenomena. Sociologists themselves have to make such decisions.

The consensus and conflict perspectives, critical theory, interactionism and ethnomethodology have been characterised as expounding their particular ways of interpreting society, its composition, how it changes and what are useful central concepts and processes. We have presented a very broad and of necessity introductory approach. While we have touched on some major divisions in their broad perspectives, there are many other variations which students of sociology will encounter.

As components of sociological perspectives, different questions are asked about social phenomena and they are investigated in different ways. The example of mental illness was used at the beginning of the chapter to demonstrate the kinds of research questions and approaches likely to evolve from different perspectives. This is typical of the diversity to be found in the way that health topics are conceptualised as well as in approaches used to study the social world more generally. There are ongoing debates around all major sociological, theoretical and research methodological approaches and these will surface in some of the ensuing chapters, most explicitly in Chapter 12 which deals with sociological methods.

It is important to grasp that in gaining a sociological understanding, sociological theory is not something to be glanced at then forgotten. It is not distinct from the research which provides us with a sociology of health and illness. Without sociological theory providing particular sociological perspectives it would be well-nigh impossible to comprehend the basis of research and the assumptions on which it is based. Yet in other disciplines there is sometimes an assumption that what is being worked with are 'the facts' without ever questioning their epistemological basis. In our everyday world, a common attempt at this is the politicians' introductory remark 'the fact of the matter is' followed by a statement that many people would consider is certainly not a fact in their book.

We have attempted to show that there is no one particular perspective in sociology nor indeed could a sociology be constructed from the 'best' bits from each theory. Sociological theorists take up far too strongly-held positions within their own camps to permit this to happen and tend to adhere to one perspective which they regard as *the* approach to sociology. Although we too have our preferences, we have tried to present a balanced description of major perspectives without advocating that overall one has more relevance or more to offer than another. Different perspectives generate research on different topics and choose different methods in doing so. As you read on you will encounter

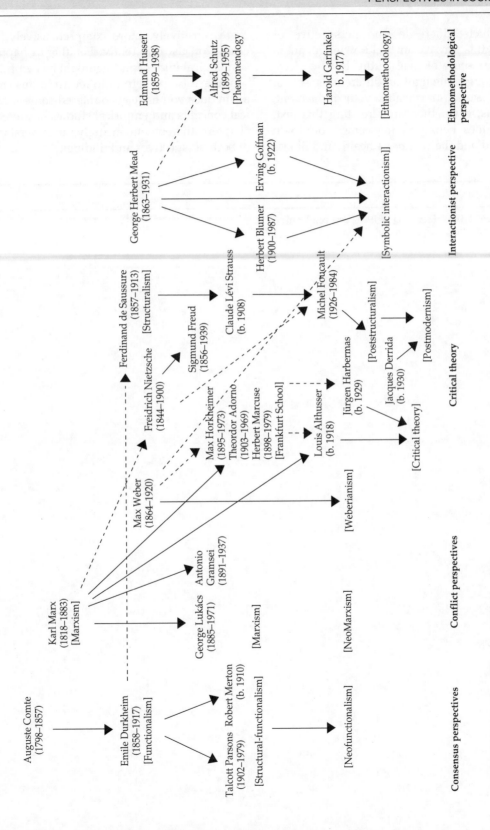

Fig. 2.3 Major theoretical perspectives in sociology.

studies which adhere to one perspective or another. In this way we amass knowledge, not in any absolute sense of final truths, but by piecemeal shedding some light on different aspects of our social world. It remains your judgement, however, as to whether, after reading this text, sociology does help you in seeing your own social world and the worlds of health and illness more sensitively, more comprehensively, more clearly or just differently. For this to happen, a sociological understanding might be helpful.

It may also be helpful to return to this chapter again once you have encountered some sociological concepts and empirical studies in succeeding chapters, thereby enhancing your understanding of both perspectives and findings.

FURTHER READING

Cuff E C, Sharrock W W, Francis D W 1990 Perspectives in sociology, 3rd edn. Unwin Hyman, London

3

Social stratification

INTRODUCTION

In the last chapter we introduced a number of different sociological perspectives. Common to all of these is a concern with the nature of social order. We shall explore this topic in a number of places throughout the book. In this chapter we look at social order from the structuralist perspective by describing the many forms of social stratification and show how the concept of social stratification relates to people's experiences, and in particular to their use of health services.

We shall examine the major structural concepts – class, status and power – and discuss their relevance to the issue of the gender order. Mobility within stratification systems will be explored and the difficulties of measuring social class identified as a preliminary to understanding data which link indicators of health, such as mortality and morbidity rates, to social structural indices. Inequalities in health are explored also.

We are all familiar with the notion of the geological stratification of rocks which are ordered according to their age. In societies there are also criteria by which social groups are stratified. In many societies, occupation is the main criterion upon which stratification is based but different cultures also use caste, as in India; 'race', most explicitly recently in South Africa; or ethnic origins, as in Nazi Germany. Concepts like 'race', age and occupation vary in importance as stratification variables in all societies and cultures. An additional dimension of the stratification system is the gender order.

Our analogy between geological stratification and social stratification could be misleading if taken too far. Worsley (1977) notes a number of ways in which the analogy is wrong. Since the principle of rock stratification is based on the age of rocks it is a permanent system. In contrast, social systems are more flexible and can change over time because the principles of social stratification are *socially constructed*. In many social strata the different levels are defined in terms of inferiority or superiority in income, prestige and power. These criteria are socially constructed. For example, some occupations which were prestigious 30 years ago are less so today; nurses and teachers both make this claim about their professions. Another characteristic of social stratification not found in geological stratification is that *conflict* often exists between different social strata, for example, between management and labour, and between ethnic and other minorities and the dominant social group. Also the principles of social stratification allow individuals to *move* from one stratum to another; for instance, the child of a labourer becomes a doctor or even a Prime Minister, or a man from the ranks gains officer status. This is called *social mobility*. Geological strata are of course static (although rock formations may move).

A distinctive feature of all social stratification is *inequality* between the strata. There are two aspects of inequality that are particularly important. The first concerns the distribution of such things as income, wealth, prestige, education, power and health. The second concerns the way individuals differentiated by such criteria relate to each other. 'Forelock tugging' is an obvious example of the way two individuals, from different social strata, relate to each other. Another common example is the differential use of first names and nicknames.

In sociology a number of different and relatively enduring systems of social stratification have been identified: slavery, caste, estates and class.

Slavery

Slavery is an extreme form of social stratification in which one person literally owns another as if he or she were their property. We tend to associate slavery with plantation economies such as in the United States, the West Indies and South America during the 18th and 19th centuries. The slaves were deprived of almost all human rights. In other societies slavery existed but was less severe, as for example in ancient Rome. Although excluded from political positions, slaves were found in most other types of occupations. A form of slavery continued to exist in Britain during the 19th century where married women and anything they 'owned' were the property of their husbands. Where slavery was based on ascribed characteristics, such as gender or 'race', postslavery inequalities continue to exist.

Caste

Caste is associated with the Indian subcontinent in which different social groups are ranked in terms of social honour. The caste system varies between different areas of the subcontinent which share certain principles. Those in the highest social group (referred to as 'varna' in India), the Brahmins, represent the most elevated condition of purity; the untouchables the lowest. The Brahmins must avoid certain types of contact with the untouchables, and it is only the untouchables who are allowed contact with animals or with substances regarded as unclean. The caste system is closely tied in with the Hindu religion and the belief in rebirth. Individuals who fail to live up to the duties and rituals of their caste are believed to be reborn into an inferior position in their next reincarnation.

The concept of caste has been applied outside of the context of the Hindu religion in societies where two or more ethnic groups are segregated from one another and where notions of racial purity prevail. Taboos against intermarriage prevail, often reinforced by legal prohibitions. In this way, the concept of caste has been used to characterise apartheid in South Africa and postslavery society in the southern United States.

Estates

Estates existed as part of the system of feudalism in Europe during the middle ages. The feudal estates comprised a number of different strata characterised by specific obligations and rights which were often reinforced in law. Three main estates were distinguished: the aristocracy, the clergy and the commoners.

Intermarriage and individual mobility was tolerated between estates although not that common. Although feudalism disappeared with the industrial revolution and subsequent establishment of democracy throughout Europe, characteristics of feudalism still exist in modern day Britain. Examples are the traditional honours system, which generates aristocracy, and the continuing role of the monarchy. Estate society, however, has developed into a class society with the aristocracy and gentry forming the basis of the 'upper' classes.

Class

The concept of class is central to modern-day theories of social stratification. It is not only used by sociologists to distinguish between different social groups, but also in Government statistics, by politicians and in everyday language. However, because it is used in so many different ways – to categorise people by income, wealth, power, prestige or occupation – it is an awkward concept.

Class systems differ in a number of respects from slavery, castes or estates. Giddens (1989) highlights four key differences:

1. Classes are more flexible than other systems of social stratification, encouraging mobility between strata.
2. Classes are achieved rather than ascribed on the basis of ethnicity or birth.
3. Classes depend on economic differences between groupings of individuals.

4. Inequalities between classes are expressed in terms of inequalities between social groups whereas other systems of social stratification express inequalities primarily in personal relationships of duty or obligation.

THEORIES OF SOCIAL CLASS

The structuralist perspective of class as a system of social stratification owes much to the writings of Marx and Weber. As we saw in Chapter 2 class was at the centre of Marx's theory of social change under capitalism. Yet Marx himself never fully defined class, although his general conceptions about social classes and their behaviour are fairly clear. Marx divided capitalist society into two classes: the bourgeoisie, who were the owners of the means of production, and the proletariat, who were not. His analysis of class struggles and conflict, which were central to his political ideology as opposed to his sociological insights, was based on this fundamental distinction between the two classes.

In contrast, Weber's use of the concept of class is somewhat wider in scope (Gerth & Mills 1948). In Weber's sense a person's class position is the location which he or she shares with those who are similarly placed in the processes of production, distribution and exchange. It includes not only the specific relationship between the bourgeoisie and proletariat but all those situations where there is a market relationship. For example, Weber would include the ownership of housing as a criterion for locating a person's class. Significant inequalities between members of the proletariat arising from home ownership would not be recognised in Marxist theory as locating individuals' in different classes.

Weber also recognised a greater variety of relationships to the means of production. Marx's dichotomy between the bourgeoisie and proletariat meant that shopkeepers and wage earners could be in a single economic and social group: the proletariat. Similarly, there is no room in this classification for the nonmanufacturing industries, ranging from the social service industries and the distribution industries to the financial service industries of banking and insurance. Weber, in contrast, recognised that individuals could be classified by class according to all of these different relationships with the processes of production, because they determined the lifestyle and life chances of different groups in society. Thus Weber argued that individuals' class positions differ because of the meaning they can and do give to the use of their property as well as because of its ownership.

The Weberian concept of class allows us to understand inequalities of class, not just in terms of the relationship between the owners and nonowners of the means of production. It allows us to understand inequalities in income, occupation and education. In this sense, class becomes a more complex social phenomenon which embraces all aspects of *economic* position in society. Inequalities of class refer to economic inequalities of income, wealth and education rather than to inequalities of prestige or power.

STATUS

Complementary to Weber's concept of class was his concept of *status*, which refers to the difference between social groups in the social honour or prestige accorded by others. To Weber, status implied not only the apportionment of prestige for some specific occupational or other role, but also involved the apportionment of generalised prestige which segregates one group from another. Both class and status are derived from different economic aspects of social behaviour. Weber placed the emphasis on styles of consumption, that is, the way income is used rather than income itself. Therefore status is determined not by income *per se* but by place of residence, type of speech, social origins, social habits and educational background.

Although there is often a strong relationship between economic class as defined by occupation and status as defined by styles of consumption, there are a number of familiar examples where high status is not matched by high occupational class. Compare the position of the poor aristocrat in a stately home with increasing debts arising from death duties, and the *nouveau riche* who may well be better placed in the economic hierarchy but are not admitted to the highest social gatherings. Many of the health professions are relatively high status occupations despite their relatively low incomes, as are the clergy.

Like class, status is a complex concept. For example, there is little theoretical discussion about the characteristics of status whose possession leads to high or low prestige. Indeed, there has been little attempt to determine the characteristics empirically. Most empirical work undertaken has consisted of surveys of occupational prestige rather than other facets of prestige. These studies have shown remarkable unanimity (Goldthorpe & Hope 1974, Runciman 1966), which suggests that status is defined by common consent.

These empirical studies do not, however, explain *how* prestige is differentially assigned between occupational groups. A functionalist explanation is provided by Davis and Moore:

If unequal rights and perquisites of different positions in a society must be unequal, then the society must be stratified, because that is precisely what stratification means. Social inequality is thus an unconsciously evolved device by which societies ensure that the most important positions are conscientiously filled by the most qualified persons. (Davis & Moore 1945, p. 243)

Rex (1961) believes that the assignment of prestige is quite arbitrary and considers the only plausible explanation is that different social positions derive prestige because they are historically important. This, however, does not tell us why they were afforded such relative prestige in the first place.

POWER

A third aspect of Weber's theory of stratification is that of power. Weber, however, is less explicit about his concept of power than he is about either class or status. Whereas he speaks of low class or low status, there is no comparable notion of low power. Yet, power is implicitly a third dimension of stratification in that Weber is concerned with the relative power of classes and status groups.

Power is a commonly used word, but what do sociologists mean by it? The holders of power need not necessarily be highly rewarded or hold a high prestige position in society. We hear regularly of the power of trade union officials and of ward domestics and nursing auxiliaries, who are neither highly paid nor hold significant prestige in the community. In order to understand the implicit notion of power we must introduce the Weberian concepts of *authority* and *legitimacy*.

Authority is the probability that a specific order, say given by a ward sister, will be obeyed by specific individuals or groups, say student nurses. The essential difference between power and authority is the continuity of the latter. Power is more often momentary: the ward sister gives an order and despite any disagreement the student nurse obeys. The exercise of this power has little continuing effect but the authority of the ward sister persists.

By *legitimacy* Weber means that people accept the authority as just and that those endowed with authority are given it rightfully. In other words, the authority of the ward sister is accepted by the student nurses as just, and the ward sister's right to issue orders, even though they might disagree, is also accepted. Student nurses would be less likely to regard the authority of a nursing auxiliary as legitimate, although at times they can exert power in the organisation of the ward.

In the same way that power need not coincide with class or status, inequality of power need not parallel inequality of status or class, although there is usually a demonstrable connection between a person's class position and his or her power position. But to the extent that power is a separate dimension of social stratification, so power is a separate dimension of inequality. In order to understand the stratifications and inequalities in our society it is probably necessary to keep in mind that all three dimensions are relevant.

Contemporary developments in stratification theory

The ideas of Marx and Weber dominate our present sociological understanding of social stratification. The contemporary Marxist and Weberian perspectives are both similar and complementary.

Marxist perspectives

The dominant challenge to Marx's concept of class was the emergence of a substantial middle class contributing to a process of embourgeoisment – the process by which the more affluent manual workers become effectively middle class. Different writers of the Marxist perspective have responded to this challenge in different ways. Westergaard and Resler (1976) in their analysis of contemporary class structure in Britain, argue that a large proportion of the new middle class are in jobs which increasingly resemble proletarian ones in terms of income and the working conditions which they offer. Their conclusion is that, although the type of jobs may be changing and society may be becoming more affluent, the labour force is undergoing a process of proletarianisation in modern Britain. In other words, the bourgeoisie in modern Britain are those who control the means of production and the proletariat are those who do not. Polarisation of society into two class groups remains inevitable.

In Europe, Poulantzas (1979) has argued that classes are structurally determined not only at the economic level but also at the political and ideological levels as well. For Poulantzas, classes continue to be defined by their relation to the means of production; in particular, whether a class is engaged in productive or unproductive labour. For Poulantzas, the true proletariat are those who are 'productive' (as opposed to 'unproductive') and engaged in 'manual' (as opposed to 'mental') labour. Poulantzas, however, recognised that a part of one class could ally itself with sections of other classes. This concept is known as a class fraction.

Elin Olin Wright has taken the Marxist perspective further utilising Poulantzas' concept of class fraction as well as some ideas from Weber (Wright 1979, 1985). In modern capitalism, Wright identified three dimensions of control over production: control over investments or money capital, control over the physical means of production and control over labour power. Those who belong to the capitalist class (the bourgeoisie in Marxist terms), he argues, have control over all three dimensions while the working class (the proletariat) have none. In between these two main classes are a number of groups whose position is ambiguous. People in these groups are in contradictory class locations, because they are able to influence to a variable extent the production process but are denied control over others. Many nonmanual workers have to contract their labour power like manual workers, however, they have greater control over the work setting than do manual workers. Wright terms the class position of such workers as 'contradictory' because the workers in such locations are neither capitalists nor manual workers although sharing features with each.

Weberian perspectives

Giddens (1973), in providing a critique of developments in Marxist analysis, outlined the process of class structuration. That is, the way that 'economic' relationships become translated into 'noneconomic' structures. The structuration of class relationships depends on two types of influence: mediate and proximate structuration. Mediate structuration includes factors like the amount of social mobility, the ownership of property or the achievement of qualifications. Proximate structuration influences are the localised factors influencing class formation, such as differences in consumption patterns.

The process of class structuration is strongly influenced by social closure. By social closure Parkin (1979) meant any process by which social groups try to maintain control over resources and limiting access to them by other social groups. Property is only one form of social closure; ethnic origin, age, gender, language or religion are other status characteristics which might be used to create social closure.

Parkin identified two kinds of process in social closure. Exclusion refers to strategies which groups adopt to separate outsiders from themselves, thus preventing them from having access to scarce resources. One feature of the professionalising of health workers was to exclude unskilled health workers from the benefits of professional membership. (We return to this aspect again in Chapter 11.) The process of usurpation refers to attempts of the less privileged to acquire resources previously monopolised by others – as are groups of radical midwives in challenging the monopoly of obstetricians in childbirth.

Where both strategies are used together Parkin uses the term dual closure. For example, where midwives are on the one hand campaigning for more clinical autonomy and on the other hand excluding nurses not qualified as midwives from working in maternity facilities. Dual closure is similar to the idea of contradictory class locations described by Wright. Both notions indicate that those in the middle of the stratification system are looking upwards while keeping a wary eye on those beneath them.

ASCRIBED CLASSES

Because of the emphasis on the economic aspects of class this has encouraged an emphasis on occupational class. We *acquire* our occupational class, whereas other strata within a system of social stratification can be identified on the basis of *ascribed* characteristics with which we are born. Age, gender and 'race' are ascribed characteristics which we implicitly or explicitly order hierarchically. This raises the question of the extent to which strata defined on the basis of ascribed characteristics also constitute a class or a status group (Fig. 3.1).

Age, gender and 'race' are natural attributes which are usually relatively easily identified. But inequalities between people in different age groups, between men and women, and between people of different 'races' are more than biologically determined – they are all social constructions. For instance, different societies construct old age in different ways: functionally, formally and temporally. In societies where old age is defined in *functional* terms, observed changes in a person's abilities to undertake the normal activities of the adult status signifies the end of active participation as an adult. The person becomes one of the 'aged'. In societies where old age is defined in *formal* terms the change in status is normally linked to some external event like becoming a grandparent or being awarded a pension. In some societies old age is related *temporally* and chronological age is used as an indicator of the status of old age. This happens in some hospitals in Britain where all 'medical' admissions aged 65 or over enter wards designated 'geriatric'.

Gender, age and 'race' in modern Britain are all ascribed characteristics which have been used to determine the division of labour in society. From a Marxist perspective, women are economically exploited by men, elderly people by young people and black people by white people. From a Weberian perspective, inequalities between men and women, people of different ages and people of different 'races' or ethnic status directly reflect the inequalities of the productive system and the hierarchy of the economic structure of society. Thus, in both these senses, men and women, young people and old people, and black people and white people can be regarded as distinct classes. Other features can equally be used as the basis for class divisions, for example occupational classes – nonmanual and manual; educational classes – graduates and nongraduates; and housing classes – owner occupiers and tenants.

Gender and class

As many feminist writers have cogently argued, both class theory and empirical research on social stratification have been gender blind (Dex 1985). Contemporary Marxist and Weberian analysts of social stratification have adopted an approach which effectively excludes women from the class structure. This has come about in empirical studies because of the tendency to treat families rather than individuals as the unit of analysis, which effectively ignores inequalities between men and women. (We shall explore the sexual division of labour within the family in more detail in Chapter 5.) Most writers on class recognise the presence of gender inequalities (Giddens 1989), but their importance to class theory has been widely overlooked. Few class analysts have attempted to justify their exclusion of gender inequalities from stratification studies.

Writing over 20 years ago, however, Parkin argues that there is a substantial overlap between class and gender inequalities:

Female status certainly carries with it many disadvantages compared with that of males in various areas of social life including employment, property ownership, income and so on. However, these inequalities associated with sex differences are not usefully thought of as components of stratification. This is because for the great majority of women the allocation of social and economic rewards is determined primarily by the position of

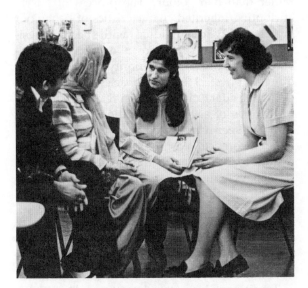

Fig. 3.1 Some Community Health Councils provide positive support to members of disadvantaged ethnic minorities to assist them obtain health care (courtesy of City and Hackney Community Health Council).

their families and, in particular, that of the male head. Although women today share certain status attributes in common, simply by virtue of their sex, their claims over resources are not primarily determined by their own occupation but, more commonly, by their fathers or husbands. (Parkin 1971, pp. 14–15)

More recently Goldthorpe (1983) has supported this view, arguing that in most families it is typically the male who has the fullest commitment to the labour market. He argues that the presence of the sexual division of labour within most families where women traditionally take major responsibility for home making and child care justifies the exclusion of women from class analysis because of their dependence on men.

We can criticize Goldthorpe's theoretical position at a number of levels. First, women in some households, nowadays, provide a major contribution to the total household resources which determines class position. Second, a wife's occupation may influence the occupation of her husband in the same way as a husband's occupation is believed to influence his wife's. Third, there exist cross-class households in which husband and wives occupy different occupational class positions. Fourth, the proportion of households in which the woman is the sole breadwinner is increasing.

In defence of the traditional approach we can see that in the past, when the proportion of women in the labour force was very small, classifying class according to the male breadwinner was pragmatic. Attempts to incorporate women into class analysis through the development of the analysis of cross-class families have been unsuccessful (Baxter 1988). The concept of class homogeneity – husbands and wives belonging to the same occupational class – is also not useful since nonearning wives continue to be classified according to their husband's occupation. Finally, much of this contemporary debate has been around issues of occupational class and takes no account of other dimensions of class. To date, attempts to add women into conventional class theory are inadequate. What is required is a substantial rethinking of class theory, which will allow women's dual experience as both unpaid home makers and members of the paid labour force to be incorporated into class analysis.

'Race' and class

Like gender, ethnic or racial origins are ascribed characteristics, which are socially constructed. A common view, however, is that 'race' is a biological category and that different biological categories of 'race' have different features. This belief was the basis of the Nazi vision of the German master 'race'. Biologists have identified any number of different 'races' depending on the traits used in classification. Many examples are to be found of characteristics of individuals which cut across any clear classifications. Developments in genetics have challenged the theory that there could have been several different lines of racial development.

Some people continue to argue that there are biological explanations for differences in the personality and behaviour of individuals based on racial and genetic origin. Why then, for example, are ethnic differences highlighted by skin colour rather than hair colour? The process of falsely attributing inherited characteristics of behaviour or personality to individuals with specific physical characteristics is known as racism. Attributing inferiority or superiority to people with different physical features is racist.

Like gender, 'race' has been relatively ignored in theories of social stratification. The relationship between class and 'race' is complex and three theoretical positions have been put forward. First, that class is the major division with 'race' having minor or secondary effects; second, that 'race' is the major division, with class being secondary; and third, that the two factors are equally important but interact in a complex way. Marxist writers tend to give supremacy to class while Weberian writers give more emphasis to 'race'.

Traditional Marxist perspectives do not distinguish individuals by 'race'. The position of black workers is no different from that of white workers, their class position being determined by their relationship to the means of production. Neomarxists, recognise that 'race' differentiates workers and have used Poulantzas' notion of a class fraction. Thus Phizacklea and Miles (1980) have used the concept of racialist class fraction to describe the position of West Indians living in Britain. They share the same class position as all workers in the same occupations but ally themselves with West Indians of other classes. The ideological category of 'race' produces different treatment, attitudes and political behaviour. Miles (1982) also recognises the presence of a racialist class fraction among the petty bourgeoisie.

The contemporary Weberian approach is to treat class position of all ethnic groups as representing their economic position in society. Ethnic minorities are disadvantaged in terms of status and power. It is the status attached to 'race' that has the potential for creating social cleavages independent of class, which at times might be more important as a basis for collective action and social closure (Parkin 1979). However, it is the underlying class positions which influence the resources available to ethnic minorities with which to engage in collective action. Hence, we cannot explain the position of ethnic minorities in society alone without focusing on their relationship with the dominant social groups in society.

In a recent analysis of class and 'race', Gilroy (1987) argues that 'race' may be seen by black people as an alternative to class as a basis for political action, but in the process be a factor in class formation. A key feature of this approach is the identification of cultural diversity between the different ethnic minorities represented in British society. This trend has been reflected during the 1980s by the development of a new form of racism, directed not at the existence of a black skin but at different physical features associated with the different cultures of ethnic minorities such as Asian dress or Rastifarian hairstyles. The value of this analysis is in highlighting the practical meaning of everyday terms like 'race', 'class', 'culture' and 'racism' as they reflect social change within British society.

SOCIAL MOBILITY

Social mobility refers to the movement of people within a stratification system. Mobility may be upwards or downwards. A nurse whose parents are from the manual classes is said to be upward mobile while a teacher's son who sweeps the road is said to be downward mobile. These are both forms of *vertical mobility*. The teacher who changes school, or the physiotherapist who changes from working in hospital to working in the community, experience *horizontal mobility* and would not, generally, be referred to as socially mobile. In everyday life we often talk of geographical mobility. The family who move to another town or city or even country are geographically mobile. If the reason for the move is to take up a better job then they are probably socially mobile as well. Social mobility and geographical mobility, however, are not synonymous.

Influences on social mobility

Within any system of social stratification there are five mechanisms which an individual might use to achieve upward social mobility. These mechanisms are related, so that one or more of them might be used by the individual consciously or unconsciously seeking upward mobility. Perhaps the most obvious means, obvious given the importance of the economic element in stratification systems, is through economic activity, such as hard work, luck or crime. By raising his or her income an individual has the means to afford the lifestyle of a higher class.

The second mechanism available in most societies is marriage. This is particularly the case for women, who are able to achieve upward mobility by marrying a man from a higher social class. Nowadays, this mechanism is not restricted to women, however, since men also marry women in higher social classes and manage to maintain their new position by the economic activity of their spouses.

Education offers the third mechanism for social mobility. Social mobility is achieved as part of an educational process which often complements the efforts of economic activity. The manual labourer's child who attends university is an obvious example.

A fourth mechanism of social mobility is political. This occurs when the social mobility of individuals or whole groups is achieved through political pressures, negotiations or guarantees. This is a particularly important mechanism in terms of group mobility. The Suffragette Movement and the Women's Movement, through mechanisms of franchise and pressing for equal employment and other social opportunity, have through political action increased the chances of upward social mobility for women.

Finally, Goffman (1971) coined the phrase *impression management* to describe social mobility achieved through the manipulation of status symbols and personal attraction. Used by itself impression management is unlikely to be a successful mechanism for upward mobility except for the small minority who have particularly attractive personalities and social skills. This mechanism, however, is important in conjunction with one or more of the four other mechanisms. The *nouveaux riches*, for example, are only acceptable to the aristocracy when they present the 'right' status images of themselves, and the person of working-class origin who, against the odds, makes it to leader of the conservative party and Prime Minister, will only succeed if he or she has learnt to conduct herself or himself socially. This does not mean, however, admission as a member of the 'establishment' (Paxman 1990).

Patterns of social mobility in Britain

It is widely argued that Britain nowadays is a more open society; in other words, that there is greater opportunity for social mobility. Since the 1940s, the favourable conditions necessary for increased social mobility have been encouraged by the social policies of successive governments, particularly in education and health. Continuous economic growth and, in the last decade, the technological revolution, have trans-

formed the occupational structure of society by increasing the proportion of nonmanual occupations, thus providing opportunities for upward mobility. At the same time, large-scale educational reforms were carried through which greatly increased educational provision and established formal equality of educational opportunity. In conjunction with other social policies educational reforms were intended to encourage a more open society.

But how successful have postwar social policies been in facilitating increased social mobility? Goldthorpe (1980) concluded, in his analysis of data collected in 1972 as part of the British mobility surveys, that there has been little increase in relative mobility rates; but because of changes in the occupational structure, there has been a general shift in absolute terms. To the average British person this is reflected in the better standard of living experienced by all strata of British society since 1940. The conclusions of this study were collaborated by analysis of new material collected about 10 years later (Goldthorpe & Payne 1986). An important change, however, was the higher proportion than before of men of working-class backgrounds who were unemployed, reflecting the spread of mass unemployment from the early 1970s onwards. The general conclusion from the British mobility studies is that, while Britain is generally more affluent, it is not a more open society than it was 50 years ago and there continues to be little relative social mobility between the various strata.

MEASUREMENT OF SOCIAL CLASS

It will be clear from the space devoted to the subject of social stratification that we consider it to be an essential ingredient to the understanding of our social structure. The concepts of social stratification, although complex, are crucial to any examination of the nature of our society. Historically, the concepts of class, status and power have played a central role in sociological theory. They have also been important concepts in public discussions of social and political change and policy.

In most empirical sociological research and in Government statistics and analysis the complex theoretical niceties discussed above are displaced by the need for pragmatic measures of 'social class'. In British research almost the sole criterion of social class which has been used is occupation. This is probably because no better empirical method of stratifying people has been found. Moreover, in the past, occupation has been shown consistently to be highly related to most other factors associated with social class, particularly income, wealth and education, and, as we show below, health.

Official measures of 'social class'

Since 1911 official statistics and studies have incorporated a measure of 'social class'. A major rationalisation of the approach to occupational classification was made in 1990 with the publication of the Standard Occupational Classification (OPCS 1990). For the national Census in 1911 the Registrar General graded occupations into eight 'classes' according to the 'social position' of the occupation. The criteria were arbitrary and have frequently been criticised. In the 1921 Census the number of 'classes' was reduced to five. Arbitrary updating of the measures continued until 1980. At the time of the 1981 Census the Registrar General used two methods of defining social class: six categories of Social Class and 17 Socioeconomic Groups. Both methods were based on occupation and both

deliberately combined the concepts of class and status. Table 3.1 gives examples of occupations which fall into each of the six Social Class categories.

Since Social Class is based on current occupation, married women, who were assumed not to work, were classified by their husband's occupation and retired persons according to their main occupation or husband's main occupation. For this reason classifications were less reliable for women and retired people.

In making comparisons between different years, particularly with years following a decennial Census, care should be taken in the interpretation of the trends because of changes in the allocation of occupations to the six Social Class categories. The most extensive changes occurred between the 1951 Census and 1961 Census but significant changes have been made at other times. Comparison between the 1991 Census and earlier years will require particularly careful interpretation given the introduction of the Standard Occupational Classification.

Standard Occupational Classification

In developing the new Standard Occupational Classification (SOC) for use by Government departments the Government Statistical Service has moved away from the somewhat tenuous link with the sociological concepts of class or status. Although occupational position is a good indicator of occupational class it is less strongly

Table 3.1 Occupations in Registrar General's social class categories

I Professional	II Managerial	III (N) Skilled nonmanual	III (M) Skilled manual	IV Partly skilled	V Unskilled
lawyer	farmer	cashier	machine tool setter	machine tool operator	builder's labourer
university lecturer	nurse	secretary	fitter	postal workers	messenger
doctor	office manager		miner (face worker)	traffic warden	railway station staff window cleaner

associated with the Marxian and Weberian concepts of class. The link with the social prestige of different occupations has been removed and the classification is more strongly associated with education and training. In the SOC, occupations are identified and aggregated with reference to the similarity of qualifications, training, skills and experience commonly associated with the competent performance of constituent tasks. From the SOC it will still be possible to aggregate individuals into the six Social Class categories and the 17 Socioeconomic Groups (Thomas & Elias 1989). The new SOC consists of the following major groups:

1. Managers and administrators
2. Professional occupations
3. Associated professional and technical occupations
4. Clerical and secretarial occupations
5. Craft and related occupations
6. Personal and protective service occupations
7. Sales occupations
8. Plant and machine operatives
9. Other occupations.

Table 3.2 gives examples of occupations which fall into each of the nine main SOC categories. The new classification has addressed the feminist criticism of the conventional approach to occupational class by making the classification applicable to paid jobs currently done by economically active persons in Great Britain. The classification does not take account of

Table 3.2   Occupations in SOC major groups

Major group	Occupations
1. Managers and administrators	General managers in NHS Production managers in manufacturing industries Managers and proprietors in service industries
2. Professional occupations	Doctor Lawyer Social worker
3. Associate professional and technical occupations	Nurses and midwifes Driving instructors
4. Clerical and secretarial occupations	Secretary Accountant's clerk
5. Craft and related occupations	Miner (face worker) Machine tool setter Fitter
6. Personal and protective service occupations	Police officer Railway station staff Traffic warden
7. Sales occupations	Cashier Roundsmen / women
8. Plant and machine operatives	Bus conductor Assembly-line workers
9. Other occupations	Postal workers Farm workers Window cleaners

women's unpaid jobs but has included additional occupational categories in areas of paid work where women predominate which lacked differentiation in previous classifications. Application of the Classification in the 1991 Census uses both the individual based and the traditional sexist household based approaches.

Social prestige measures of social class

Many sociologists were unhappy with the Registrar General's classification of Social Class and wanted a classification more firmly based on the social perceptions of occupational prestige. For the seminal study of social mobility (Glass 1954) a seven-category scale was developed, and this was modified subsequently to include the following eight categories:

1. Professionally qualified and high administrative.
2. Managerial and executive with some responsibility for directing and initiating policy.
3. Inspectional, supervisory and other nonmanual higher grade.
4. Inspectional, supervisory and other nonmanual.
5. Routine grades of nonmanual work.
6. Skilled manual work.
7. Semi-skilled manual work.
8. Routine manual work.

Table 3.3 gives examples of occupations which fall into each of these eight categories.

Like the Registrar General's classification of Social Class this categorisation of occupations is somewhat arbitrary, since it is impractical to invite samples of the population to rank 20 000 or more occupations. In the further development of this measure Goldthorpe and Hope (1974) used a basic 20 occupations and related these to the ranking of a further 860 by asking subsamples of people to rank two groups of 20 occupations: the basic 20 and a variable 20. In order to extend the concept they also asked each respondent to rank both groups of occupations on four separate dimensions:

- standard of living
- prestige in the community
- power and influence over other people
- value to society.

This approach tied the final classification closer to the Weberian perspective on social stratification rather than the pragmatic needs of the Government Statistical Service. It also achieved more consistent grading of occupations on the basis of prestige but at the cost of distinguishing a large and cumbersome number of grades. It adopted the conventional approach to the issue of gender and class.

Emphasis on status aspects of occupation has been criticised for its *normative* emphasis on the measurement of social class. Writers like

Table 3.3   Occupations in eight social classes used in British Social Mobility Study

Professionally qualified and high administrative	Managerial and executive	Inspectional, supervisory, and other nonmanual higher grade	Inspectional, supervisory and other nonmanual	Routine nonmanual work	Skilled manual	Semi-skilled manual	Unskilled manual
lawyer	headmaster	colliery engineer	accountant's clerk	tax officer	taxi driver	bus conductor	builder's labourer
doctor	missionary	social worker	shop manageress	receptionist	slater	farm labourer	railway station staff
surveyor	nurse administrator	qualified nurse			miner (face worker)	postal workers	window cleaner

Townsend (1979) have argued that, because they emphasise status rather than economic class, the classifications developed are more suitable for measuring the inequalities of occupational prestige than inequalities of class. He argues that this approach conditions society to interpret and accept inequality as one involving differences in the absolute distributions of occupations. Thus some inequalities, which are avoidable, are regarded as unavoidable and aspirations for social equality are interpreted only as aspirations for upward occupational mobility and not equality. Despite these criticisms, Townsend himself has been able to show gross inequalities between occupational classes (Townsend 1979) and it is to some of these to which we will turn to below.

Marxist measures of class

One response by sociologists in different countries to the normative approach of measuring 'social class' has been to utilise Wright's empirical operationalisation of Marxist categories of class (Wright 1979). As we have seen above, Wright distinguishes between two types of class locations – basic class locations and contradictory class locations. Basic class locations are those groups who either have control over the three spheres of production (control over investments or money capital, control over the physical means of production and control over labour power) or do not; in classical Marxism the bourgeoisie and the proletariat. Contradictory class locations, however, are not defined by such a simple polarisation of interests. Individuals are able to influence the production process to a variable extent but are denied control over others.

Wright (1979) also identifies contradictory class locations between different modes of production. These are small employers who own sufficient capital to hire workers but must work, and self-employed individuals who own sufficient capital to work for themselves but not enough to hire workers. On the basis of this framework Wright (1985) identified seven class locations (Fig. 3.2). Empirically, the bourgeoisie and small employers are defined in terms of self-employment and number of employees;

managers and supervisors defined in terms decision-making, authority and formal hierarchical position; semi-autonomous employees in terms of autonomy in the workplace; the petty bourgeoisie are defined as self-employed individuals with one or no employees; and the proletariat are defined as wage-labourers who do not fit into any of the above categories.

Empirically, Wright's classification was criticised because of the so-called boundary effects between different class locations and in particular that of the middle class. At a theoretical level Roemer (1982) criticised the emphasis that Wright placed on various aspects of control and in separating domination from exploitation. Despite these criticisms the classification has been used in stratification studies in the USA (Wright et al 1982), Britain (Marshall et al 1988) and Australia (Baxter 1988).

In his more recent work Wright (1985) has redesigned class locations in terms of exploitation. Ownership of the means of production remains the dominant asset to individuals. For nonowners other forms of exploitation also exist, however, in the form of preferential access to organisational positions and exploitation of credentials or skills to restrict entry to lucrative positions, such as the professions. Using these theoretical ideas and assuming three levels of assets, Wright's new class model is set out in a matrix of differentiation in terms of ownership and for employees, organisational position and skill or credentials level (Fig. 3.3). The distribution of British socioeconomic groups within this matrix using the empirical work of Marshall et al (1988) is also indicated.

Owners are differentiated in a crude way. The bourgeoisie are owners with 10 or more employees; small employers have from two to nine employees; and the petit bourgeoisie one employee or none. Organisational assets are defined in terms of an employee's relation to decision-making in his or her organisation. Three categories have emerged: managers who have direct involvement in decision making and real authority over subordinates; supervisors who lack involvement in real decision making but who have authority over others;

and nonmanagers who have neither decision-making powers nor authority over others. Categories of skill level or credentials are not straightforward. Skills or credentials are meaningless unless they can be used to exploit others. Wright identifies three categories: 'experts', 'skilled' employees and 'unskilled' employees. The experts are all professionals, and managers and technicians with college degrees. 'Skilled' employees include teachers, craftworkers, managers and technicians without degrees, and sales and clerical workers with both degrees and high autonomy. The 'unskilled' are all other sales and clerical workers and all manual and service workers. The categorisation of some occupational positions appears somewhat arbitrary. Wright's new class model is conceptually superior to his earlier one but suffers like all approaches to the measurement of class from the arbitrary nature of the classification of occupations, particularly at the boundary of different categories.

SOCIAL CLASS DIFFERENCES IN BRITAIN

Differences between social classes, however they are defined, and other important aspects of life

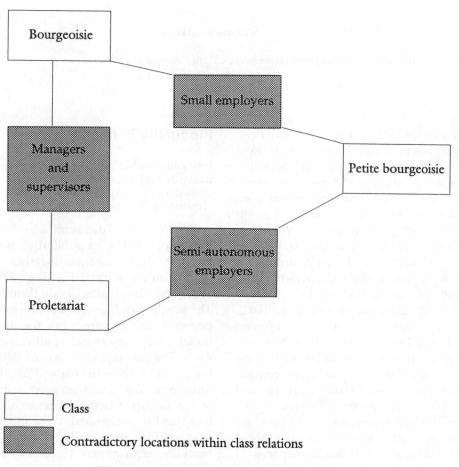

Fig. 3.2 Wright's class locations (after Wright 1985).

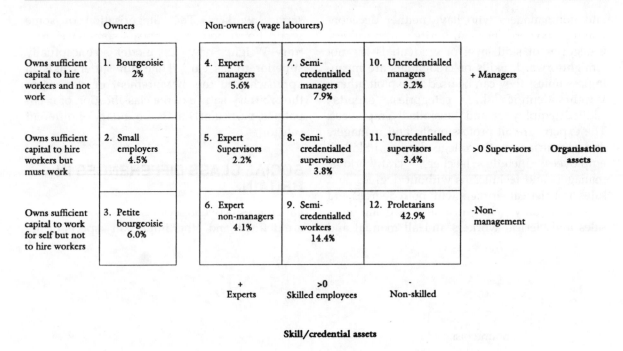

Fig. 3.3   Distribution of respondents into revised class categories (after Marshall et al 1988).

are well documented. British studies have been brought together in a useful source book (Reid 1989). Class differences have been found in the economic sphere – income and resources, occupational pensions, expenditure and employment (Townsend 1979); in health and the use of health services (Townsend, Davidson & Whitehead 1988; Townsend, Phillimore & Beattie 1988) in the nature of families and family formation (Newsom & Newsom 1965, Cartwright 1970, Haskey 1988, Haskey & Kiernan 1989, Haskey 1990a, 1991); in education (Foster et al 1990); and in politics, religion, leisure and opinion (Heath & Evans 1988). To reproduce here evidence of these differences would be duplicating the work of other writers who have concentrated specifically on social class differences and inequality. We will, however, given the importance for health professionals of understanding inequalities in health, identify some of these and the differential use of health services in Britain.

Inequality in health

Inequalities in health are of concern to the whole nation and represent one of the biggest possible challenges to the conduct of government policy. (Townsend, Davidson & Whitehead 1988, p.1)

In this way, Townsend and his colleagues introduced their joint publication Inequalities in Health which brought together two major reports on the subject: The Black Report (DHSS 1980) and The Health Divide (Whitehead 1987). The simple conclusion of both reports is that the poorer health experience of the lower occupational groups are found at all stages of the life cycle. The data reported showed that whereas in the 20 years up to the early 1970s the mortality rates for men and women aged 35 and over and in the Registrar General's Social Class I and II had steadily diminished, those in IV and V had changed little or even deteriorated. 10 years on from the publication of The Black Report, Davey Smith and colleagues concluded:

- Social class differences in mortality are widening.
- More sophisticated measures of socioeconomic position show greater inequalities in mortality.
- Health inequalities have been shown in all countries that collect the relevant data.
- Social selection and measurement artefacts do not account for mortality differentials.
- Social class differences exist for health throughout life, as well as the length of life.
- Trends in the distribution of income suggest that further widening of mortality differentials may be expected. (Davey Smith, Bartley & Blane 1990, p. 373)

Measuring inequalities in health

The World Health Organization has defined health as 'the state of complete physical, mental and social well-being and not merely the absence of disease or infirmity' (WHO 1983, p. 1). This perspective of health emphasises the necessity of individuals to identify and define their own health. In Chapter 1, we used the example of the elderly lady who was found by routine examination to have anaemia but who felt fine and therefore unwilling to receive a blood transfusion. This illustrates the sometimes conflicting perspectives of health professionals and patients.

The art of measuring individuals' perceptions of their health is relatively embryonic. At the same time, conceptions of health and illness vary among different groups of people within the same society (for example, between people in different social strata) and between different societies, as well as in any single society over time (Morris 1975). As a result, in the analysis of inequalities in health analysts have been forced to rely on a medical model of health which, in theory, can claim to have a number of standardised and universal measures of health.

Infant mortality

A common set of indicators of a nation's health are mortality statistics. Infant mortality is seen as a particularly good indicator both of the health of the population and living conditions. The infant mortality rate is the proportion of stillbirths and deaths of children under one year of age per 1000 live births. The national rate has fallen from as high as 150 per 1000 live births at the turn of the century to about 10 in the last decade of the century. Despite this decline, during this century the relative disparity between the social classes has remained: the higher the social class the lower the death rate.

Tables 3.4–3.6 show these data for England and Wales and for Scotland for the period 1939–1990. Table 3.4 shows that the stillbirth rate declined in England and Wales and in Scotland, but inequality remained marked. Indications in the late 1970s that the relative position of the lower classes might be improving have recently been discounted by analysis which suggests that this trend was largely due to the exclusion of children born outside of marriage (Pamuk 1988).

Table 3.5 shows that the neonatal death rate (deaths in the first 4 weeks of life) has also declined over the same period. Inequality persists between social classes I and V. Table 3.6 shows that postneonatal death rates (deaths after the first 4 weeks but in the first year of life) have also declined in the same period. These data suggest that up to 1990 the mortality differences between classes I and V have been wider after, rather than during, the early weeks of life. Thus we see that social class is related somewhat to infant death rates, but we need to go beyond these data to discover the specific factors which cause the inequality.

Adult mortality

Similar disparities between the social classes are evident if we look at the mortality of men aged 20–64. Table 3.7 shows the standard mortality ratios of men aged 20–64 for the period 1930–1983. The standard mortality ratio is the number of deaths, either total or cause-specific, in a given occupational group expressed as a percentage of the number of deaths that would have been expected in that occupational group if

Table 3.4   Stillbirths by social class in England and Wales and Scotland
(Rates per 1000 total births)

| Social class | England and Wales | | | | 1979-80 | |
	1939	1949–50[1]	1964–65[2]	1975–76[3]	1982-83[4]	1990[5]
I Professional	–	15.9*			4.5+	3.6#
			11.8	7.8		
II Managerial	–	19.4*			5.4+	3.4#
III Skilled manual and nonmanual	–	21.0*	15.6	9.8	5.8+ 6.8+	4.1# 4.4#
IV Partly skilled	–	22.9*			8.0+	5.7#
			17.2	12.0		
V Unskilled	–	25.5*			8.0+	5.6#

| Social class | Scotland | | | | | |
	1939[6]	1949[6]	1964[6]	1975[6]	1980[6]	1990[7]
I Professional	33.9	17.3	9.3	7.8	5.1	3.4
II Managerial	37.8	21.4	12.3	7.7	5.5	4.4
III Skilled manual and nonmanual	44.5	26.5	17.6	11.2	6.7	5.6 5.1
IV Partly skilled	38.0	28.7	19.9	12.9	7.9	5.1
V Unskilled	42.4	35.0	23.7	14.4	6.6	7.2

*   Single legitimate births only
+   Legitimate and jointly registered illegitimate births
#   For births within marriage only

Sources:
1. Heady J A, Heasman M A 1959 Social and biological factors in infant mortality. Studies on Medical and Population Subjects, No. 15. HMSO, London, Table 5A

2. Spicer C C, Lipworth L 1966 Regional and social factors in infant mortality. Studies on Medical and Population Subjects, No. 19. HMSO, London, Table 13

3. Officer of Population Censuses and Surveys, Medical Statistics Division 1978 Social and biological factors in infant mortality, 1975–76. Occasional Paper No. 12. OPCS, London, Table 6

4. Officer of Population Censuses and Surveys 1988 Occupational mortality: childhood supplement. The Registrar General's decennial supplement for England and Wales, 1979–80, 1982–83. Series DS No. 8. HMSO, London, Table 2.7

5. Office of Population Censuses and Surveys 1992 Mortality Statistics. Perinatal and infant: social and biological factors. Review of the Registrar General on deaths in England and Wales, 1990. Series DH3 No. 24. HMSO, London, Table 1

6. Registrar General for Scotland 1982 Annual Report, 1980. HMSO, Edinburgh, Table D1.3

7. Registrar General for Scotland 1992 Annual Report, 1991. HMSO, Edinburgh, Table D1.6

Table 3.5 Neonatal death rates by social class in England and Wales and Scotland
(Rates per 1000 total births)

		England and Wales				
Social class	1939	1949–50[1]	1964–65[2]	1975–76[3]	1979–80 1982–83[4]	1990[5]
I Professional	–	12.2*			5.0+	3.6#
				9.2	7.9	
II Managerial	–	14.2*			5.7+	3.3#
III Skilled manual and nonmanual	–	15.9*	11.8	9.3	6.2+ 6.6+	4.0# 4.1#
IV Partly skilled	–	17.9*			8.3+	4.8#
				13.2	11.7	
V Unskilled	–	19.1*			8.6+	5.8#

		Scotland				
Social class	1939[6]	1949[6]	1964[6]	1975[6]	1980[6]	1990
I Professional	25.9	13.7	9.5	7.6	3.9	–
II Managerial	25.1	17.9	10.9	8.7	5.8	–
III Skilled manual and nonmanual	38.6	22.6	15.8	11.2	7.7	–
IV Partly skilled	34.8	24.4	18.0	10.8	6.6	–
V Unskilled	39.9	31.3	21.9	14.6	8.6	–

* Single legitimate births only
+ Legitimate and jointly registered illegitimate births
# For births within marriage only

Sources:
1. Heady J A, Heasman M A 1959 Social and biological factors in infant mortality. Studies on Medical and Population Subjects, No. 15. HMSO, London, Table 5B (i)

2. Spicer C C, Lipworth L 1966 Regional and social factors in infant mortality. Studies on Medical and Population Subjects, No. 19. HMSO, London, Table 10

3. Office of Population Censuses and Surveys, Medical Statistics Division 1978 Social and biological factors in infant mortality, 1975–76. Occasional Paper No. 12. OPCS, London, Table 6

4. Office of Population Censuses and Surveys 1988 Occupational mortality: childhood supplement. The Registrar General's decennial supplement for England and Wales, 1979–80, 1982–83. Series DS No. 8. HMSO, London, Table 2.7

5. Office of Population Censuses and Surveys 1992 Mortality statistics. Perinatal and infant: social and biological factors. Review of the Registrar General on deaths in England and Wales, 1990. Series DH3 No. 24. HMSO, London, Table 3

6. Registrar General for Scotland 1982 Annual Report, 1980. HMSO, Edinburgh, Table F1.4

Table 3.6 Post neonatal death rates by social class in England and Wales and
Scotland (Rates per 1000 total births)

| | England and Wales | | | | 1979–80 | |
Social class	1939	1949–50[1]	1964–65[2]	1975–76[3]	1982–83[4]	1990[5]
I Professional	–	4.8*			2.9+	2.0#
			3.5	3.0		
II Managerial	–	5.7*			3.1+	2.0#
III Skilled manual and nonmanual	–	10.3*	5.4	4.0	3.1+ 3.9+	2.3# 2.4#
IV Partly skilled	–	13.7*			5.2+	3.5#
			7.6	6.1		
V Unskilled	–	17.0*			6.9+	5.4#

| | Scotland | | | | | |
Social class	1939[6]	1949[6]	1964[6]	1975[6]	1980[6]	1990
I Professional	7.6	4.9	2.9	1.8	4.8	–
II Managerial	14.8	9.1	3.8	3.8	2.6	–
III Skilled manual and nonmanual	30.2	16.2	6.8	4.7	3.8	–
IV Partly skilled	33.4	22.9	8.5	5.1	3.5	–
V Unskilled	44.9	30.8	13.5	10.8	7.5	–

* Single legitimate births only
+ Legitimate and jointly registered illegitimate births
# For births within marriage only

Sources:

1. Heady J A, Heasman M A 1959 Social and biological factors in infant mortality. Studies on Medical and Population Subjects, No. 15. HMSO, London, Table 5B (ii)

2. Spicer C C, Lipworth L 1966 Regional and social factors in infant mortality. Studies on Medical and Population Subjects, No. 19. HMSO, London, Table 11

3. Office of Population Censuses and Surveys, Medical Statistics Division 1978 Social and biological factors in infant mortality, 1975-76. Occasional Paper No. 12. OPCS, London, Table 6

4. Office of Population Censuses and Surveys 1988 Occupational mortality: childhood supplement. The Registrar General's decennial supplement for England and Wales, 1979-80, 1982-83. Series DS No. 8. HMSO, London, Table 2.7

5. Office of Population Censuses and Surveys1992 Mortality statistics. Perinatal and infant: social and biological factors. Review of the Registrar General on deaths in England and Wales, 1990. Series DH3 No. 24. HMSO, London, Table 4

6. Registrar General for Scotland 1982 Annual Report, 1980. HMSO, Edinburgh, Table F1.4

the age-and-sex-specific rates in the general population had been obtained. Table 3.7 suggests that between 1949–53 and 1959–63 the risk of premature death of adult men of different social classes appear to have become more unequal and, between 1971 and 1981 the difference between the manual and nonmanual groups appeared to increase. During this period social class differences in mortality in people over retirement age were noticed for the first time (Fox et al 1985).

When individual occupational classes are considered these show even greater inequalities. The Decennial Supplement 1979–80, 1982–3 on occupational mortality reports that the standardised mortality ratios for men aged 20–64 in Great Britain were: 48 for university lecturers; 81 for sales managers; 84 for bread, milk and laundry roundsmen; 154 for chemical gas and petroleum process workers; 180 for steel erectors and riggers; 234 for fishermen; and 243 for general labourers (OPCS 1986, Appendix IV).

Morbidity

Deaths are usually registered and therefore mortality statistics are fairly reliable. By contrast morbidity data (data on the presence of illness) are less reliable because of the difficulties surrounding its measurement. The annual *General Household Survey* has provided regular information about morbidity since 1970. The types of morbidity data collected, however, are difficult to interpret. Whether people report illness differs according to their customary expectations of their own state of health, and according to the degree of inconvenience and cost attached to being sick.

Data from the *General Household Survey* suggest that morbidity is greater amongst the socially and materially deprived, especially during middle and old age. In 1987 the rate of self reporting of 'long-standing illness' among 16–64 year old men ranged from 27% in Social Class I to 41% in Social Class V. Davey Smith and

Table 3.7 Mortality of men by social class in England and Wales (standardised mortality rates)

Social class	1930–32[1]	1945–53[*1]	1959–63[1] Unadjusted	(Adjusted)[+]	1970–72[1] Unadjusted	(Adjusted)[+]	1979–80[#2] 1982–83
			Men aged 15–64				
I Professional	90	86	76	(75)	77	(75)	66
II Managerial	94	92	81	(–)	81	(–)	76
III Skilled manual and nonmanual	97	101	100	(–)	104	(–)	94 106
IV Partly skilled	102	104	103	(–)	114	(–)	116
V Unskilled	111	118	143	(127)	137	(121)	165

* Corrected figures as published in Register General 1971 Decennial Supplement, England and Wales, 1961: Occupational mortality tables. HMSO, London, p. 22
+ Occupations in 1959–63 and 1970–72 have been reclassified according to the 1950 classification of occupations.
# Men aged 20–64 (Great Britain).

Sources:
1. Townsend P, Davidson N 1982 Inequalities in health. Penguin, Harmondsworth, p. 67

2. Office of Population Censuses and Surveys 1986 Occupational mortality. The Registrar General's decennial supplement for Great Britain, 1979–80, 1982–83. Series DS No. 6. Part 1 Commentary. HMSO, London, Appendix IV

colleagues (1990) reviewed *ad hoc* enquiries which have been published since the Black Report, and conclude that these are a more valuable source of information about the relationship between a wide range of measures of health state and socioeconomic position. For example, they report data from the British regional heart study (Pocock et al 1987) which indicated that the prevalence of angina was almost twice as high in manual compared with nonmanual middle-aged men, and that systolic blood pressure was on average 6 mm Hg higher.

The *Health and Lifestyle Survey* (Blaxter 1990) undertaken in 1984/85 surveyed some 9000 individuals in England, Wales and Scotland and measured health in a number of complementary ways: physical fitness, psychosocial health, perceived health status and absence of medically-defined disease. On each of the four dimensions of health people from lower social classes had higher age-standardised health ratios. The study also highlights the different patterns of health for men and women of different social classes confirming the cruder data collected as part of the General Household Surveys.

Use of health services

Ever since Richard Titmuss (1908–73) first wrote: 'higher income groups know how to make a better use of the service; they tend to receive more specialist attention; occupy more of the beds in better equipped and staffed hospitals' (Titmuss 1968, p. 196) there has been considerable interest in the use or consumption of health services by people of different social classes.

Use of services, however, is related to their availability. For instance, in Aberdeen, Knox (1979) found that the location and accessibility of general-practitioner surgeries favoured the long established middle-class areas of the city. The difficulties of access are compounded by the availability of public and private transport. In particular, car ownership and easy access benefited middle-class patients living in the outlying owner-occupied areas of Aberdeen. In a separate study, Whitehouse (1985) indicated that difficulties with travelling to surgeries were a deter-

rent to the use of primary health care services. These findings confirmed a national survey undertaken in 1977 which investigated access to primary health care services. Difficulties in using services were experienced most often by elderly people and women from lower social classes. People in Social Classes IV and V were also less likely to use ophthalmic, dental and chiropody services (Richie et al 1981). Legislation instituting charges for eye tests and changes in the charges for dental care are likely to increase these differences.

Of course, differential use of services is not only a function of access or costs. It is also not simply a matter of analysing data about the use of services by different social classes. Such an analysis shows that, for children, no large differences in the likelihood of consulting were found between social class groups. For adults under 65, however, there was a steady increase in the likelihood of consulting according to social class, with those in Social Classes IV and V more likely to consult than those in Social Classes I and II (McCormick et al 1990). But because of real inequalities in health, the use of services must be related to the need for services. Both Brotherston (1976) and Forster (1976) have used *General Household Survey* data to look at the relationship between health, service use and social class. Brotherston calculated a 'use-need ratio' for general-practitioner consultations and the number of days with restricted activity. He found that the ratio declined from the highest to the lowest socioeconomic group showing that lower socioeconomic groups consulted less than higher socioeconomic groups in relation to need. Forster used aggregated data for the years 1971 and 1972 and also found statistically significant trends with social class for a consultation rate/morbidity ratio where the morbidity measure took into account both chronic sickness rates and sickness absence rates. There are weaknesses in this method (see Townsend & Davidson 1982, pp. 77–80 for a comprehensive review) and therefore the conclusions can only be accepted as tentative.

Qualitative studies of general practice suggest that middle-class patients receive longer consultations than working-class patients (Buchan & Richardson 1973, Cartwright & O'Brien 1976) and that more problems were discussed at consultations with middle-class patients than with working-class ones. These data suggest that middle-class patients are receiving a better service when they consult their general practitioner (Fig. 3.4).

Social class differences in the use of hospital services have been reviewed by Carstairs and Patterson (1966). Using hospital admission rates and data about length of stay in hospital in Scotland for 1963 they found clear evidence of increased use from Social Class I to Social Class V. More recent data reported in *Inequalities in Health* (Townsend, Davidson and Whitehead 1988) confirmed these trends.

Perhaps one of the most striking conclusions of the *Inequalities in Health* report was that social class differences are greater in the use of preventive services. Routinely collected Scottish data about antenatal booking show that, although there has been an increase in the proportion of women in all social classes booking by 20 weeks gestation, the proportion of married women making a later antenatal booking, that is after more than 20 weeks of gestation, increased for lower social classes (Table 3.8). We have some difficulty in interpreting the marked increase in the proportion of women booking by 20 weeks, but the data is only for married women, and we refer to this example again in Chapter 12 when discussing the use of official statistics in research.

Similar class differences have been found in presentation for postnatal examination, immunization, antenatal and postnatal supervision and uptake of vitamin supplements (Gordon 1951). Cartwright (1970), in her study of family planning services, found a clear relationship with social class of the proportion of the mothers having an antenatal examination, attending a family planning clinic and discussing birth control with their general practitioners. Sanson and colleagues (1972) found that women from Social Class IV and V were less likely to be screened for cervical cancer, though this disease is more prevalent among women of the lower social classes.

Differential use of preventative services by adults and their children was also documented after the analysis of the second national morbidity survey of general practice (Blaxter 1984, Crombie 1984). Nutbeam and Catford (1987) recorded differential use of screening and preventative services in Wales. Fisher and colleagues (1983) reported differential attendance at local authority developmental assessment clinics for preschool children. Social class differences have also been reported for the frequency of attendance for dental services (Todd & Dodd 1985, Eddie & Davies 1985); orthodontic clinics

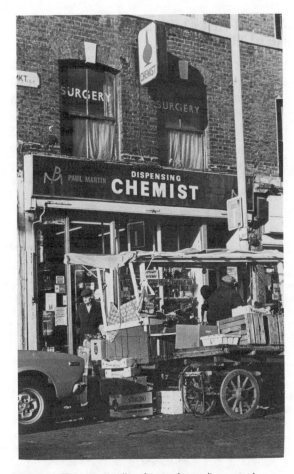

Fig. 3.4 The poor quality of some inner-city general practitioner services could be reflected in the quality of surgeries (courtesy of City and Hackney Community Health Council).

(Jenkins et al 1984) and attendance at well-women, well-men and cytology clinics (Marsh & Channing 1986).

The data reported in this chapter, and other studies reviewed elsewhere (Townsend, Davidson & Whitehead 1988, Fox 1989, Davey Smith et al 1990), show quite convincingly that, despite the overall increased affluence of Britain, there remains a strong relationship between social stratification and health. Why do such inequalities persist? How can professionals assist in reducing these inequalities to improve the health of those worst off? We need to understand clearly the reasons for inequality before we are in a position to do much about it.

CLASS-RELATED DIFFERENCES IN HEALTH

In this chapter we have tried to emphasise the importance of the difficult concept of social stratification for understanding society as a whole and for understanding the health of members of societies. To this end we have introduced concepts of class, status and power, and have indicated how social class in particular is associated with inequalities in health. One obvious

danger of this strategy will be that readers, in common with other health professionals, will leap to the conclusion that social stratification is the *cause* of health problems and inequalities. The oversimplification of social class has led many notable analysts to reduce their statements to a trite comment that some human action is 'due to social class.' In Chapter 2 we used the example of late booking for antenatal care in our discussion of fact and theory. The example is relevant again here. One might be tempted to think that women are late attenders for antenatal care because of their social class. Such a conclusion is not only misleading but can also be positively harmful to individual mothers. What is important is not social class *per se* but what lies behind the classification in terms of the social processes which link individuals' actions to their occupational classifications. Women are likely to attend late for antenatal care not because their occupational classification is Social Class V but because Social Class V women tend to live some distance away from clinics; to have heard too many unpleasant stories about antenatal clinics; or to be unable to find a baby sitter while they attend. McIntyre (1980), in interviews with women having first babies, found that few had

Table 3.8 Percentage of married women making a late antenatal booking (after more than 21 weeks gestation)

	Scotland	
Social class	1971[1]	1981[2]
I Professional	28	11
II Managerial	35	12
III Skilled manual and nonmanual	36	12
IV Partly skilled	39	15
V Unskilled	47	18

Sources:
1. Brotherston Sir J 1976 Inequality: is it inevitable? In: Carter C O, Peel J (eds) Equalities and inequalities in health. Academic Press, London, p. 85

2. Information Services Division 1983 Unpublished Tables.

ever given any thought to, or been given specific information about, the purpose of antenatal care. Midwives and obstetricians took this for granted. Reasons for late booking will depend on a number of social and environmental factors which are related to social class but do not themselves constitute social class.

Studies like that by Blaxter and Paterson (1982), described in Chapter 6, begin to explain something of why class differences exist. Blaxter and Paterson found that mothers and daughters in Social Class IV and V, who were themselves products of disadvantaged social and medical histories, lacked a concept of positive health and showed scepticism and even fatalism about the benefits of preventive medicine or dentistry. Their attitude was: 'If your kids are healthy, they're healthy. If they're going to be ill, they'll be ill.' If such a fatalistic belief system is widespread in Social Class V families, it is not surprising that differences exist between social classes in the use of preventive services. Cultural or behavioural explanations of differences in the use of services is, of course, only one reason for differences in morbidity and mortality.

Another explanation of inequalities in health due to social selection processes has been provided by Illsley (1955; 1980). In an investigation of women with one child, at the time living in Aberdeen in 1951–4, he found that women who were upward socially mobile tended to have a higher intelligence quotient (IQ) (a measure of environment rather than a genetic predictor), higher education and occupational skills. These women also tended to be taller, in better health, and to have lower rates of prematurity, infant and maternal mortality. Conversely, Illsley found that the women who were downward socially mobile at marriage tended to have the opposite characteristics (Illsley 1955). More recent data indicates that the same processes were still operating in Aberdeen some 20 years later (Illsley 1980).

Of course, one explanation of this selective mobility at marriage is to attribute it to postmarital social, economic and environmentalconditions. Illsley, however, found that even some of the women who were living in the poor housing of the 1950s, or living in their parents' homes, or even those who were conceived prenuptially, were upward mobile and shared the more positive characteristics. These data also showed that the experiences of children in similar social classes, as measured by the social classes of their fathers, were varied. Variations in diet and environmental factors are all positively correlated with such factors as education and intelligence, more so than fathers' occupation. These predispose to occupational attainment. Thus it would appear that social mobility differentiates between the fit and not so fit. As one early sociologist put it:

Physical superiority has been the condition which has favoured the social promotion of individuals and has facilitated their social climbing, while physical inferiority has facilitated the social sinking of individuals and their location in the lower social strata. (Sorokin 1959, p. 275)

This type of explanation has often been advanced in strongly eugenic terms (Himsworth 1984) and therefore received considerable criticism. More recent data on social class from the 1971 and 1981 Censuses used in the national study of occupational mortality (OPCS 1986) has made it possible to explore the relationship between social mobility and mortality. These analyses suggests that downward social mobility does not account for the differences in mortality (Goldblatt 1988; 1989).

A further explanation of the relationship between health and social inequality is that observed differences are an artefact of the way that different studies have chosen to measure social phenomenon. Artefact explanations take two forms. The first suggests that both health and class are artificial variables thrown up by attempts to measure social phenomena and that the relationship between them may itself be an artefact of little causal significance (Townsend, Davidson & Whitehead 1988). The second suggests that official statistics are socially constructed by official agents who process new items of information through their preexisting interpretative frameworks (Bloor et al 1987). We explore this explanation about the appropriateness of official statistics in more detail in Chapter 12.

The first, and simple, artefact explanation suggests specifically that mortality differentials between social classes are due to numerator-denominator bias arising because social class may be assigned differently on the death certificate (numerator) than at the Census (denominator). Bloor and colleagues (1987) cite a number of examples of studies where this may have happened. The problem has been overcome, however, in the national study of occupational mortality (OPCS 1986) by using social class as assigned to them at the 1971 Census also to categorise individuals at death. Eliminating numerator-denominator bias in this way was found to have no effect on the differences in mortality of different social classes (Fox & Goldblatt 1982).

Changes in the classification of social class at each Census has also been highlighted as a potential artefact. The national study of occupational mortality (OPCS 1986) again shows that these changes have not affected the relative mortality rates of different social classes. The decline in the proportion of the population in Social Class V due to the changing occupational structure has also been identified as a potential artefact in apparently widening class differences. This suggests that as the size of Social Class V decreases those remaining within it represent those at high risk of dying. The use of an alternative measure of socioeconomic status allowing for larger groups has, nevertheless, found similar differences in mortality between the groups (Davey Smith et al 1990).

Whatever the most valid explanation of health inequalities, it follows that the greatest contribution that health professionals can make toward their reduction is to have a positive approach to the problems facing the lower social classes. It is not a matter of attributing blame to the patient for his or her lifestyle and using the excuse that the poor health or unequal use of service is 'due to social class'. Attention needs to be given to finding out what factors, which happen to link with social class, lie behind observed differences. These are matters which require sociological investigation. Only in this way, by beginning to understand what causes inequalities in health, can we provide socially appropri-ate services to complement advances in other applied sciences and so promote health.

The relevance of social stratification will be taken up again, particularly in relation to social causes of illness (Ch. 4), professional-client inter-action (Ch. 9) and in relation to death and dying (Ch. 10).

SUMMARY

In this chapter we have discussed social stratification from a structuralist perspective. In particular we have outlined differences between the Marxian and Weberian approaches to social class. Marx divided society into two social classes: the bourgeoisie and proletariat, and emphasised that the inequality between them was based on the exploitation of the proletariat by the bourgeoisie. Weber identified a number of social classes which were based on the shared experiences of people who are similarly placed in the processes of production, distribution and exchange. Class embraces all aspects of economic position in society. Contemporary theoretical approaches to class continue to be influenced by both Marx and Weber as reflected in the Marxist approach of Wright, and the identification of contradictory class locations and the approach of Parkin and his emphasis on social closure.

We described the common methods of measuring class and identified the different ways that class can be categorised in the Government statistics used to influence health policy. We saw that official definitions of occupational position relate more closely to Weber's concept of status, which focuses on the social estimation and prestige of a particular social group. Thus we saw that the official definitions of class are based on the relative prestige of different occupational groups rather than their economic position. The new Government Standard Occupational Classification is also linked to educational and skill dimensions of social stratification.

A third aspect of social stratification highlighted in this chapter is power. In order to understand this concept we introduced Weber's concepts of authority and legitimacy. We saw that authority was more enduring than power which is often momentary and not always legitimated. Legitimacy means that people accept the authority as just and those endowed with authority are given it rightfully.

We explored the mechanisms by which people move between different social strata and identified influences on social mobility. We reported the findings of Goldthorpe's studies of social mobility in Britain which suggest that there has been little increase in relative mobility rates; although, because of the changes in occupational structure, there has been a general movement upwards in absolute terms.

The chapter concluded with a summary of data on inequalities in health highlighting the relative disadvantages of people in the Registrar General's Social Classes IV and V. Individuals in these social groups were shown on a variety of mortality and morbidity indicators to be less healthy. Relative to their need for health services they also used these services less frequently than people in Social Classes I, II or III. Finally, we suggest that health professionals should seek explanations for such inequalities beyond the observation that poor health or unequal use of service is 'due to social class'.

FURTHER READING

Giddens A 1989 Sociology. Polity Press, Cambridge, Ch 7, pp. 205–241

Hamnett C, McDowell L, Sarre P 1989 Restructuring Britain: The changing social structure. Sage, London, Chs 3–4, pp. 78–157

Runciman W G 1966 Relative deprivation and social justice. Routledge & Kegan Paul, London, Ch 3, pp. 36–52

Townsend P, Davidson N, Whitehead M (eds) 1988 Inequalities in health: The Black Report and the Health Divide. Penguin, Harmondsworth

4

Social influences on health and the role of prevention

INTRODUCTION

Our discussion in the last chapter concerning inequality in health indicated a number of social influences on illness and health. In this chapter we develop this theme by outlining what sociologists mean by the social causes of illness. Then we will discuss what McKinlay (1979) has called the 'manufacture of illness': those aspects of the social, economic and political structure, the individuals, groups and organisations which, in addition to producing material goods and services also produce, as inevitable by-products, widespread morbidity and mortality. *We review some of the evidence which supports* the general hypothesis that stressful life events, like bereavement or unemployment, have a role in the aetiology of illness. Social conditions similarly have physical or psychological consequences, like depression. We examine one model to explain the relationship between life events and health, and why individuals' experiences differ. Finally, we raise the topic of prevention.

All of us will be aware of some social influences on illness aetiology. Smoking increases the risk of a person acquiring lung cancer, bronchitis and heart disease. Excessive alcohol consumption in association with driving, cycling or walking increases the likelihood of a person sustaining injuries from road traffic accidents. Living in areas of the world where poor sanitation, overcrowding and inadequate nutrition is rife increases the chance of contracting infectious diseases such as TB or cholera. Working as a coal-miner increases the risk of many lung diseases but particularly pneumoconiosis. Needle sharing among injecting drug users increases the risk of HIV infection and AIDS. These examples, and numerous others, indicate the ubiquity of social influences on the aetiology of illness and disease. There are few illnesses which have not been linked to some kind of human behaviour or another, yet health professionals make limited use of this information.

A story of a doctor trying to explain the dilemmas of modern medical practice, related by the sociologist Irving Zola, suggests why this might be:

'You know', he said, 'sometimes it feels like this. There I am standing by the shore of a swiftly flowing river and I hear the cry of a drowning man. So I jump into the river, put my arms around him, pull him to the shore, apply artificial respiration. Just when he begins to breathe, another cry for help. So I jump into the river, reach him, pull him to shore, apply artificial respiration, and then just as he begins to breathe, another cry for help. So back into the river again, reaching, pulling, applying, breathing and then another yell. Again and again, without end, goes the sequence. You know, I am so busy jumping in, pulling them to shore, applying artificial respiration, that I have no time to see who the hell is upstream pushing them all in.' (Quoted in McKinlay 1979, p. 9)

This simple story usefully sums up the theme of this chapter.

SOCIAL CAUSES

In Chapter 1 we described two different general models of health – the medical model and the social model. We also introduced Lalonde's health field concept to show the complementary nature of the two approaches.

The medical model is a limited one, although it is also an effective one. We know that social factors – the environmental and lifestyle elements of Lalonde's model – influence health: smoking, alcohol consumption, drug use, poor sanitation and coal-mining as an occupation. Thereafter it is essentially physical means – the human biology element of the health field con-

cept – which play a major role in the aetiology of lung cancer, road traffic accidents, AIDS, TB and pneumoconiosis. Sociology is not only concerned with the link between smoking and cancer, alcohol consumption and road traffic accidents, drug use and AIDS, sanitation and TB, and coal-mining (Fig. 4.1) and pneumoconiosis. It is also concerned with why people smoke, drink, share needles during drug use, live in poor housing and engage in coal-mining. Sociological answers to these questions are not straightforward and the answers we provide by way of illustration may be partly speculative and not based on a full reading of the sociological theory and empirical data.

Both smoking and alcohol consumption afford examples of social actions which have symbolic meaning to the individual and the social group of which he or she is a member. School children will often take up smoking not because at first they enjoy the activity, but because of its symbolic value in the adolescent subculture. The symbolic value is reinforced by one 'manufacturer of illness': the tobacco industry. Some adolescents sniff glue because of its symbolic significance in certain deviant subcultures.

The association between needle sharing among drug users and the prevalence of HIV infection has been clearly documented yet the cultural context in which needle sharing occurs is not clearly understood. One early explanation attributed the behaviour to the practise of local police officers who confiscated needles and syringes from individuals suspected of drug use. The subsequent reduction in the availability of the necessary equipment for drug use increased the extent of needle sharing (Mulleady 1987). Although the availability of clean injecting equipment is clearly associated with reduced needle sharing, the phenomenon is more complex with notions of risk, risk avoidance and individual and group relationships among drug users being important. In a subculture in which the sharing of material goods is a dominant feature of social life, the sharing of injecting equipment has little *particular* symbolic significance (McKeganey 1990).

Inadequate sanitation and coal-mining as an occupation are not social actions and therefore have no symbolic significance. They are, however, important structural characteristics of a stratified society. People tend to get TB if they live in overcrowded housing with poor sanitation and contract pneumoconiosis if they work at the coal face. Whether or not one lives or works in these kinds of environment depends on one's position in society. As we saw in Chapter 3, inequalities in health are often explained in structural terms by sociologists.

A social model of the causes of illness and disease focuses on the individual and his or her relationship to the social structure of society. It takes as its concern how individuals perceive and react to their structural position in society and why they perceive and behave in the way they do. We will describe a model of the social causes of illness and disease, which relates the physical and biochemical factors in the development of disease to the way that individuals perceive and react to their way of life.

Illness and social structure

From the structural perspective we can all identify those elements of the way society is organised which appear to be directly related to the aetiology of illness. At the broadest level the social, economic and political structure of capitalist society can be identified as a major contributor to illness in Britain. A dominant characteristic of modern industrial societies, both Western capitalist and state capitalist societies, is their preoccupation with economic growth. Social and economic policies practised in pursuit of the single goal of greater growth invariably neglect a variety of health hazards (McKinlay 1984), not least those associated with environmental pollution.

We do not have to look far to find examples of what McKinlay calls 'the manufacturers of illness'. From the economic perspective of growth, cigarette production is wealth producing – to the tobacco industry, to the workers in that industry and to governments who levy taxes on tobacco

products. Yet we are all aware of the good scientific evidence about the relationship between smoking and ill health. The promotion of tobacco products is also a major wealth-producing activity for the advertising agencies, not to mention the corner and tobacconist's shops. To expand their markets and increase their production of wealth 'the manufacturers of illness' promote their products in other countries and cultures. Thus, a high proportion of the wealth in the Developing World is being spent on tobacco products with the consequent cost to health (Doyal & Pennell 1979).

The example of tobacco is not, however, the best illustration of the ubiquitous nature of the goal of growth. The production and consumption of food, which everyone is involved with, in our view better illustrates the extent to which the economic structure of society influences health.

Production

A number of disabling conditions have been related to the nature and organisation of the pro-

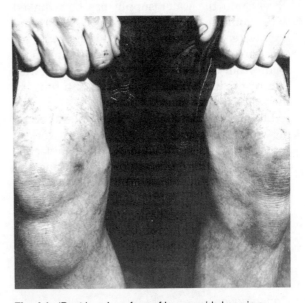

Fig. 4.1 'Beat knee' – a form of housemaids knee in a coalminer. Results from kneeling in narrow seams with limited working height (courtesy of Department of Environmental and Occupational Medicine).

duction of food. Occupational diseases related to farming are less often reported because of insufficient cases concentrated in one place for a connection to become clear. The effects of chemicals and pesticides used in modern farming on health are not clearly understood, yet the prophetic work of Rachel Carson (1963) on the relationship between pesticides and the natural food chain in lower order species indicates the likelihood of health hazards to both food producers and consumers. The long-term effects of slight poisoning, like the long-term effects of smoking, are subtle and will probably only be noticed after many years of exposure. Some of the effects of the use of modern chemicals in farming have been discovered by chance. In 1967 five workers on a Derbyshire farm reported being impotent. The disability disappeared after they were taken off crop spraying (Smith 1977). In 1977 over half the male workers in a California pesticide factory were found to be sterile or had very low sperm counts (Whorton et al 1977).

Agricultural chemicals are a potential danger, not only to those who manufacture and use them but also to the public at large. The presence of high levels of nitrates seeping from fertilisers into the water supply has been linked with stomach cancer (The Lancet, 1977), and high water nitrate levels are a constant cause for concern. So far these conclusions have only been made from observational data and require further research before the full effects of nitrates in the water supply are known.

Like agricultural workers, many food processing workers are poorly paid. They also work in some of the worst conditions of the manufacturing industry. Many aspects of food handling and packing are probably hazardous to the workers' health. The dust from cardboard and paper, the dyes, plastics and resins on the boxes, the noise in bottling plants and the fumes from cutting and sealing film wrapping have all been identified as potential health hazards (Kinnersley 1973).

Consumption

Whereas the health hazards related to the production of food are limited to a relatively small number of agricultural and food processing workers, the health hazards related to the consumption of food affect the whole population. Diet is directly related to the changing pattern of disease in modern industrial societies. We can illustrate this proposition by looking at the pattern of sugar consumption. Sugar is probably the only known serious dietary cause of tooth decay (Sheiham 1983). In Norway, Finland, Austria, the Netherlands, Denmark and Britain the rate of tooth decay fell by half during World War II when sugar was rationed (Sognnaes 1948). In Britain, in 1952 (at the end of rationing) on average a 15-year-old had four teeth decayed, but by 1959 the average had increased to 10. During the same period the consumption of sugar had increased markedly (James 1965).

Processed sugar is not the only dietary change which has influenced our health. Changes in the consumption of roughage (the fibre content of the diet) have been related to changes in the pattern of diseases affecting the digestive system. In particular, highly processed foods like modern white bread usually contain very little roughage. As the consumption of roughage has decreased

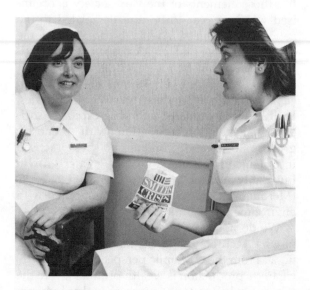

Fig. 4.2 'Junk food' for lunch can easily become the norm (courtesy of Rik Walton).

there has been an increase in the incidence of diseases of the digestive tract (Burkitt & Trowell 1975).

Lack of fibre also encourages obesity because, without the fibre, the food is less bulky (Van Itallie 1978); to compensate one tends to eat more food, and as a result end up eating an excess of calories (Fig. 4.2). Obesity is also related to an increase in the consumption of sugar and fat (Royal College of Physicians of London 1983). This increase in obesity has been associated with an increased risk of heart disease, high blood pressure, diabetes, and arthritis (Chiang et al 1969, Tansey et al 1977, Royal College of Physicians of London 1983).

The level of consumption

Like tobacco consumption, food consumption is considered to be a relatively free choice, putting the onus on individual lifestyle. Yet like tobacco consumption it is affected by a variety of social pressures. Perhaps the greatest influence on individual consumption is advertising, which is determined by the manufacturers' need to sell their products. Manufacturers are also concerned with making a profit. The manufacture of meat products, wheat products and sugar products is encouraged because they are more profitable – they cost less to cultivate and transport than, for example, fresh vegetables. The Politics of Health Group (1980) have described the incentive to manufacturers to develop these products in the following way:

White flour is more profitable than brown, because the bran and the germ can be sold separately, so people tend to eat more of them. Sugar can make products more satisfying to taste, particularly if we were encouraged as children to enjoy highly sugared products. As we have seen, sugar and white flour are among foods causing ill health. Animal fats have been associated with cancer of the bowel and the breast, and with heart disease. Yet some of the most profitable products of the meat industry, such as sausages and pies, are particularly high in fats.

The food industry has a particular problem. It cannot expect us to consume more of their products when our incomes rise. There is, after all, a limit to the amount we can eat, so that with a rise in real wages we do not buy more and more of the same sort of food. So in order to keep up their profits, the industry encourages us to shift our purchasing of food with less profit to food with more profit. (The Politics of Health Group 1980, p. 7).

The impact of the food industry has also had a great impact on the health of people in the Developing World. Perhaps the most serious has been the export of formula milk for babies. With a static home market, dried milk producers can only expand their markets by selling to the Developing World. Although health professionals tend to support the view that breast milk is best for a newborn child, there is less evidence, nowadays, that babies born in Britain and *fed correctly* on formula milk are seriously disadvantaged (Thomson & Black 1975). This is not the case in Developing World countries, where bottle feeding has been lethal. In the West Indies to feed a 3-month-old baby on formula milk can take up to a third of a family's income. Often mothers resort to watering down feeds, which causes malnutrition. In contrast to modern industrial societies, feeds are usually prepared in conditions which are far from ideal and which encourage gastroenteritis. In Africa a combination of gastroenteritis and malnutrition is known as the *lactogen syndrome* (Jellife & Jellife 1978).

Diet and social stratification

In Chapter 3 we reviewed inequalities in health and found that people from lower social strata in Britain had a shorter expectation of life, higher rates of infant mortality and higher rates of acute and chronic sickness.

A number of researchers have emphasised the importance of diet on the health of individuals. McKeown (1979), in his review of the role of medicine, describes the historical determinants of improved nutrition and relates this to the decline of mortality from infectious diseases. Lord Taylor (1975), from a review of the factors influencing the rate of infant mortality, concluded that maternal and infant nutrition were the most important. Wilkinson (1978) has shown that diet is probably the main factor responsible for class differences in life expectancy. He made a number of dietary comparisons for the decade 1964–74 and found that there were marked differences in the consumption of fruit, fresh vegetables, cheese, milk and meat. People from lower socioeconomic groups consumed far less of these than people from higher socioeconomic groups but consumed more sugar and refined wheat.

Studies of food consumption taking a structuralist perspective do not alone provide an adequate explanation of patterns of food consumption. For example, they do not explain differences observed between middle-class and working-class households. Calnan (1990) has briefly reviewed the ways in which sociologists have approached differences in food consumption. In line with a structuralist perspective, Blaxter and Patterson (1982) identify the material constraints of food consumption highlighting the effect of the purchasing habits of low-income families on the availability of certain food stuffs, such as fresh fruit, which is not often available from corner and mobile shops. In contrast, Murcott (1983) has examined patterns of food consumption within the context of the social organisation of households and has shown that the traditional division of labour within families means that women do most of the cooking and are responsible for food preparation. However, they are constrained and influenced by such factors as the competing demands of other tasks, including child care and paid work. Women are also likely to provide meals according to the tastes and preferences of their male partners rather than themselves, although the influence of advertising, particularly TV advertising, on the preferences and choices of children should not be underestimated.

Eating habits have also been examined in relation to their social and cultural context. Dietary patterns can be explained in terms of culturally defined rules and codes of conduct which shape the time and setting of meals, the content of the meals and the serving order of different dishes served. Douglas and Nicod (1974) report that meals are highly structured events and that any attempt to change patterns of food consumption would have to take into account the rules that govern the social and cultural context in which eating takes place. Working-class meals were shown by Charles and Kerr (1985) to have the dual functions of ensuring that children eat properly and healthily every day and of teaching them about the social relations which characterise food consumption within families.

Calnan (1990) reports on differences in the ways different social groups define the importance of food in relation to their health beliefs. Both Pill (1983) and Calnan (1987) conclude that although diet is perceived by working-class families to be of little relevance in the causation of illness, it was important in maintaining health. In trying to explain these differences Calnan (1990) suggests that the greater discrepancy between working-class women's health beliefs and patterns of food purchase and consumption may be influenced by beliefs, tastes and preferences which have little to do with health. Health may not be seen as a priority or even considered when deciding what food to buy. Even when healthy food is considered as important, working-class women are constrained by other family members' choices and the lack of material means.

Our discussion of the effects of food and nutrition on the health of individuals has been somewhat speculative, since much of the data are based on observational studies alone. However, nutritionists are convinced of these data (NACNE 1983). The possibility of comprehensive prospective data being collected on the relationship between food policy and health is slight. Unlike health care, where evaluation of new treatments, particularly medicines, before their widespread use by health professionals is accepted practice, the introduction of new food lines or new food additives is not usually the subject of full-scale evaluation. These data do, however, indicate some of the ways in which the structure of society can be said to be a cause of illness because of its association with diet.

ILLNESS AND THE INDIVIDUAL

We now focus our attention on the question: why is it that individuals from similar social backgrounds and lifestyles have differential morbidity and mortality experiences? Genetics probably provides a partial answer to this question but not a complete one. In the behavioural and social sciences one fruitful line of research has been life-events research. The basic premise of life-events research is that the incidence of stressful life change, such as bereavement or unemployment, is related to the onset of illness. A causal relationship between life events and illness is postulated. This relationship has been confirmed by a number of studies. For a review of these we suggest you consult Brown and Harris (1989). In this section we consider three kinds of stressful life events: bereavement, social change and unemployment.

Bereavement

It is now reasonably well established that there exists a causal relationship between bereavement and subsequent ill health. Parkes (1986) catalogues the numerous cross-sectional studies which report the strong association between mortality and bereavement. One explanation of these data is that couples who have shared a similar life style for a number of years would be expected to experience similar patterns of morbidity and mortality. While this could explain the increase in the mortality rate among the widowed population as a whole, it does not explain the peak of mortality in widows and widowers during the first year of bereavement, first observed by Young et al (1963). A number of small studies have confirmed these findings. Of course they do not indicate that bereavement is the *cause* of death of the remaining spouse. They do not even tell us whether bereavement causes the illness which causes death or simply aggravates an existing condition.

Other studies have identified recently bereaved people and collected data at a later time about the period since bereavement. Marris (1986) interviewed widows 2 years after the event and asked them to report their general health during that period. These women reported a high proportion of headaches, digestive upsets, rheumatism and asthma. Similar data have been collected by other researchers and are reported by Parkes (1986). From these studies Parkes concludes that bereavement does influence the pattern of physical illness but as yet the causal mechanisms are not fully understood.

Many of these studies suffer from what is called *retrospective bias*. Since data about an event are collected after the event has occurred, the choice of data to be collected and the way the data are recorded and interpreted can be unconsciously influenced by the scientist's ideas about the relationship between the event, that is, bereavement, and the outcome, that is, the death of the remaining spouse. *Retrospective studies,* in which data about the event are collected after the event has occurred, however, provide scientists with a simple and effective method of identifying possible relationships. *Prospective studies,* in which data are collected longitudinally from the point where an event is first identified, provide a sounder basis on which to test relationships between the event and its outcomes but are often more complicated and expensive to undertake.

Social change

In his book *Loss and Change,* Marris has described a number of similarities between bereavement and other types of social change. He applies the concept of grieving to situations of change where people suffer loss: a woman losing her husband; a household being evicted by a slum clearance scheme; the son of a peasant farmer launching a modern wholesale business in his village; and a new plan of action setting out to challenge the jurisdiction of established bureaucracies. In each of these situations, a familiar pattern of relationships has been disrupted and in each of them the disruption seems to provide similar reactions. Whenever people suffer loss their reactions express an internal conflict, whose nature is fundamentally similar to the working out of grief.

We can understand broadly how this is so. When a sudden change occurs there is a need to deny and also a need to accept that the change has occurred. This ambivalence generally inhibits straightforward adjustment. Adjustment to a major change involving loss is likely to be both painful and erratic. Our ambivalence at times of change reflects what Marris terms our *conservative impulse*. We depend on the fact that the meanings we give to daily events are essentially predictable. The loss of someone close to us can strike at this very sense of purpose or meaning. Of course, this loss is not necessarily only the loss of the object, but will also involve a loss of *role*. As we shall see, this loss of role can also be applied in the context of unemployment, and it applies to bereavement when the remaining spouse must alter his or her role.

Marris does not claim to have discovered the causal link between social change and health. His hypothesis is based on selective evidence from his own research. It would be an impossible task to review all the relevant evidence. The diversity of his examples, however, illustrates the possible wide application of his theory, which deserves more formal testing.

Unemployment

It is generally accepted that unemployment is not only undesirable but has detrimental effects on health (Colledge 1982, Miles 1987, Smith 1987). A number of writers have postulated that unemployment is a stressful life event which is causally related to ill health. At times of relatively low levels of unemployment following the 1939–1945 war, research about unemployment and health was unable to establish whether unemployment caused ill health or ill health caused unemployment. During that time most of the research about unemployment was concerned with the characteristics of the unemployed rather than on the effects of unemployment.

Technological innovation and the recession in the world economy during the 1980s have provided a unique opportunity to study the effects of unemployment on health, since unemployment levels have been so high that living without work is the experience of young and old people, men and women, black and white people, and manual and nonmanual workers.

Studies of unemployment comprise three types: studies of the unemployed, econometric studies, and studies of factory closure or redundancy (Mullen & Illsley 1981). The majority of the descriptive studies of the unemployed make little attempt to compare the health status of unemployed people with employed people. They generally show that unemployed people are unhealthy mentally and, less conclusively, physically. They are unable to indicate, however, whether ill health is caused by unemployment. People may be unemployed because they were less healthy. They may also be less healthy because of the conditions in which they live so that it is difficult to identify which of the many social deprivations, such as unemployment, bad housing, poverty or geographical location, are the cause of ill health. A major problem with these studies is that they are usually too small to account for all the possible explanations.

Some researchers have used econometric models similar to models used by economists in predicting the state of the economy. These models have attempted to relate unemployment to macro health indicators like psychiatric admission rates, health trend data, and mortality statistics. This approach is similar to the social epidemiological approach used by Durkheim in his classic study of suicide which we have already mentioned in Chapter 2. Of course nowadays, with the help of computers, complex multivariate statistical models, which can take account of more than one variable at a time, are used. This approach to the relationship between unemployment and health is surrounded by controversy. An advanced knowledge of statistics is required to understand many of the nuances of the arguments. Two kinds of conflicting explanations have emerged. Some writers claim that unemployment causes increased mortality while other writers, using apparently similar models and data, suggest that economic booms are the cause of increased mortality and psychiatric illness, not unemployment. Such disagreements are not unknown between economists using similar econometric models. Further studies of this kind will be necessary before we have an indication of who is right. Recent data from the OPCS longitudinal survey of mortality, however, suggests that the mortality of men who were seeking work was raised for reasons other than initial poor health (Moser et al 1987).

The third group of studies of unemployment, which focus on factory closures, suggest a more fruitful line of approach than descriptive and econometric studies. Unfortunately studies of redundancy or factory closure have been few in number. The advantage of such studies is that they afford the opportunity to examine the health status of workers over time: before and after termination of employment. Prospective or longitudinal enquiries are really the only way of establishing causality. Longitudinal studies, however, are not without their problems. In the case of unemployment, the unemployed person can be reemployed or move to another area. Both starting a new job and moving home have been identified as potential stressful life events. In such studies we therefore need to examine both the effects of unemployment *and* other life events together.

The emphasis on the association of unemployment with health status in unemployment research ignores the social context in which employment and unemployment takes place and has led to the medicalization of unemployment. Unemployment-related problems are sometimes isolated from their social roots by health professionals. They may see unemployment as a personal characteristic that renders the individual prone to illness rather than as a risk factor in people's lives. A second danger of ignoring the social context of unemployment is the normalisation of unemployment. During the 1980s unemployment remained higher than in any other decade since the 1930s. As long-term unemployment becomes institutionalised into everyday life, professionals focus on ways

of making this experience more comfortable. Sometimes this involves challenging the work effort and educating for leisure rather than encouraging the creation of jobs or finding ways of sharing jobs. Greater emphasis in the future on the cause of ill health – unemployment – rather than its cure is something we take up again later in this chapter when discussing prevention.

In this section we have tried to examine the evidence that stressful life events such as bereavement, social change and unemployment are causally related to ill health. Another way of exploring this relationship is to take a single medical condition or group of conditions and seek explanations for these conditions in terms of stressful life events. To illustrate this approach let us consider depression among women.

The social origins of depression

Our heading for this section is taken from the important study undertaken by George Brown and Tirril Harris in the early 1970s. In Chapter 3 we discussed differences between the social classes in their experience of illness. The prevalence of clinical depression is one condition which was found to be significantly higher among 'working-class' women than among 'middle-class' women. Brown & Harris (1978) discuss why this might be. They studied women from an inner-city area in London (Camberwell), using detailed accounts of women's daily lives and recent experiences and systematic descriptions of any psychiatric symptoms. Their data suggest that certain kinds of severe life events, especially losses, and major long-term difficulties are significant in the aetiology of depression. Other psychosocial factors also emerged as important determinants of women's vulnerability to such events and difficulties, and of the severity of the depression. The nature of these other factors help account for the higher prevalence of clinical depression among 'working-class' women and help us understand some of the inequalities in health discussed in Chapter 3. Although much of the work on depression has been done with women, the few studies to include men, who have a lower prevalence, have reached similar conclusions about the social causes of depression (Brown & Harris 1989).

The essential features of the model used by Brown and Harris (1978) in their study of women are shown in Figure 4.3. It identifies two important components of the model: provoking agents and vulnerability factors. These data suggested that severe life events occurring at a particular time, such as losing a job, and severe long-term difficulties, such as a partner's alcoholism, were both causally related to depression. Yet a number of women who experienced severe life events or long-term difficulties did not develop depression. The data were used to identify a second component of the model: vulnerability factors, such as low intimacy with a partner or loss of a mother before the age of 11 years. Vulnerability factors were found only to be capable of increasing the risk of depression in the presence of a provoking agent.

Although the model identifies the negative role of vulnerability factors, Brown and Harris emphasise the importance of the positive role of what they call protective factors. High intimacy with partner and no loss of mother before the age of 11 are examples of such factors.

A third set of factors identified by the model are symptom formation factors. Such factors appear only to influence the severity of depression once established. Previous history of psychiatric illness, the age of the woman and past loss were all identified as important symptom formation factors.

Recent studies using similar methods have confirmed the usefulness of the model in other contexts: among older people (Murphy 1982), Gaelic speaking women living in the Outer Hebrides (Brown & Prudo 1981), working-class women with children living in Oxford (Campbell et al 1983) and working-class women with at least one child living in London (Islington) (Brown et al 1986).

In summary: there are three major components to the model. The provoking agents influence when the depression occurs, the vulnerability factors influence whether these agents will have an effect, and symptom formation factors influence the severity and the form of the depressive disorder itself. The model itself tells us only that in some way the factors are causally linked to the disorder – it does not tell us how and why.

HEALTH, STRESS AND COPING

Much of the life-events research has focused on the causal relationship between a stressful life event and illness. This research has contributed little to the explanation of why stressful life events should be a cause of illness. Another way of looking at the relationship between stressful life events and illness is to seek explanations about why some people who experience stressful life events remain healthy while others become ill. This has been the central concern of Aaron Antonovsky over a number of years, which is embodied in his search for the origins (*genesis*) of health (*saluto*). An explanation of why people remain healthy is provided by the *Salutogenic Model* (Antonovsky 1979, 1987). A simple outline of the model is shown in Figure 4.4. Let us run through each of the components in turn by first defining the sense of coherence, which Antonovsky presents as the

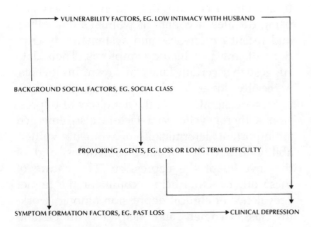

Fig. 4.3 A simple causal model of depression (adapted from Brown & Harris 1978).

core of his answer to the question of the origins of health *(salutogenesis)*.

Sense of coherence

The *sense of coherence* is a global orientation that expresses the extent to which one has a pervasive, enduring though dynamic feeling of confidence that one's internal and external environments are predictable and that there is a high probability that things will work as well as can reasonably be expected. (Antonovsky 1979, p. 123)

We can see *similarities* here with Marris's concept of *conservative impulse*. Both are concerned with the predictability of life experiences, but a sense of coherence implies something more: that we are in control of our own situations.

Life experience

Our *life experiences* are crucial in shaping our sense of coherence (arrow A). Throughout life, from birth to death, we experience a variety of social situations. When such experiences are

characterised by consistency, then the meanings and purpose we give to events are predictable, and we see the world as coherent and predictable. When people's lives are characterised by total predictability, however, they are likely to have a weaker sense of coherence than people experiencing some unpredictable events, which force the individual to adapt and maintain a more flexible approach to life. There is therefore benefit in a degree of unpredictability; too much of it and, on the other hand, total consistency, are both harmful.

Our sense of coherence develops at different stages of our lives. In childhood individuals are to some extent protected from unpredictable events. They experience a limited number of relationships with others and therefore get feedback from relatively few people. In adolescence a sense of coherence is reinforced by similar experiences but at this stage there is a far greater choice of experiences available. As individuals reach adulthood there are more changes in store for them: marriage, employment and new relationships. Usually these provide a fairly stable life experience which further strengthens the sense of coherence.

Major life events, such as divorce or unemployment, will force individuals to modify their sense of coherence. How we adapt to these life experiences will depend on our ability to cope or our generalised resistance resources.

Generalised resistance resources

At the most general level the generalised resistance resources (GRR) are the resources at our disposal which enable us to resolve tension. More specifically Antonovsky defines the GRR using the following mapping sentence:

Source of GRRs

Antonovsky identifies two primary sources of GRRs: child-rearing practice, and the roles assigned to us in particular cultures (arrow C). The kinds of social roles, whether they be gender, occupational or family roles, will be a major

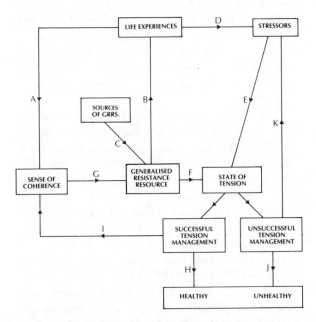

Fig. 4.4 Simplified diagram of the Salutogenic Model (adapted from Antonovsky 1979).

A GRR is a $\left\{\begin{array}{l}\text{physical}\\\text{biochemical}\\\text{artifactual-material}\\\text{emotional}\\\text{valuative-attitudinal}\\\text{interpersonal-relational}\\\text{macro sociocultural}\end{array}\right\}$ characteristic of an

$\left\{\begin{array}{l}\text{individual}\\\text{primary}\\\text{group}\\\text{subculture}\\\text{society}\end{array}\right\}$ that is effective in combating a wide variety

of stressors and thus preventing tension from being transformed into stress. (1979, p. 103)

influence. The importance of chance and serendipity also should not be ignored. Thus the sociocultural and historical context in which individuals live will influence the development of their GRRs.

Stressors

Stressors are a part of life. They will depend not only on biological forces but on our own life experiences. As a response to stressors we develop a state of tension (arrow E). What are stressors? One definition suggests that stressors are 'demands that tax or exceed the resources of the system or, to put it in a slightly different way, demands to which there are no readily available or automatic adaptive responses' (Lazarus & Cohen 1977, p.109, emphasis in original). We must not forget that different individuals will perceive stress in different ways. To many people normal activities of daily life like going outside in the open or using an escalator are stressful. In terms of the Salutogenic Model, however, this may not be particularly important, although it makes prediction of stressful life events about some of us more difficult. Stressors, therefore, affect each of us in different ways.

Tension management

As we can see from the model, how we manage the tensions created by stressors (arrow E) will depend to a large extent on our generalised resistance resources (arrow F) which in turn are mobilised by our sense of coherence (arrow G). Successful tension management may lead not only to a healthy outcome (arrow H) but will also reinforce our sense of coherence (arrow I). In contrast, unsuccessful tension management will lead to an unhealthy outcome (arrow J) and will increase the stressors affecting each of us (arrow K).

This is a much simplified summary of the Salutogenic Model, which itself may even be too simplistic. However, the full model is too complex to explain adequately here. We can only direct you to Antonovsky's book *Health, Stress and Coping* which is devoted entirely to an explanation of the model. Since writing this book Antonovsky (1987) has acknowledged the existence of similar models of health which support similar concepts to that of the sense of coherence (Kobasa 1979, Boyce 1985, Moos 1984, Werner & Smith 1982, Reiss 1981). These models still require empirical testing, a not insubstantial task! They do, however, provide a theoretical framework in which the individual might find a solution to the *private troubles* of how to promote personal health. For society it highlights the *public issue* of how to prevent stressors.

PREVENTION

It is now appropriate to recall the short story which we quoted at the beginning of the chapter. The moral of the story is, of course, that *prevention* is better that cure. If we can stop people being pushed in upstream then we will not need to expend so much effort in pulling people out downstream. The relevance of this story to many health professionals, however, is that they have little time for prevention because they spend most of their time caring and curing; that, rather than a health service, we have an illness service. What we do we mean by prevention?

Prevention of ill health can be classified as primary, secondary or tertiary (Report of the Royal Commission on the National Health Service 1979). Primary prevention involves taking measures which prevent disease or injury occurring. Discouraging smoking, encouraging participation in safer sexual practices, legislation to enforce the use of car safety belts in motor vehicles and providing adequate sanitation and nutrition are good examples of primary prevention. Secondary prevention refers to health care measures which are concerned with identifying and treating ill health. The early detection of disease through screening programmes, such as antenatal care, breast and cervical cancer screening, or through hypertension clinics, are common examples of secondary prevention. Tertiary prevention is concerned with mitigating the effects of illness and disease which have already occurred. Surgery to remove cancerous tissues, rehabilitation following a stroke and the aftercare of diabetics are examples of tertiary prevention. Health services have concentrated on tertiary prevention and, to a lesser extent, secondary prevention. In contrast, primary prevention, for reasons illustrated by the story, has virtually been ignored, and usually for economic and political reasons.

The focus of this chapter has been on those features of social life which contribute to health or ill health. From the examples cited, primary prevention is much more a social and political activity than the other two kinds described. We might then be justified in thinking that primary prevention is outside the sphere of health professionals' work. Certainly the historical evidence suggests that changes in the standard of living conditions, such as the provision of clean water supply and an efficient sewage system, and improved nutrition and standards of food hygiene, were responsible for the improvements in the nation's health (McKeown 1979). Medical advances may have little effect on mortality rates and there is little clear evidence that the health services are markedly improving our experience of disease or illness. We make this point not to belittle the achievements of the National Health Service or those professionals working in it but to put their role in primary prevention into perspective.

Our way of life, we have argued, is a central contribution to the development of illness and disease. This has been recognised in recent years by a number of official publications which have emphasised specific targets for primary prevention. The Report of the Royal Commission on the National Health Service (1979) advocates that *society* should act to discourage smoking, prevent accidents and encourage the 'right' kinds of foods. In 1988, the King Edward's Hospital Fund for London in collaboration with The Health Education Authority (formerly The Health Education Council), The Scottish Health Education Group and the London School of Hygiene and Tropical Medicine published *The Nation's Health* (Smith & Jacobson 1988). This report, prepared by an independent multidisciplinary committee, outlines a strategy with detailed health targets for individuals and society. But how might we achieve such ends? For example, this report, like many before, has implicated the role of tobacco in the development of poor health and identified four general objectives:

1. To create a physical and social environment where nonsmoking is the norm.
2. To support the creation of a generation of nonsmokers.
3. To maximise public awareness of the risks of smoking across all sectors of the community.
4. To support the efforts of those who wish to stop smoking.

In order to identify how these general objectives might be implemented we need to understand tobacco consumption from a sociological and psychological perspective.

The literature on smoking indicates that psychosocial factors influence whether an individual starts smoking, but it is psychological and pharmacological ones that play a part in its continuance (Raw 1978). It is in the explanation of why people *start* smoking that sociological factors are paramount. Smoking has come to be interpreted as a form of rational action by individuals under certain circumstances, even though it may have some negative consequences (Calnan 1982). Bynner (1969) describes a recruitment model which identifies barriers to taking up smoking and factors which increase the chances. Major barriers are negative parental and school attitudes toward smoking and perceived health risks. On the other hand, factors influencing young people to smoke include the availability of cigarettes, curiosity, rebelliousness, a desire to appear tough, anticipation of adulthood, social confidence, and parents, older siblings and friends smoking. It is young people's social environment that plays a crucial part in influencing whether they start smoking.

McKennell and Thomas (1968) demonstrated that a large proportion of young regular smokers persist in the habit when they grow up. An analysis of types of adult smoker suggests that the career of the smoker starts off with socially oriented motives and then moves to the stage where smoking is nicotine motivated (Russel 1976). Nicotine dependence is then crucial but it is supported by the social environment in which the smoker lives, including images created by tobacco advertising.

Calnan (1982) points out that present models of cigarette smokers fail to explain why people have different levels of cigarette consumption and why it is that many smokers state that they smoke when under stress (Schachter 1978). We already indicated that stressors include a number of life events as well as continuing long-term difficulties (Brown & Harris 1989). If smokers smoke heavily because they believe it relieves tension, anxiety or stress, then smoking can be interpreted as not only meeting a person's perfectly rational need for coping with stress but also indicating that stress is generated by events outside the smoker's control. If, as advocated by the Royal Commission and *The Nation's Health*, society should act by discouraging smoking then, by Calnan's argument, policies would require either to provide a substitute or alternative coping mechanism, or attempt to eradicate the sources of stress. In making recommendations for the implementation of the general objectives for tobacco consumption the multidisciplinary committee fail to make such recommendations about the solution of individuals' long-term difficulties (Smith & Jacobson 1988). They do, however, address the wider role of health authorities, Government, employing organisations and the tobacco industry. Perhaps it is unrealistic for us to expect the resolution of long-term difficulties since *the* primary goal of society is not health. We would live in a very different kind of society if *the* primary goal was health. Some health professionals, as well as other members of society, may consider health to be *the* primary goal, but we suspect that they are a very small minority.

As it is, health education remains the major vehicle for attempts by the State to achieve a healthier society (Secretary of State for Health 1991, 1992). Health education is typically based on the belief that responsibility for health lies with the individual, and therefore health education involves changing individuals' attitudes and knowledge. Health education is important but in emphasising the individual's responsibility the State is individualising the problem so that there is often a tendency by the State and health professionals to blame the individual for their own ill health. Recent evidence from *The Health and Lifestyle Survey* (Blaxter 1990) suggests that it is only individuals in the higher social classes who are likely to improve their health through changes in exercising, smoking, drinking and eating habits. The survey found that individuals who are disadvantaged through poverty or lack of local support, for example, are unlikely to improve their health status by changing their consumption of tobacco, alcohol and certain types of food or by engaging in regular exercise.

The State appears unwilling to acknowledge the wider structural characteristics of a modern industrial society which impinge on health where *the* primary goal of society appears to be economic growth in increasing material prosperity for some members of society. Thus the resources devoted to changing individuals' attitudes and behaviour towards lifestyles for health, let alone the broader structural and environmental changes which influence health outcomes, are a very small proportion of the total resources devoted to health and education. They are far less than the manufacturers of tobacco products use to advertise their products.

Froggatt (1989), in a review of the United Kingdom's Governments' policy on smoking, identifies the political and economic obstacles to increased State intervention. The objection of the British Government to the European Commission's proposed ban on advertising except at the point of sale is the most recent contradiction in the State's policy on smoking since the link between smoking and ill health was first established in the early 1950s.

Health education is central to the health professional's role. But in providing health education, our sociological understanding will identify that different social groups respond to it in different ways. Take the issue of tobacco consumption again. Once doctors had taken the lead in reducing their personal consumption of tobacco products, there was a slow reduction among similar professional groups. Although considerable numbers of people from the professions and other high socioeconomic groups have stopped smoking, this has been matched by an increased consumption among people from lower socioeconomic groups, particularly women (Foster et al 1990). For health education to be effective it would appear, from these data, that new ways of influencing smoking behaviour among people from lower socioeconomic groups are required, especially among young people. We have noted that the major influences on smoking behaviour among young people are parents, peers and friends. Thus for health education to become more effective it must use social networks for social change, or at least recognise that health education measures need to take account of the social context in which people live.

When certain groups of people behave in ways which are detrimental to their own or other people's health there is a tendency to blame them. People who have bronchitis and smoke, mothers of unvaccinated children with whooping cough, gay men who are HIV positive, and women who have difficulty when delivering their babies, may be blamed by health professionals for their behaviour. Clearly, they are all theoretically in a position to alter their life styles and influence their own or their children's health by not smoking, by getting their children vaccinated, by using safe sexual practices or by attending antenatal care. In this chapter, however, we have identified both structural and personal constraints which make it difficult for some people to adopt standards of behaviour considered acceptable to some health professionals.

SUMMARY

This chapter has raised what we consider to be important issues about the relationship between social factors and health. Our discussions on diet and tobacco consumption and the relationship with health and illness are examples of the ways in which social, political and economic forces, as well as patterns of production and consumption interact to influence the health of the population. Unfortunately in attempting to prevent illness related to lifestyle factors, the government has emphasised individuals' responsibility to look after their own health without tackling the structural factors which also influence lifestyle and health (Secretary of State for Health 1991, 1992).

The link between events which individuals find stressful and ill health was explored with reference to studies of a range of such events. There is now a large body of evidence pointing to a causal relationship between stressful life events and illness, and evidence is developing from studies of life events and illness that it is causally linked to social factors (Brown & Harris 1989). Why some people should become ill while others do not when exposed to objectively similar circumstances is explained by Antonovsky (1979, 1987) in terms of the coherence individuals are able to attribute to their life

and what happens to them. This model is one attempt to explain the processes at work but it remains to be empirically tested. Given the current interest in health, stress and coping, it is likely that other models will be developed which will influence ideas about prevention of stress and facilitating coping strategies.

It is evident that while individuals are in a large part responsible for their health, their health related actions, which permeate most of their daily lives, are inexplicably linked with social processes. It is by understanding these processes that health professionals will appreciate and relate to the difficulties that many of us have in conforming to a lifestyle which maximises our health.

FURTHER READING

Antonovsky A 1979 Health, stress and coping. Jossey Bass, San Francisco

Brown G W, Harris T (eds) 1989 Life events and illness. The Guildford Press, London

Froggatt P 1989 Determinants of policy on smoking. International Journal of Epidemiology, 18: 1–9

Smith A, Jacobson B (eds) 1988 The Nation's Health: a strategy for the 1990s: Report from an independent multidisciplinary committee chaired by Professor Alwyn Smith. King Edward's Hospital Fund for London, London

5

Family and life career

In Chapter 3 we introduced the concept of social stratification and indicated the importance of social class and other similar concepts in the development of a sociological understanding. We saw how a sociological understanding extended and modified conventional interpretations of health inequalities. In Chapter 4 we described how illness was caused and prevented by social factors and how these could be interpreted in relation to social structure. Before turning to a fuller discussion of health-related concepts in the next chapter we wish to focus on another important aspect of social structure, namely, family.

We shall introduce different definitions of what constitutes *family* and consider how family has been handled by different sociological perspectives. Placing family in a broader social context, we introduce the concept of life career and discuss processes of socialisation as well as transition points. Finally, we turn to more generalised aspects of social change.

Almost all of us have an intimate knowledge of at least one family. Family is often acknowledged to be one of the most universal of human institutions but it takes many forms both within one culture and between different cultures. All of us will have experienced, at some time in our lives, differences between the way our own families and those of acquaintances are organised: families which are mother-centred, or what sociologists call the *matriarchal family*; families which are father-centred – the *patriarchal*

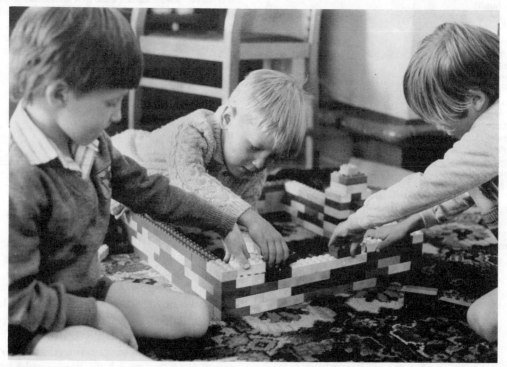

Fig. 5.1A

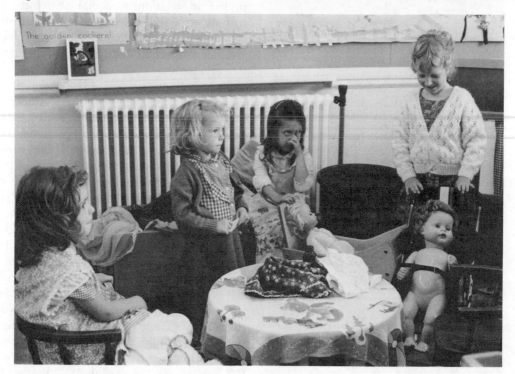

Fig. 5.1B A,B: 5-year-olds already showing stereotyped roles in their play (courtesy of Rik Walton).

family; families which are neither mother nor father centred; and single-parent families. Think of your close acquaintances and see whether you can identify an example of each of these. Of course, many of the families we each know will exhibit characteristics which are due not to the social structure of the group but to differences in the personalities of family members.

Much of what we know about the family we take for granted. Our intimate knowledge of our own families makes it difficult to step outside of all that we already understand about them. In making a study of *the* family as an institution we must confront a major problem of sociological research – this is learning to understand our own values while gaining an understanding of the way others define their situations. But there is a third obstacle to a sociological understanding of family. In our culture we define family relationships as intimate and private. People are not always willing to respond to detailed study of their family life and those who do respond to questions are likely, as are the sociologists studying them, to couch their answers to conform to society's normative expectations.

Family, therefore, is a concept which has significant personal meaning; it also has a variety of distinct sociological interpretations, which we shall turn to shortly.

A second concept we want to develop in this chapter is *career*. This has both everyday and sociological interpretations.

We generally use the word 'career' to refer to a person's advancement through life, especially in relation to her or his profession or occupation. In sociology the concept of career has been applied to a number of very different situations, although retaining the general meaning of progression through life. In this book we shall use the concept in relation to the *life career*, the *patient career* (Ch. 8) and the *professional career* (Ch. 11). Common to each of these careers are a number of related sociological concepts. In this chapter we focus on two – *socialisation* and *social change* – and, in the process, introduce a number of others.

Everyone, everywhere, is subject to the process of socialisation by virtue of being born into and continuing to learn the ways of a given society or social group (Fig. 5.1A, B). Children learn the meanings of different ways of dressing for social events like going out to play, going to church or going to school; patients learn when and in what terms it is appropriate to talk about their illness to different kinds of hospital staff, to other patients and to their families; and students learn the expected ways of acting in front of hospital consultants, senior members of their own profession and their peers.

Like socialisation, social change is not only a common but also taken-for-granted feature of social life and exerts influence on different kinds of career. Social change affects us all, both in the short and in the long term. In the short term, technological innovations like the telephone and the personal computer have revolutionised many aspects of everyday life: at home, at work and at leisure. In the long term, changing patterns of social behaviour influence the development of our life careers. Employment patterns, leisure activities and family life have been influenced markedly in the last 30 years by social changes such as the changing pattern of female employment and the shorter working week.

In this chapter we shall illustrate the variety of forms the family can take in the context of the life career, and we shall describe the related concepts of marriage and kinship. We shall look at changes in the role of the family in contemporary society, describing two contrasting sociological explanations of the functions of the family. We reserve our discussion of the role of the family in health care until Chapter 6.

THE FAMILY

The term 'family', like the term 'career', is widely used in everyday speech. People may refer to their relatives as 'the family' and may use it to include or exclude their relatives through marriage. Sometimes it is used in a more restrictive sense to refer to parents and their offspring, while on other occasions the term will refer to the household. What do sociologists understand by the term 'family'? Like other sociological concepts its use will depend on perspective. From a broadly structuralist perspective Worsley (1977) identifies three central elements of family: marriage, parenthood and residence. The important thing about these three elements is that they are neither necessary nor sufficient parts of the definition but do, in var ous combinations, delineate a definition of the family. Let us examine each of these three elements in turn.

Marriage

Traditionally, *marriage* has been seen as a relatively unitary concept consisting of a relationship between two adults, one male and one female, which is legally recognised through participation in a religious or civil marriage ceremony. In Britain, the Royal Commission on Marriage and Divorce (1956) defined marriage as a 'voluntary union for life of one man and one woman to the exclusion of all others' (p. 7). That is a union which is voluntary, permanent and strictly monogamous. Nearly 40 years on, since the publication of this Report, marriage remains very popular. In 1987, 93% of men and 95% of women by the age of 50 were or had been married (Haskey 1988, p. 22). Traditional monogamy, that is having one spouse for life, is relatively less common than it used to be. Increasingly, modern Britain is characterised by serial monogamy – the practice of having a sequence of spouses, one at a time. In 1965, 11% of marriages involved a divorced bride or groom; this increased to 22% in 1972 (Leete 1976, pp. 6–7) and 33% in 1987 (Haskey 1988, p. 22). More difficult to enumerate (Brown & Kiernan 1981, Haskey & Kelly 1991) is the increasing trend toward common-law marriages – cohabitation. In 1986–87 12% of men and 14% of women aged 16–59 were cohabiting (Haskey & Kiernan 1989, p. 24). Cohabitation is often short-term (median length of time in 1986–87 was 24 months), and such liaisons are regularly legalised at the appearance of the first child

(Haskey & Kiernan 1989, p. 27). Even more difficult to enumerate is the not insignificant increase in the number of stable homosexual relationships.

Traditionalists may well argue that some of these modern trends do not constitute marriage. But from a sociological perspective what *would be* the characteristics of a particular form of social organisation which can be embraced by the term 'marriage'? To help answer this question let us consider an early sociological definition. Westermark defined marriage as a relation 'of one or more men with one or more women which is recognised by custom or law, and which involves certain rights and duties, both in the case of the parties entering the union and in the case of the children born of it' (Westermark 1926, p. 1).

Westermark's definition is useful because it highlights the fact that marriage has wider social implications than merely biological mating. An important feature is the emphasis on rights and obligations of marriage, which are common to many societies. Thus marriage may exclude casual sexual relationships and other social relationships not approved by the particular society. Westermark excluded homosexual 'marriages'. But in the 70 years since this definition was penned homosexuality has become more widely accepted and in some cultures 'marriage ceremonies' take place. Arguably, then, given the breadth of his definition, he would have included homosexual relationships if he had been writing in the 1990s.

We can see that traditional monogamy is just one of many patterns of marriage embraced by Westermark's definition. Group marriage, either polygyny – where a man has more than one wife – or polyandry – where a woman has more than one husband – are included. Marriages can be either permanent or, by divorce or death transitional, the latter also permitting serial monogamy. Marriages can be involuntary, as well as voluntary. In many societies, including subcultures in our own, marriages are arranged by parents.

Britain, nowadays, experiences a great many different cultural traditions, and so many of these different patterns of marriage exist. British law, however, decrees polygyny and polyandry illegal, while group common-law marriages are not sanctioned in law. Serial monogamy, as we have already noted, is increasingly common and among some ethnic minorities marriages are still arranged in accordance with the normal customs of the subculture, causing some young women to ask to be made 'wards of court' in order to avoid having to enter a marriage. Marriages of convenience provide a means of overcoming immigration laws.

Parenthood

Parenthood is also socially constructed. Biological parenthood is the basis of many types of families in different cultures. The identification of the biological father, however, can often be a matter of conjecture. As a result, fathers will assume paternity without necessarily being the biological father. Recognition that a parent is not the biological parent takes a number of forms in modern society. Being a step-parent, an increasing likelihood nowadays, has rights and obligations almost identical to those of parenthood. Similarly, step-children have rights and obligations similar to those of biological children but, until recently, illegitimate children were deprived of many of these. Adoptive parents, foster parents and grandparents acting as adoptive or foster parents are further examples of social parenthood.

Similar problems of definition surround a number of taken-for-granted relationships. 'Brother' and 'sister' are both kinship terms used to describe offspring of the same parents. They are also used by the black power movement in the United States and the trade union movement, for example, to signify comradeship, as is sister in the feminist movement. The term 'uncle' has been used in at least three ways: a brother of a person's mother or father; an adult friend of a person's parents; and a mother's lover. In studying family relationships we must be careful to be aware of these taken-for-granted uses of the terms, and to remember that other cultures will describe the family in different ways.

Residence

We have already introduced the idea of *residence* in our discussion of marriage. Childless common-law marriages or 'living together' illustrate the importance of residence in defining family. Parents may be married but not living together, for instance, in families where one or other parent is at sea, in prison or working away from home, or where parents have temporarily separated. Laslett (1965) describes how, in preindustrial societies, families would include not only close kin but also servants and other workers – in other words, all those living in the same household. A similar emphasis on residence rather than marriage or parenthood as a definition of family is used by the Census Office, who categorise 'family groupings' into households defined as follows:

A household is either: (a) one person living alone; or (b) a group of people (who may or may not be related) living, or staying temporarily, at the same address, with common housekeeping. (OPCS & General Register Office for Scotland 1992, p. 10).

Figure 5.2 attempts to illustrate the overlap between the three elements of the family identified by Worsley (1977). Sociologists studying family have often followed traditional ideas. They have most often focused on family as man, woman and their offspring. To some extent this conception of family is an *ideal type*. It masks considerable variations which are highlighted in Figure 5.2 and which are indicated in the Rapoports' collection of essays on the family in modern Britain (Rapoport et al 1982). But as Gubrium and Holstein (1990) suggest family is also a good example of a social construction which has wider meaning than the structuralist perspective emphasised here.

Kinship terms

Conjugal family

Sometimes the terms *conjugal family* and *nuclear family* are used to define a social group consist-

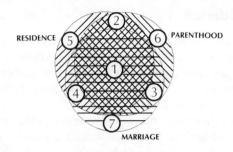

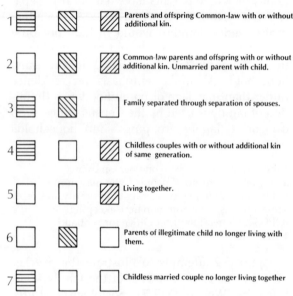

1 — Parents and offspring Common-law with or without additional kin.

2 — Common-law parents and offspring with or without additional kin. Unmarried parent with child.

3 — Family separated through separation of spouses.

4 — Childless couples with or without additional kin of same generation.

5 — Living together.

6 — Parents of illegitimate child no longer living with them.

7 — Childless married couple no longer living together

Fig. 5.2 Overlap of the three elements of the family showing seven possible combinations of marriage, parenthood and residence (adapted from Worsley 1977).

ly of origin, the family of marriage, ego's kinship core, the T-core and the near kin. We illustrate these in Figures 5.3–5.5, using normal anthropological notation. Three symbols are used – a triangle represents the male of the group, a circle the female and the equals sign between them represents marriage or common-law marriage. The person who is defining the situation is called the ego.

The family of origin

This is the first of two ways of looking at the conjugal family. The family of origin, sometimes referred to as the family of orientation, refers to the kin grouping of ego, including parent(s) and sibling(s) (see Fig. 5.3).

The family of marriage

This is the second way of looking at the conjugal family. The family of marriage, sometimes referred to as the family of procreation, refers to the kin grouping of ego, including spouse and their children (see Fig. 5.3).

ing of a man and woman and their dependent offspring. The term 'nuclear family' is limited to this grouping which subscribes to the view that this is the 'nuclear' unit of social organisation. The term 'conjugal family', while including the above social group, is sufficiently inclusive to describe four of the seven categories defined in Figure 5.2 (categories 1, 2, 3 and 6). The central element of the conjugal family is parenthood. Marriage and residence are not necessary for the species to survive.

Family sociologists have generated a confusing list of terms. Their ambiguity led Harris and Stacey (1969) to identify five key terms: the fami-

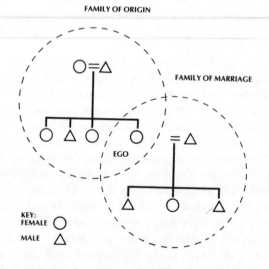

Fig. 5.3 Family of marriage and family of origin.

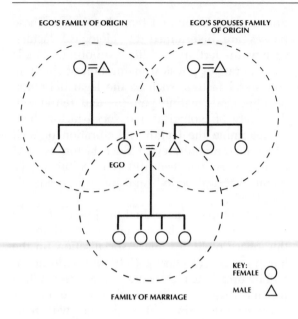

Fig. 5.4 The T-core.

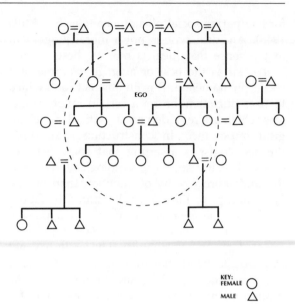

Fig. 5.5 Ego's near kin

Ego's kinship core

The kin grouping consisting of both the family of origin and the family of marriage is called ego's kinship (see Fig. 5.3).

The T-core

This kin grouping consists of the couple's kinship core: ego's family of origin, the spouse's family of origin and their common family of marriage (see Fig. 5.4).

Near kin

This term refers to ego's *first and second degree kin,* in other words, the kinship cores of ego, ego's spouse (the T-core), ego's children, ego's father, ego's mother and ego's siblings (brothers and sisters). Figure 5.5 shows the kinship universe within which ego's kin exist.

While there are different structural family arrangements and families have different degrees of permanence, the family is an enduring institution. Any one of us in our lifetime is likely to be a member of more than one family. We progress through life, engaging in different kinds of family relationships, in what can be termed our life careers.

THE LIFE CAREER

All of us are born and in the end we all die. Some people survive in this world for only a few minutes while others last a century. The concept of *life career* embraces this time span representing one way in which we can look at our collective biographies. Figure 5.6 shows the various stages of the life career starting with birth and ending with death. Along the way, typically, the individual will be socialised as a child (and subsequently at all stages of the life career), be educated, raise a family, work, become a patient, and live through old age. At different points in the career the typical individual will pass some important milestones: reaching the age of majority, obtaining a job, getting married and retiring.

Ideal type

This illustration of the life career exemplifies the notion of *ideal type,* which was used by Weber for comparing social phenomena (Gerth & Mills 1948). An ideal type is not a moral judgement in the sense that ideal is morally best; neither is it ideal as the best or average example of a social phenomenon. It is an abstract tool, which focuses our attention on a certain range of factors which are regarded as of particular sociological importance. In constructing ideal types the sociologist is asserting that some features of social reality are more sociologically interesting and more worthy of attention than others. Our concept of life career illustrated in Figure 5.6 is not the average life career of a person, or indeed the best, but an ideal type constructed as an explanatory device. It has not included features like moving home or being made redundant, which are important to the individual but of less sociological importance for understanding life careers.

Family cycles

In the context of the family, the life career is concerned with the family cycle, sometimes referred to as the family life cycle or the cycle of family development. Individual families change in structure: an ideal type would be courtship to marriage, to procreation, to child rearing, to chil-dren leaving home and then dissolution. These phases are determined by biological factors, such as the fertility and life span of individuals and the rate of physical maturation of children, and social factors, such as the legal definition of adulthood, mating patterns and retirement. A variety of biological and social factors help to determine the length and duration of each phase of the family cycle. Such factors will, of course, vary between different cultures, different historical periods and different economic conditions.

For the typical individual the first experience of the family will be the family of origin. At this phase of life, primary socialisation (in the family) and secondary socialisation (education) will be prime characteristics of the career. When the individual reaches adulthood he or she may leave the family of origin and, with marriage, enter the family of marriage. This transition will be followed by the period of 'having a family' and child rearing. This phase ends when all offspring have reached adult status and have left their family of origin, ego's family of marriage, to begin a new family life cycle. The original family of marriage will then enter a phase of independence, probably during middle age, when both work and leisure are predo-

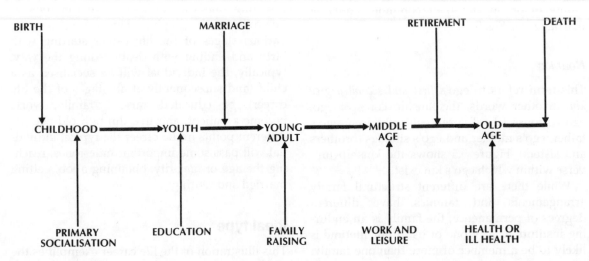

Fig. 5.6 The life career.

minant aspects of the life career. Old age and retirement from work and other major life roles signal the final drama of the life career and the family cycle.

Socialisation

Our individual social biographies begin with our birth. At this point, and continuously through our lives, we are subject to the process of *socialisation*. Elkin has defined it 'as the process by which someone learns the ways of a given society or social group so that he can function within it' (Elkin 1960, p. 4).

In the first few months of life infants experience numerous stimuli. They experience hunger, thirst, pain, discomfort and pleasure. Although these are physical experiences they are mediated through social interaction. Infants learn when and where to eat, sleep and defecate according to a set of predefined rules adhered to by their parents. Of course, such rules will vary between different societies and between different social groups (cultures and subcultures) within a particular society. Even within our own society childrearing practices, for example, vary between different social groups (Newsom & Newsom 1965). Young babies will experience and learn, for example, the different rules of demand feeding and regular scheduled feeding according to the social group of their mothers and the feeding policies of different maternity hospitals.

Primary and secondary socialisation

We call the socialisation of an individual in early childhood *primary socialisation*. Learning more complex social rules in later childhood and adulthood is known as *secondary socialisation*.

Secondary socialisation is experienced throughout the life career. In order to function in a socially appropriate manner we have to learn new rules when we enter any new and strange situation. How many of us would know how to behave when presented to the Queen? When we begin training for a profession, when we start working in a new organisa-

tion, when we travel abroad on holiday or enter hospital as a patient we are learning the rules appropriate to the social setting in which we are currently interacting. From the cradle to the grave we are being socialised.

Anticipatory socialisation

How does socialisation proceed? Socialisation is often referred to as *anticipatory socialisation* because during the learning of new social rules we anticipate our future behaviour when we have learned these rules. In the socialisation of young children a crucial step is what Mead (1934) called 'learning to take the attitude of the other'. Children will not only learn to recognise a certain attitude in someone else and understand its meaning, but will learn to adopt the attitude themselves. This is readily observed in young children who engage in games of mothers and fathers with their dolls. When the doll 'wets' its clothes the child will imitate both verbally and nonverbally the expressions and gestures of parents in the real-life situation.

Similarly, during training student nurses and medical students will anticipate their future roles by acting out that role during training. They will at first 'play nurse' or 'play doctor' rather than be a 'real nurse' or 'real doctor' and hope that those watching will approve the performance. Through time and with practice students gain the conviction that the practices are authentic because others respond in ways indicating that they are competent and legitimate in the role. Try to think how you yourself have behaved when you were faced with a new situation and had somehow to manage through it. How did you react, for instance, the first time you had to break bad news to a family, or the first time a patient had an extreme emotional outburst or you encountered death?

Definition of the situation

As part of the socialisation process individuals learn particular ways of defining the situations in which they find themselves. In other words, 'it all depends on how you see it'. The basis of any definition of a situation described by individuals is rooted in their past social experiences. It is affected by the norms and values of their social groups which have been learnt through socialisation. Thus, the *definition of the situation* is the typical meaning which members of a social group attach to any given social event. For example, people define social roles according to their social experience so the role of husband in relation to child rearing practices varies between social groups (Newsom & Newsom 1965). This has the potential for generating conflict in some working-class women when they receive advice from middle-class professionals about the role their husbands *should* play as fathers-to-be, because they hold different normative expectations of what is appropriate. Therefore in order to understand how men and women will act their social roles it is necessary to know and understand how they define a given situation, and to do this we need to know something about what they take for granted. If a nurse's and a patient's definition of the situation, say the patient's normal bathing patterns, are different, then unless the nurse is willing to appreciate the patient's point of view social understanding and consequently social interaction will be impaired. A patient who is used to bathing once a week may find it difficult and distressing to comply with hospital routines which expect a daily bath. Similarly, the male patient suffering from a myocardial infarction who is washed and shaved by a nurse may resist this attention because he feels it reflects adversely on his manliness, and feels distaste at being attended by a young girl carrying out such personal tasks. He does not understand or appreciate the nurse's attempts to do everything to help him rest. Their definitions of the situation are entirely at odds. They need to be given the opportunity to clarify their varying perspectives to each other and to agree about what is appropriate for care to proceed more effectively.

Norms, values and attitudes

What people learn and the way that they are socialised into a particular mode of behaviour will depend on a variety of factors: where they live, with whom they live, to whom they talk, and where they work. The socialisation process will be influenced by the *norms, values* and *attitudes* of the people with whom they engage who are their agents of socialisation.

Norms

'Norms' refer to those patterns of behaviour in society which are more or less taken for granted. When we meet people we greet them in different kinds of ways; if we want something we say 'please' and when we receive it we say 'thank you'. Similarly, men will normally wear trousers and we would not expect them to wear skirts, although in Scotland we would not be surprised if they were wearing kilts. Female physiotherapists, nurses and teachers now often wear trousers at work. Norms are dependent on given social situations. In hospital, professional staff are expected to look at and touch parts of the body of the same and opposite sex as they carry out their professional functions (Lawler 1991). The same behaviour outside hospital, or out of context in hospital, would be a gross violation of society's norms. Male doctors and nurses have been disciplined for having sexual relationships with female patients in the patients' own homes but no action would have been taken had the women not been *their* patients.

Values

Values may also be taken for granted but they differ from norms in that they are ideas which we hold to be right or wrong. So, for example, in some social groups it would be regarded as wrong to break into someone's house and remove their possessions, but those same people might consider it all right to use an employer's telephone to make private calls or 'borrow' the odd envelope, paper tissues or bandage. In an absolute sense, all are forms of theft.

Within British society there are variations in both norms and values. In some areas it is taken for granted that women do not frequent certain public houses or areas within them, whereas in other parts of the country it is taken for granted that women may visit any bar or public house. Similarly, different social groups hold different values. In some families where the man is the main wage-earner and does manual work, it is not thought right that men should tell their wives how much they earn, whereas among nonmanual workers the opposite generally holds.

Attitudes

Attitudes are more specific than values and often less enduring; like values they are always present but not necessarily taken for granted. Thus, it is taken for granted that doctors, teachers, lawyers and similar people will have what we call 'middle-class values'. They will have certain tastes in food and drink, for example they may have a preference for whole-meal bread rather than white or for Brie rather than Cheddar cheese; they may see an importance in school work which other parents might not. Although we shall not always be able to predict the values of middle-class individuals we know something of the group's values. Their attitudes, however, are something quite different. These are more likely to change over their lifetime and are more likely to be specific and unpredictable – for example, their attitudes towards nuclear weapons, classical music, euthanasia or abortion. We must also remember that attitudes are more likely than values to be highly emotional issues, both in the sense of being irrational and illogical and in the sense of arousing powerful defences.

Agencies of socialisation

We have suggested that a person's norms, values and attitudes are influenced by the norms, values and attitudes of their *agents of socialisation* – those people or groups who parti-cipate in the socialisation process. If we look again at Figure 5.6, depicting our ideal type of life career, we can identify a number of phases in the career where major socialisation processes will take place. The prominent agents of socialisation in our society are the family, school, peer group, mass media and institutions, such as the church, the pub or the discotheque. At different points in the life career other institutions, such as hospitals, prisons and old people's homes, may teach us new rules to follow.

All of us, as well as being socialised, are also agents of socialisation at some time in our lives. In the family the parents teach their children a set of roles appropriate to their age, gender and social class. Further on in the life career the teacher will guide pupils towards ways of acting, while peers will lead in other and sometimes conflicting ways. In hospital the staff and other patients teach new patients the role of patient, while students learn the role of the professional group towards which they aspire. Perhaps, with the exception of professional teachers, the role of socialisation agent is not obvious to those acting it, but informal teaching or role modelling is often a far more important mechanism of socialisation than what is formally taught in classrooms.

Culture and subculture

Perhaps one of the most striking influences on the individual through the socialisation process is the effect on an individual's *culture* or *subculture*. In sociology the term 'culture' is often used in such a way as to include almost every aspect of entire patterns of beliefs, attitudes, values, ideas and knowledge that members of different social groups hold about themselves.

Within any society there are a number of distinctive smaller cultures called subcultures. These develop their own particular cultural patterns. A true subculture develops when its members as a group work or live in relative isolation, such as a village of coal miners or fishermen; when a group perceives external threats to its welfare, for example, battered wives or homosexuals; or when a group has a common interest to defend against others, such as black minorities in European societies. As subcultures develop their members may acquire preferences for different kinds of material objects such as clothes or music, and they may develop norms, values and attitudes of their own. Sometimes these involve a rejection of the norms, values and attitudes of the larger culture. We have only to look at many teenagers to see how their subcultures reject traditional modes of dress and behaviour. In some subcultures values are reversed. Petty crime and drugs use which would be termed delinquent by the larger society may be admired among subcultures.

Ageing

Throughout the life career individuals also undergo a process of ageing. Ageing is both a biological and a social process: it involves interaction between the social and physical environment and the individual's biological state. From a biological perspective ageing in individuals can be defined as a deterioration process through which the resistance of the organism to the pressure of the environment progressively diminishes, until it can no longer withstand them and dies. Thus, throughout an individual's life, there will be a decline in biological functioning: in basic metabolic rate, in cardiac output, in the vital capacity of the lungs, in breathing capacity, in nerve conduction velocity, in body water content, in kidney plasma flow and in the filtration rates of the kidney. A similar dynamic set of processes, which operate at all stages of the life career, can be seen from a sociological perspective. However, from a sociological perspective ageing does not necessarily imply social *decline*; rather it is an example of social change.

Social change

Social changes are experienced at various stages throughout our life careers. We get married,

we move house, we divorce and we retire. A number of important changes occur to many of us in our lives and the socialisation process prepares each of us for some of them, although inevitably we are left unprepared to deal with others.

Status passage

To describe major changes in our life careers we use the concept of *status passage*. A status passage is a significant event in the life career which marks the change from one social position to another. Thus birth, graduation, marriage, divorce, redundancy and death are all examples of status passage.

Rites de passage

In traditional African and South American cultures these may take the form of ritual dances and feasts. In contemporary Britain the presentation of the hospital badge to newly qualified nurses, the graduation ceremony, and the lavish presentation of gifts at the birth of a new baby and marriage are common examples. Perhaps the best illustration of the status passage and its associated *rites de passage* is retirement. People's experience of retirement and their reactions to the process will be numerous. Changes for the individual throughout the life career, like retirement, are often predictable, however, and represent persistent patterns of action.

Retirement

We tend to use the concept of retirement in two complementary ways: to describe the transition from the role of worker to the role of retired person and to describe the social status of the retired person. In the first sense retirement is a *rites de passage*. In many traditional societies the various *rites de passage* provide a smooth transition from one social status to another. Three kinds of rites can be distinguished for any given status passage: rites of separation, rites of transition and rites of incorporation (Van Gennep 1960). Crawford (1973) has described the experiences of a small number of men before and after retirement. She suggests that in British society retirement includes rites of both separation and transition but not of incorporation.

Rites of separation

The experiences of workers during their last week at work may be described as *rites of separation*. For a time they would be expected to leave their normal tasks and spend much of the time saying farewells to their colleagues and other workers. The time spent participating in this ritual will be determined not only by the size of the establishment and the individual's role in it but its significance to other members of the organisation.

Retirement not only means relinquishing the status of worker but also implies giving up the status identity associated with a particular kind of job – electrician, driver, lawyer, speech therapist or whatever. This identity will have more chance of continuing where a job is taken over by someone else. Thus an important aspect of the rites of separation includes handing over the job to someone else.

Rites of transition

The retiring worker will signify the 'sacred' status of the transition by not being subject to the ordinary disciplines of the work place. For example, blue-collar workers may wear more formal clothes which would normally be inappropriate for the job done. The *rites of transition* may include a number of symbolic acts such as visits, exchange of gifts, final drinks or special meals and outings away from the work place. In contemporary retirement ceremonies the presentation of gifts from colleagues and employers appears to be the most common *rite*. Gifts, as well as other ways of showing real appreciation of the retiring colleague, also provide a focus for the leaving ceremony.

Rites of incorporation

The social group to which retired workers are incorporated is the family. In retirement they will spend more time with the family and it is the family which will be most closely identified by the rest of the community. Such *rites of incorporation* would include celebration meals or retirement parties for family and friends. Rites of incorporation do not appear to be such a common practice among retiring workers in Britain (Crawford 1973). Since the rites of incorporation are an important part of a *rites de passage* in helping the individual to adjust to a new role, the absence of such rites during retirement might be greeted with some concern.

In the second sense in which we commonly use the term 'retirement' it represents a social status often identified as synonymous with old age. In the life career described earlier in this chapter we have constructed an ideal type which implies this synonymity. It is more appropriate, however, to talk about 'old age' and reserve the term 'retirement' to describe the process of transition between the status of worker and status of retired person. It is particularly inappropriate to use the term retirement to describe the status of elderly women if they have never been formally employed. Increasingly, however, elderly women are retired from employment within the labour market (Phillipson 1990).

Characteristics of contemporary social change

Not only do we face change throughout our individual life careers but we must also learn to recognise and adapt to structural changes in society. Before concluding this chapter with a discussion about social changes and the contemporary family we shall identify a number of common characteristics of change.

Social change influences all aspects of our lives. In contrast to earlier periods of history the 20th century has experienced dramatic social changes, and according to writers like Toffler

(1970) changes are becoming even more rapid. The rate at which changes occur influences our sense of time. Yet the strength of ancient Islamic traditions in the Middle East, the revival of African culture among American blacks and the continuing importance of the family in contemporary European societies might suggest that social change in the world at large has not been very rapid. Relative to other historical periods, however, there is little doubt that for most societies more rapid social change is now occurring, sometimes bringing strife as new and old values clash.

Social changes in contemporary Europe are generally piecemeal rather than revolutionary or utopian, with the exception of the political changes in Eastern Europe resulting from the dissolution of the Soviet empire, which have unleashed social forces not experienced since the revolution which created the Soviet empire and two World Wars. In Western Europe, institutions such as the family, the Church or Government, are constantly subject to minor changes but they are neither sudden nor violent. The changes which have taken place in the reorganisation of the National Health Service since it was established in 1948 show that while change is not revolutionary, the rate at which changes have been introduced has increased over time and when changes are regarded as occurring too frequently this can cause social unrest. Usually, in our society, changes are piecemeal, evolutionary, less dramatic and therefore less obvious. There is also inherent conservatism built into higher levels of decision-making (Paxman 1990).

In the past social change was usually unplanned. Nowadays, much social change is planned, as in, for example, the introduction of information technology into the health service. The wider introduction of silicon-chip technology has led to increased automation and information processing is changing dramatically. Technological innovations can have profound social consequences – higher residual unemployment, early retirement, shorter working weeks and longer holidays. The obsolescence of some procedures and forms of organisation in our worlds of work has been matched by new ways of working, with people increasingly working from their homes (Handy 1989). In addition, new forms of employment and leisure activities have been established.

The consequences of current social change to the individual can be severe. Families are uprooted; people change occupations and homes more frequently; new relationships have to be established. We all need to learn ways of adapting to our changing social environment or milieu. Social change affects every feature of modern life and every stage of the life career.

SOCIAL CHANGE AND THE FAMILY

In Chapter 2 we identified a number of sociological theories. Three of these, all in the structuralist tradition, are relevant to our discussion of social change and the family: structural functionalism, which provides a consensus perspective, and Marxism and feminism, both of which provide a conflict perspective. Each perspective has focused on the family as central to its theories about society and, not surprisingly, offers different interpretations of the relationship between social change and the family.

The study of the family presents a number of theoretical difficulties. As we have described in this chapter, the individual family is a constantly changing structure, moving from courtship to marriage, to procreation, to childrearing, to children leaving home, and then to dissolution and the birth of new families. A study of the same family cannot easily be made over its natural life cycle since the sociologist undertaking such a study might not survive that long! Sociologists attempt to overcome this difficulty by comparing different families at various stages of the life cycle, in other words, using a cross-sectional rather than a longitudinal approach. This method is not without its own problems, however. It is difficult to distinguish between differences in study families which are due to the various stages of their life-cycles from those which are due to more general changes in the structure of modern families over time; this is typical of problems which particularly haunt students of social change.

Most institutions, such as hospitals or schools, have clearly identifiable boundaries, formal structures and a set of clearly specified functions. Whereas hospitals are usually defined by a physical boundary, have explicit structures and exist for the cure and care of patients, the family is more difficult to define, has little formal structure and functions variously as a vehicle for procreation and as an agency of socialisation and social control. Indeed, different theoretical perspectives identify different structures and functions as being differentially important.

Structural functionalism

Parsons (1951, 1954, 1964) provides the fullest account of the functionalist perspective of the family. His analysis identifies two major functions of the conjugal family. First, families exist to facilitate the procreation of children and to socialise them into adult roles of the kind which are accepted and expected by the social group in which they live. For example, the Western family plays a major role in teaching adult gender roles. This is achieved in the way children are dressed, the games they are allowed to play, how they are spoken to and the different attitudes of parents toward their children's behaviour. Children are socialised into identifying with a gender role.

Second, the family acts to reinforce primary and secondary socialisation and is used to stabilise adult behaviour to adopt the stereotyped roles of husband and wife. Thus, in traditional conjugal families, men and women not only influence the way their children identify adult gender roles as described above but they also act as role models for their children. In industrial societies men often have as their primary duty earning money to support the family, and as a result their activities and interests are more often focused outside the home than are those of women, whose main occupations are domestic and therefore home-centred.

Thus the functionalist perspective views the relatively autonomous conjugal family, with its emphasis on free mate selection and relatively weak kinship ties, as the family structure most appropriate for modern industrial society. This kind of structure facilitates free mobility of labour, on the one hand, which is essential for economic growth and, on the other hand, a supportive relationship for men and women which acts as an emotional balance to the stresses and tensions of modern life (Parsons 1964).

Marxism

Marxist theory also stresses the importance of the relationship between the family and the functioning of the economy. The emphasis, however, is different. In Marxist theory the family is the institution within capitalist societies by which capitalism reproduces itself. In addition, as a unit of consumption, the family reinforces capitalism. The family provides workers to operate the system and also provides the mechanism for the socialisation and social control of both men and women. A similar view of gender roles is described for both functionalist and Marxist theories. The feminine role consists of one which supports the male worker by fulfilling various physical, sexual, social and emotional needs. The masculine role is one which disciplines individuals to sell their labour to the capitalist system. The influence of the Marxist perspective is evident in the feminist critique of the family.

Feminism

The feminist critique of the family identifies the inherent contradictions of the family. On the one hand, the family unit has been established to serve the function of procreation and to provide practical and emotional support to male workers. On the other hand, the family is a major source of emotional tension between men and women. Whereas the Marxist perspective blames the oppression and exploitation of women on the class system in capitalist societies, the feminist perspective identifies the importance of *patriarchy* in modern capitalist societies and therefore blames both the class system and the family (Segal 1983).

Weaknesses of functionalist and Marxist theory

There are three important differences between the theoretical approaches we have described above. First, whereas functionalism emphasises the needs of industrial society, Marxism emphasises the needs of capitalism and feminism stresses the power of men. Second, from a functionalist perspective the relationship between the family and the economy is one of reciprocity whereas from both the Marxist and feminist perspectives it is a relationship in which the economy is the dominant partner. Third, as we described in Chapter 2, the functionalist perspective postulates a relatively stable equilibrium within the social system, while the Marxist perspective postulates conflict between two antagonistic social classes which will lead to social change. The feminist perspective also sees change occurring through women's struggles to overcome oppression by men and has emancipation as a goal.

None of these theoretical traditions have been substantiated through the collection of empirical data. As we have shown above, although there exists no generally recognisable family unit other than the conjugal family in these theories, the variations in the basic structure are numerous. Neither perspective really explains, for example, the emergence of the dual-career family (Rapoport & Rapoport 1971) or the single-parent family (Hardey & Crow 1991). Nor do they explain the changes in the relationship between the family unit and other sectors of society, particularly the economy. For example, there has been little attempt to accommodate within the theories the increasing involvement of women, particularly women who have children, in the labour market.

Although we are unhappy with these theoretical contributions to the study of the family they are important to our understanding of modern society. In particular, they are important to our understanding of the family in a changing society and the debate over gender roles.

The family in a changing society

In our discussion of what constitutes a family we indicated substantial changes in the prevalence of different family structures. The traditional conjugal family still dominates, but the increase in divorce and remarriage, in single-parent families and in other family forms fuels the ideological debate about changing values of the family.

At the centre of this debate are three areas of family life which have been the subject of rapid social change since the Second World War, namely gender roles, family planning, and child-care practices and rights.

It is maintained by many commentators that within the family there has been a marked change in gender roles. Bott (1971) in her seminal study of gender roles noticed that in small conjugal families partners substituted for each other when either was ill or away from home. It is much easier to maintain gender differentiation in a larger family unit when someone of the same gender is usually available to perform duties of a member who is not present. Young and Willmott (1973) in their study of *The Symmetrical Family* report an increase in the substitution of partners' roles. More married women are working in paid employment and their husbands are sharing more domestic tasks. Young and Willmott note, however, that it is still the women who made household decisions and lived with the pressure of 'two jobs'. How many truly egalitarian families do you know? Even among examples of dual-career families there will be few in which traditional gender roles are fully shared (Brannen & Moss 1991). Observed changes in gender roles are another example of evolutionary social change, in this case toward a more egalitarian family structure.

The increasing availability of abortion and contraception means that women, who are more in control of their own fertility, are less likely to spend such a large proportion of their lives bearing and rearing children and are more likely, therefore, to seek employment outside the home.

As well as changes in the relationship between men and women, it is argued that there have been similar changes in relationships between adults and children; child care has become more 'permissive' so children can play some part, albeit a small one, in the decision-making processes of the family. Ideological debates about the permissiveness of current child-rearing practices have been encouraged by changes in the behaviour of adolescents. Yet there are no strong data to show actual levels of change in permissiveness.

Data from the Newsom's study of infant care (now 30 years old) suggest that changes have been subtle: from physical to emotional means of controlling children (Newsom & Newsom 1965). While there certainly has been a development of a prominent youth culture, this may be largely independent of child-rearing practices and due to, for example, changes in the economy, peer-group influences or even television.

The interpretation of these three examples of social change and their relationship to the family varies enormously between the two sides of the feminist ideological debate. Traditional feminist rhetoric focuses on egalitarian gender roles. They demand 'equal rights' for all in the public sphere. This ideal is based on the assertion that all differences in occupational positions are the result of discrimination, in other words, they are socially constructed by a male-dominated or patriarchal society. Much feminist rhetoric denies any innate differences between men and women, while a minority of feminists believe that, far from being equal to men, women are superior. We suspect, however, that a majority of women who would consider themselves to be feminists would adopt a 'differential-egalitarian position' (Berger & Berger 1983). That is, they would demand equality of opportunity but accept some innate differences between men and women, such as physical strength.

Traditional rhetoric has opposed these views, arguing strongly that a woman's role is first and foremost in the home 'servicing' husband and family. Ideologically, this approach is probably widely approved by both men and women but, in practice, the economic needs of families are an incentive for them to become more egalitarian.

Abortion and contraception are probably taken more for granted than is gender-role egalitarianism. Yet the issue of abortion galvanises far more passion than any other issue concerning the family – even than divorce. This is perhaps not surprising, given the gulf in ideals between the groups on either side of the divide. Feminists argue that it is the fundamental right of a woman to have control over her own body and her own life. Others defend the right of society to protect even its weakest members – in this instance, unborn children. The debate centres on the issue of whether the fetus is a person with rights. One side argues that the fetus is just a part of a woman's body and that she should therefore decide on its future, while the other side argues that the fetus is a separate being. The only definite statement we should wish to make is that the views adhered to in this particular debate will be socially constructed, with different cultures and subcultures taking up different positions.

The third area of family life which has also attracted bitter argument is that of child-rearing practices. We look at this issue in some detail in the next chapter when we consider the role of the family in the maintenance of health. For the present it is probably sufficient to say that the black-and-white dichotomy which summarises the position of the feminists and traditionalists is, as with our other two examples, too oversimplified. In between, there are various shades of grey representing a large number of viewpoints.

SUMMARY

This chapter has introduced a number of new concepts, each of which helps us to understand our ideal type of life career and the family. We have indicated the methodological difficulties in studying family, and highlighted the extent to which different groups in society take up ideological positions based on different definitions of the situation.

It is our assumption that human beings in all societies arrange themselves into families. Different societies, however, have constructed the family in different ways and, indeed, in modern Britain individuals modify and interpret their own families in the light of their own experiences, expectations and perceptions. Therefore for us the meaningful question is not *whether* the family will survive but, rather, *what kinds* of family will occur in the future. We do not think that the rhetoric of either the feminists or the traditionalists can provide an answer to this question. Consideration of their debates should, however, encourage you to think carefully and question your own fundamental and taken-for-granted ideas about *family*.

In this chapter we described the interrelationship between the family and the life career. We saw that for all of us our experience of family life will change as we move through life from childhood, through adolescence, young adulthood, child rearing, middle-age and old age. Of course, as we proceed along our life career we will also have different experiences of health and ill health. The chapter was also concerned with showing the effects of social change on the structure of the family and identifying the various competing explanations of the function of the family.

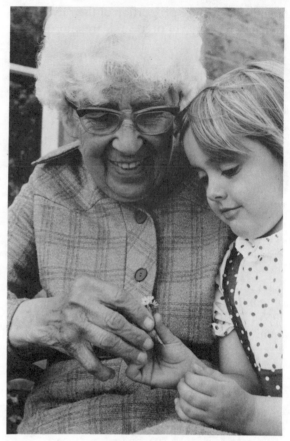

Fig. 5.7 Two ends of the life career (courtesy of Rik Walton).

FURTHER READING

Rapoport R N, Fogerty M P, Rapoport R 1982 Families in Britain. Routledge & Kegan Paul, London

Worsley P (ed) 1987 The new introducing sociology. Penguin, Harmondsworth, Ch 4, pp 125–165

6

Health and the family

Arguably, the family provides the most important social context within which health is maintained and illness occurs and is resolved. The manner in which individuals react to illness, and the nature of the family's response to it, may influence the course of the illness and the health and happiness of the family as well. The effects that illness has on family life will depend on the characteristics of particular families, including factors such as the allocation of roles, the extent of emotional support available, and financial stability or vulnerability. A long-term illness of the mother in a single-parent family is likely to have different effects on the family than would the same illness on a nonemployed mother in a traditional conjugal family. These considerations led Litman (1974) to argue that the family serves as the primary unit in health and medical care.

The interrelation between the family and health is a highly dynamic one which has a number of facets. In this chapter we shall explore this relationship in three ways:

1. The family in the maintenance of health.
2. The family at times of illness.
3. The role of the family in community care.

We will also discuss competing explanations for family roles. But before we do this we need to think about the question, 'What is health?'

WHAT IS HEALTH?

In Chapter 1 we reviewed the distinction often made in social and behavioural research between the medical and social model of health. This distinction underpins the dichotomy between a biomedical or 'scientific' model of health and a model which includes personal and social factors. The biomedical model is one where medical knowledge is grounded in universal and generalisable science. Medical knowledge constitutes a particular *scientific paradigm*, a shared agreement among scientists often based on taken-for-granted and unexamined assumptions about social life. We examine this concept in more detail in Chapter 12. The biomedical model has highlighted the concept of disease which is defined as deviations of measurable biological variables from the norm, or the presence of defined and categorised forms of pathology. In contrast, the social model of health is grounded in lay concepts of health.

Lay concepts of health

In industrialised societies lay concepts of health are likely to include biomedical explanations of health since people have been taught to think, at least in part, in biomedical terms. Yet although 'educated' lay people may accept and take for granted biological knowledge like the germ theories of disease, it is clear from a number of studies that lay explanations of health are often complex, subtle and sophisticated and based on other data.

One approach to the study of lay perceptions of health uses the Durkheimian notion of *social representation* (Durkheim 1964a). An important influence on this approach has been the work of Claudine Herzlich who for some 20 years has carried out lengthy interviews with French people in order to explore the ways in which people make sense of ideas like 'health' and 'illness'. In her first study, Herzlich (1973) interviewed middle-class Parisians and a few rural respondents from Normandy. Herzlich concluded that different understandings and explanations for health and illness are not polar opposites to each other but are quite discrete conceptions. Respondents distinguished between illness which was produced by ways of life and the positive concept of health which came from within. Health was identified as having three dimensions: 'health in a vacuum', 'reserve of health' and 'equilibrium'.

Health in a vacuum was the term Herzlich used to describe the idea of health being the simple absence of disease, a lack of awareness of the body or not being concerned about the state of the body.

Reserve of health represents health as an asset or investment rather than a state. She highlighted two aspects: physical robustness or strength which enables one to work and play, and resistance to illness which enables one to defend oneself against disease or recover from illness.

Equilibrium was used by Herzlich to highlight the notion of positive well-being described by her respondents to include notions of internal harmony and balance.

The descriptions of illness provided by Herzlich's respondents were less clear. They were able to distinguish between four classes of illness: serious illness which may be fatal; chronic conditions; trivial illnesses and childhood ailments. From her data Herzlich provides three metaphors for illness which clearly distinguish between three social representations: illness as 'destroyer', illness as 'liberator' and illness as 'occupation'.

Illness as destroyer was an image held by people who were particularly engaged or active in life and for whom illness interfered with their lives by limiting their ability to continue with their daily activities and responsibilities.

Illness as liberator reflects the ability of individuals to be freed from the responsibilities of life and to receive the privileges of sympathy and care from others.

Illness as occupation describes the reaction of individuals who respond to illness as a challenge to overcome. In responding to the challenge of illness all other activities and responsibilities are relegated while the individual concentrates on recovery.

Herzlich has continued her exploration of the meaning of health by studying illnesses and ill people from ancient times until the present day. Herzlich and Pierret (1987) conclude that people's experiences and conceptions can only be properly understood in relation to the cultural context of their lives. Lay perceptions of health go well beyond biomedical explanations of health.

In the United Kingdom a number of studies have been influenced by these analyses or independently have found rather similar distinctions. A study of 41 working-class mothers of young children in South Wales (Pill & Stott 1982) found that about half the sample held fatalistic views about illness and causation and did not accept they were morally responsible for their own health outcomes. The remainder were prepared to recognise that individual behaviour had *some* part to play in illness causation. This broad dichotomy of health beliefs reflected the level of education of respondents. Those whose education had extended beyond the minimum school leaving age were likely to conform to the biomedical explanation of illness and accept the current official view that individuals should take responsibility for their own health.

In a study of 24 people from a working-class community in East London, Cornwell (1984) concluded that respondents provided two contrasting accounts of health – the public and the private. In early interviews with respondents, before Cornwell had become accepted and trusted by those being interviewed, they provided public accounts of health and illness based on lay interpretations of expert opinion. At later interviews private accounts were offered, based on personal experiences and the feelings and thoughts which accompany them. For most respondents the idea of personal responsibility for health was unacceptable, and respondents vociferously denied that they could control their lifestyles. Ill health was more often blamed on others, such as people with colds and other infections not staying away from public places.

Table 6.1 Lay definitions of health

Definition	Sample response
Health:	
as not ill	Someone I know who is very healthy is me, because I haven't been to a doctor yet.
despite disease	I am very healthy despite this arthritis.
as a reserve	Both parents are still alive at 90 so he belongs to healthy stock.
as 'the healthy life'	I call her healthy because she goes jogging and doesn't eat fried food.
as physical fitness	There's tone to my body, I feel fit.
as energy or vitality	Health is when I feel I can do anything.
as social relationships	You feel as though everyone is your friend, I enjoy life more, and can work, and help other people.
as function	She's 81 and she gets her work done quicker than me, and she does the garden.
as psychosocial well-being	Well I think health is when you feel happy.

Source: Blaxter M 1990 Health and lifestyles. Tavistock/Routledge, London, Ch. 2.

Blaxter and Paterson (1982) and Williams (1983) in their separate studies of people in Aberdeen showed that health can be defined in very similar ways to Herzlich's respondents. Health was perceived negatively, as the absence of illness; functionally, as the ability to cope with everyday activities; or positively, as fitness or well-being. Since, within the modern world, health continues to have a moral dimension, ill health and moral wrongdoing are interconnected. Nowhere is this more evident than in HIV infection. Health can therefore be seen in terms of willpower, self-discipline and self-control (Blaxter 1983).

A common problem of all these studies is that they are culturally specific and based on small samples so it is difficult to estimate how generalisable they are to the wider population. Blaxter (1990) has observed that there are several areas of agreement, however, which has led to four concepts of health being commonly identified: freedom from illness, ability to function, fitness and the idea of health as a reserve. In a study of *Health and Lifestyles* Blaxter was able to ask a cross-section of some 3000 people from different parts of the United Kingdom for their ideas about health. A content analysis of their open-ended responses generated nine different lay definitions of health (Table 6.1).

Most respondents offered multiple concepts of health. The kinds of definitions reported, however, varied by gender and life-cycle position. Thus younger men tended to describe health in terms of fitness, whereas younger women identified energy, vitality, and being able to cope. In middle age people's responses became more complex, with greater emphasis on overall physical and psychological well-being. In later life the focus was on function, particularly among elderly men, although ideas about contentment and happiness were common place.

Stainton Rogers (1991) in her book *Explaining Health and Illness*, drawing on the theoretical perspectives of anthropology and psychology as well as sociology, has attempted to synthesize many of these ideas about health. From her own studies of health she has presented a number of accounts of the meaning of health using the notion of social presentation. These eight accounts are summarised as follows:

1. 'Body as machine' – operating within the modernist world view of science, within which illness is regarded as naturally occurring and 'real'. Modern biomedicine is seen as the only valid source of effective treatment for any kind of serious illness.
2. 'Body under siege' – in which the individual is regarded as under threat and attack from germs and diseases, interpersonal conflicts and the 'stress' of modern life acting upon the body through the agency of 'mind'.
3. 'Inequality of access' – convinced of the benefits of modern medicine, but concerned about the unfair allocation of those benefits and their lack of availability to those who need them most.
4. 'Cultural critique' of medicine – based upon a 'dominance' sociological worldview of exploitation and oppression and a postmodernist analysis of knowledge as socially constituted and ideologically mediated.
5. 'Health promotion' – which recognises both collective and personal responsibility for ill health, but stresses the wisdom of adopting a 'healthy lifestyle' for good health to be achieved and maintained and illness to be prevented.
6. 'Robust individualism' – which is more concerned with the individual's right to a 'satisfying life' and their freedom to choose how to live their lives, than with the aetiology of illness.
7. 'God's power' – within which health is a product of 'right living', spiritual well-being and God's care, and recovery from illness a matter of regaining spiritual wholeness, attained by intercession to some form of Deity or spiritual power.
8. 'Willpower' – puts the individual preeminently in control, and stresses the moral responsibility of individuals to use their 'will' to maintain good health.
   (Stainton Rogers 1991, pp. 208–209)

THE FAMILY AND THE MAINTENANCE OF HEALTH

Given the increasing interest in the meaning of health to individuals, empirical studies of the role of the family in the maintenance of health have been relatively few. A World Health Organization report observed:

In spite of its central position in society, the family has been infrequently studied from the public health point of view. The complex interrelationships between health and the family virtually constitute *terra incognita*. In the form presented or available, statistics too often tell very little about the family setting although this is undoubtedly a major factor, in, for example, the rearing of children and the development and stabilisation of adult personality. Many of the strains and maladjustments which place an increasing burden on paediatric, general medical and psychiatric services can be understood and efficiently tackled only after due attention has been given to the family setting. The fact that the family is a unit of illness because it is a unit of 'living' has been grossly neglected in the development of statistical tools suitable for coping with this set of problems, and in the provision of statistical data essential for an investigation of the individual as part of the family in illness as well as health. (WHO 1971, p. 2)

Those studies which have looked at the role of the family in maintaining health have tended to focus on the family as a social *cause* of illness. The negative effects of family life on physical and emotional health are increasingly well documented (Haavio-Mannila 1986). In contrast, there are few studies examining the positive effects of family on health and well-being although recent research is now addressing this issue (Backett 1990). In Chapter 4 we identified a number of social causes of illness. Here we deal only with the relationship between family structure and health and illness and, in particular, we focus on the role of the family in the aetiology of psychiatric illness, on parental and maternal deprivation, on family breakdown and intergenerational influences on health and illness behaviours. Finally, we will examine the role of the family in maintaining health and identify the challenges facing sociologists trying to study this aspect of family life.

Psychiatric illness and the family

In Chapter 8 we develop the concept of *labelling* which refers to a social process by which individuals or groups classify the social behaviour of other individuals. Labels are social constructions which change through time. For example, in 1980 the American Psychiatric Association decided that homosexuality was no longer a psychiatric illness. Patients are no longer admitted to hospitals for people with learning difficulties as 'morally defective'.

The psychiatrist Laing in studying schizophrenia used a labelling perspective. He argued that schizophrenia is not so much an illness as a label given to people who react to family life in a specific way (Laing 1965). Such a view is not in accord with the majority of psychiatrists who seek organic causes for schizophrenia. Nevertheless, Laing (1967) argues that case studies of families of people regarded as schizophrenic show that the apparent irrationality of the individual is quite rational when interpreted in the context of the schizophrenic's family. By living in particular families we all absorb our own family's system of role-relationships. In other words, 'to be in the same family means having the same family inside oneself' (Laing 1967, p. 119). To establish individual autonomy in certain family situations, Laing argues, individuals will reject their family role systems and exhibit what conventional psychiatrists interpret as 'schizophrenic behaviour'.

Through Laing's case study of Jane we can get some idea of how this happens. Jane experienced a change in her personality from an active, friendly, involved 17-year-old, to an inactive, self-absorbed and silent figure. During psychotherapy she described herself as a tennis ball being passed to and fro in a game of mixed doubles. This fantasy, Laing argues, is derived from her role relationships in her family in which she acted as the message carrier between different family members: father, mother, mother's father and father's mother. For weeks at a time all communication would pass through Jane. 'Mother would turn to Jane and say, "Tell your father to pass the salt", Jane would say to her father, "Mother wants you to pass the salt" and so on' (Laing 1967, p. 122). The purpose of psychotherapy would be to establish for Jane the connection between her game of 'mixed doubles' inside her head and the world of her family outside. The aim would be to get Jane to understand that her response was an essentially *rational* reaction to her family situation.

While Laing's analysis of his case studies challenge the assumptions of mainstream psychiatry, we must be careful not to reject radical reinterpretations out of hand. To reject novel ideas could be like our forbears continuing to accept the notion that the earth is flat. However, as with Freudian psychology, we have only a series of case studies to support Laing's theories and, as always, the case studies may be open to other interpretations. For example, it could be that Jane's behaviour was in some sense causing the 'tennis-ball' effect on other family members. Also thinking of all the families we know with adolescent members, including our own, we are surprised that there is not a greater prevalence of schizophrenia! In other words, our sociological concern is not so much one of why Jane was labelled schizophrenic but why so many other Janes are not.

Brown et al (1972) were also concerned with the part the family plays in schizophrenia, not in its aetiology, but in the course of the illness. They studied a group of patients already diagnosed with different forms of schizophrenia and their families. The hypothesis being tested was that families in which there was a high degree of *expressed emotion* were likely to cause a florid relapse of symptoms independently of other variables, such as length of history of the illness, severity of previous behaviour disturbance or type of symptoms. The concept of expressed emotion among relatives was constructed from a number of measures, including critical comments about others at home, expressed hostility towards other family members, expressions of dissatisfaction about several areas of family life and emotional overinvolvement of parents with

the patient. It is a measure with mainly negative connotations.

Brown and his colleagues examined the course of the illness over 2 years, and observed particularly whether patients relapsed. Relapse was related to major family and other variables, shown diagrammatically at Figure 6.1. A high degree of emotion expressed by relatives at the time of a key hospital admission was found to be strongly associated with subsequent symptomatic relapse in the 9 months following discharge from hospital. Previous work impairment and behavioural disturbance were also associated with relapse. This was because of their high association with the level of expressed emotion. No other factor was able to predict symptomatic relapse. Two factors, however, could mitigate the effects of high expressed emotion by family members. One was regular phenothiazine medication for the patient, and the other was reducing the amount of contact between the patient and a highly emotional relative. Social withdrawal from the family could, therefore, be a protective mechanism for some patients.

Expressed emotion within families is one factor which influences relapse. So too does previous history and type of schizophrenic condition. However, expressed emotion is strongly associated with patients' behaviour and work record and the direction of cause and effect is inter-

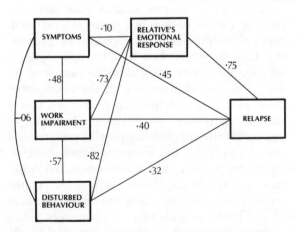

Fig. 6.1 Relationship of main variables to each other and to relapse (Brown et al 1972).

preted by Brown and his colleagues as mutually dependent, i.e.

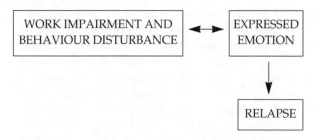

They relate the deleterious effects of living in a family with high expressed emotion to patients experiencing high levels of arousal over long periods. When a critical life event occurs (see our discussion of life events in Chapter 4) and patients are already in a state of high arousal, then they are particularly likely to suffer relapse. While elements of the environment other than family life are likely to influence arousal, they have not yet been systematically studied. However, the interaction between biological and social factors in the course of illness in this context adds to our developing stock of knowledge about the complex nature of illness and its management. A major recommendation of Brown and his colleagues' study is that 'The optimum social environment would be structured with clear-cut roles, only as much complexity as any individual can cope with and with neutral but active supervision to keep up standards of appearance, work, and behaviour' (Brown et al 1972, p. 256). The implications of this are evident for current policies to provide mental health care out of hospitals and for the traditional view of 'asylum'.

Parental and maternal deprivation

Other social abnormalities have also been attributed to aspects of family functioning. Many of these hypotheses focus on *parental deprivation* and, in particular, on *maternal deprivation*. A wide range of social abnormalities have been attributed to parental deprivation, including developmental retardation, affectionless psychopathy, delinquency, growth failure, and depres-

sion in adults (Rutter 1972). Many of these hypotheses make certain assumptions about parenting.

First, the family provides stable bonds or relationships which may serve as the basis for the child's growing circle of relationships outside the family (Bowlby 1971). Second, as we described in Chapter 5, the family is a primary agent of socialisation, so that parents will provide children with a set of values and attitudes which they may accept or reject. Third, the family will provide the necessary life experiences which children require for 'normal' development. Finally, the family provides a secure background to act as a base from which children can explore their world (Rutter & Madge 1976).

Such expectations of the family have what Rapoport et al (1977) have called a *biological emphasis* suggesting that parental behaviour is biologically rather than socially rooted. This view implies that it is mothers who are the primary nurturing parent; fathers are peripheral and, while they are expected to protect and provide for the mother and child, substitutes are more acceptable for them than for mothers. The domestic division of labour that reflects the above is regarded as the most natural and appropriate one (Rapoport et al 1977). The reader will note a number of similarities between this view of parenting and the functionalist theories of the family described in the previous chapter.

Functionalist theories also form the basis for the *systems emphasis* on parenting. Parenting behaviour mirrors social structure and adapts responsively to social values. Thus the functionalist view of the family emphasises the gender-linked division of labour which fits the environment and is functional both for individual family members and for wider society. From a functionalist perspective it is logical to attribute the wide range of social abnormalities to changes in family structure and parenting behaviour. The conjugal family with stereotyped gender roles would satisfy the requirements of modern industrial society: labour mobility, stability of income and reliability of personal relationships. This view of parenting and the family has come under increasing attack both ideologically and theoretically. In addition, Rapoport et al (1977) have shown that many of the theoretical assumptions do not stand up to empirical investigation.

Another way of considering parenting is to use a *cultural emphasis*. The family is considered to be the universal social institution for reproduction and socialisation of infants, but its structure and norms for parenting vary according to the cultural context. Thus the experience of the Israeli *kibbutzim* suggests that maternal deprivation as such does not exist in all societies (Oakley 1976). Indeed, it is probable that maternal deprivation as strictly defined does not truly exist in contemporary British society. If it did, with the increasing proportion of mothers working, we would expect a corresponding increase in maternal deprivation and its consequences. It is now apparent from a number of studies 'that working mothers have children with no more problems than the children of women who remain at home' (Rutter & Madge 1976, p. 213). In addition, as Oakley (1976) has pointed out, the empirical evidence of the concept was based on the juxtaposition of maternal child care, which was regarded as inevitably good, with institutional child care, which was interpreted as bad. Of course, this is too simple an analysis.

The evidence that parental deprivation makes an individual extremely vulnerable has been examined by Chen and Cobb (1960). They found that tuberculosis patients, accident victims and parasuicides reported being parentally deprived. A common factor linking the backgrounds of these vulnerable groups was found to be social isolation. However, Chen and Cobb advise caution in the interpretation of these data since they only suggest that certain individuals are at risk; we cannot conclude that parental deprivation is a *cause* of these illness events.

Intergenerational influences and health

In Chapter 3 we looked at inequalities in health which persist between different social groups in society. One explanation for the persistence of such inequalities, which has gained accep-

tance among health professionals because of its common-sense usefulness, is what Lewis (1964) termed the *culture of poverty*. Lewis argues that in anthropological usage the term 'culture' implies a design for living which is passed down from generation to generation. (This is a slightly different meaning of the concept which we described in Chapter 5.) 'In short, it is a way of life, remarkably stable and persistent, passed down from generation to generation along family lines' (Lewis 1964, p. xxiv). Both Rutter and Madge (1976) and Townsend (1979) have criticised the culture of poverty thesis, but does it have any credibility in regard to the transmission of health attitudes between generations?

Blaxter and Paterson (1982) set out to examine the hypothesis that an individual's health experience might, in poor socioeconomic circumstances, create attitudes of apathy toward health care and conflict with health professionals. These attitudes might be transmitted through generations among female members of the family. From an older generation of women (the grandmothers) information was obtained about their past and present perceptions of the structure and functions of health services. These are compared with the attitudes of the daughters (the mothers) to see to what extent values and beliefs are transmitted or recur throughout generations.

Of major importance are the behavioural consequences of attitudes, since it is behavioural variables which will influence the health of the next generation of children. The health care behaviour of the mothers was therefore documented over a 6-month period by obtaining regular reports from them of illness among their children and their response to such episodes. The focus was on women because there is some agreement about the central role of the mother in coping with illness in the family (Locker 1981), about her role in the transmission of attitudes (Pratt 1973), and about the continuing importance of the mother-daughter relationship (Young & Willmott 1957, Litman 1974).

In this study the effect of social change was minimised by excluding upwardly mobile families. The study was therefore confined to 58 three-generation families from the Registrar General's Social Classes IV and V living in one Scottish city. The interview data obtained from grandmothers and mothers was supplemented by data on health behaviour of the grandmother group from an extension study carried out when they were having their first babies in 1950–1953 and followed up 5 and 10 years later.

Analysis was carried out to determine the mothers' and grandmothers' perceptions of health, illness and disease. Detailed analysis of all reported illness episodes among children and of the use of health services was completed. Mothers' perceptions of, and behaviour toward, symptoms of acute illness among their children, was documented. Data were also collected about chronic and handicapping conditions, accidents, dental care, immunization, fertility control, infant feeding and child nutrition and the pattern of lay remedies and lay referral.

Grandmothers' and mothers' attitudes toward available health services were examined. Of course, the relationship between attitudes and behaviour is complex and other influences on the use of health services, like economic constraints, transport, location of services and other practical contingencies, as we discussed in Chapter 3, were included in the study. While the emphasis was on the womens' attitudes, it is important to remember that how professionals respond to patients and clients is influential in shaping these attitudes.

To what extent is the conventional wisdom – 'like mother, like daughter' – upheld? There was some evidence that lay remedies and methods of child care in illness were passed on. However, it appears that only in the area of the early introduction of solid foods to young babies were the grandmothers particularly influential. When comparisons were made between grandmothers' and mothers' accounts of advice given, they were very consistent. Only two out of 47 comparisons showed contradictory accounts. Most respondents agreed that, although there was often discussion between grandmothers and mothers, the mothers usually went their own way. The advice grandmothers most often gave

was to go to the doctor. Grandmothers helped in emotional and practical ways but demonstrated little overt influence on health care or child-rearing practices.

Both grandmothers and mothers were characterised by early child rearing and high rates of youthful, illegitimate and prenuptial pregnancies. The grandmothers, however, were likely to have large and unplanned families while mothers had no intention of following this example. The norms of behaviour in relation to family size and to other aspects of child health have so changed that intergenerational comparisons mean little. This is certainly so in such areas as contraception and infant feeding.

Thus, in a community characterised by close family networks, no consistent relationships were found between the attitudes of grandmothers and mothers. More important than direct family transmission were intergenerational changes bound up with changes in lifestyle and circumstances, service provision and more widespread changes in public attitude – that is, wider social change.

The examples of 'health-deprived' children were often in part associated with the mother's behaviour. Of more major importance, however, were aspects of a disadvantaged environment and organisation of services. It was in circumstances where the environment had changed least and the young mothers were in the most disadvantaged positions that their attitudes resembled those of their mothers. Both generations exhibited a disorganised and apathetic approach to preventive care.

Thus intergenerational continuity is present only in some ways and under some circumstances. The study has been reported in some detail to demonstrate the complexity of family studies and the need for sophisticated methods of data collection and analysis. These complexities indicate some reasons why only a few such studies exist.

Positive health and the family

These three examples – mental health, parental deprivation and intergenerational influences on health – illustrate the predominant approach to understanding the family and the maintenance of health from a negative perspective. The dominance of the biomedical model and hence an emphasis on ill health is evident. There has been a paucity of studies concerned with positive aspects of health and Backett (1990) highlights another reason for this paucity. Studies of health in families involve two aspects of social life with which we all have personal experience and which therefore we take for granted. Prior to radical critiques of health and society, most studies were grounded in consensus theories and tended to be superficial in their provision of 'public accounts' of health in families. Family life related to health was not considered as problematic or worthy of serious academic study.

How might we study the role of the family in the maintenance of health in order to avoid such pitfalls? Since quantitative studies are likely to reflect public accounts of health maintenance and the role of the family, small-scale qualitative studies are advocated. An important feature of such studies would be the study of families as social groups and not as individuals within families. This would enable gender and generational differences in the meanings given to health and illness to emerge. Those advocating qualitative methodologies highlight the advantages of researchers becoming closer to their respondents than would data-collectors for quantitative studies of illness. Only by researchers becoming accepted by the families being studied will there be any likelihood of gaining access to private accounts of health and health behaviour.

Qualitative studies also are able to approach the everyday nature of health from the respondents' perspectives. They move beyond the taken-for-granted interpretations of health and health behaviour to uncover the variety of meanings given to health and illness. The influence of family life on positive health behaviours is difficult to unravel. Health behaviours, like much of family life, are open to conflicting demands, compromises and negotiations. They include taken-for-granted aspects of every day life such as eating, sleeping, sex, physical exercise, emotional support and hygiene. Whereas there might exist some agreement within individual family groups about what influences positive health it is not necessarily matched by a shared commitment to change individual behaviour. This is readily observed in relation to dietary preferences and the complexity of feeding a family.

THE FAMILY'S RESPONSE TO ILLNESS

Few studies of the family's response to illness have highlighted the different ways in which men and women or adults and children react. Indeed, many of the early studies focused on the family as a unit. One classic study is Davis' study of 14 child victims of spinal paralytic poliomyelitis (Davis 1963). Even though polio has now ceased to be a prevalent illness in European countries, this study provides major insights into the way that families identify and react to a life-threatening illness and subsequent chronic disability.

Following the initial appearance of symptoms the 14 families exhibited a common pattern in the process of identification, interpretation and reaction. Davis identifies four stages in this process: *prelude, warning, impact* and *inventory*. In the prelude stage, the family will perceive the symptoms as an ordinary childhood illness. Unusual symptoms will be ignored when they do not fit into a common-sense explanation, such as the diagnosis of colds or 'flu. The warning stage usually commences with some dramatic change in symptoms or the behaviour of the child. For example, the cue to something more serious was read by one father at the sight of his 3-year-old winning a fight with his 6-year-old son. The differential perception of such cues affects the timing of consultations with the medical profession. During the impact stage many families had difficulty in accepting a diagnosis of polio. This may have been affected by the doctor's reluctance to provide a definite diagnosis, encouraged by a desire not to be seen to make a mistake, combined with a protective attitude toward the family. The impact stage is characterised by extreme reactions of fear, grief and loss. The inventory stage emerges once the acute condition has abated. It is a period of taking stock and reappraising the situation in readiness for the long-term effects of the disease.

A diagnosis of leukaemia or of genetic disorders like cystic fibrosis, in common with disorders like polio, will have both immediate and long-term consequences for the families of affected children. One approach to understanding the implications of having such a severe illness has been to consider their diagnosis as a particular form of stressful event or crisis (Kaplan et al 1973). Vincent (1967) states that the family is uniquely organised to carry out its stress-mediating responsibility and is in a strategic position to do so. Given our early discussion of the variety of forms that family units now take (see Ch. 5), it is noteworthy that Venters (1981) found that single-parent families of cystic fibrosis children functioned less well through the course of the illness than did 'intact families'.

Recent feminist writings on women's health have highlighted gender differences in the way that men and women respond to illness. Miles (1991) suggests a number of reasons why women may respond to illness in a different way to men. First women's experiences of pregnancy and childbirth, and menstruation and menopause, cause them to think about their bodies and their bodily sensations routinely whereas men do not. Second, primary and secondary socialisation of gender roles encourages men to think about health in masculine ways and women to think about it in feminine ways. Third, structural differences in the lives of men and women, which lead to expectations that it is the women who will take responsibility for the caring and supporting roles in families, forces women to think about health and illness differently. Finally, as we saw in Chapter 3, their experience of illness is different from that of men and this will inevitably influence the way they perceive health and illness.

Responding to chronic illness

In responding to acute illness the family is able to cope in the knowledge that the effects of illness on the family should be short lived and that a return to normality is guaranteed. Life can be very different in the event of chronic illness or disability in the family. Unlike acute illness, chronic illness or disability has to be reckoned with in terms of months and years, not weeks. Miles (1991) highlights the differential response of men and women to chronic illness within the family. Women, who in their life time are likely to experience more long-term illness than men, are expected to respond more stoically than men. Within families they are perceived to 'hold' the family together and they therefore cannot afford to be ill. Thus, women who suffer from debilitating conditions, such as a psychiatric illness or arthritis and chronic pain, are under more pressure than men in similar circumstances not to make demands on the family. Both Miles (1988) in her study of psychiatric illness among women and Robinson (1988) in his study of the management of multiple sclerosis report examples of other family members exhorting female sufferers to 'keep going'.

The effect of chronic illness on other family members can be considerable irrespective of gender or the social position of the sufferer. Venters (1981) reviews a range of consequences in families where a child has cystic fibrosis, including financial strain, increased communication difficulties between husband and wife as well as other family members, accentuation of preexisting marital problems, increased social isolation of the family unit and disorganisation of family routines resulting in role disorganisation. Such negatives only occur in certain families, as it appears that some are more vulnerable than others. Harrisson, in her study of the long-term medical treatment of children and associated parental stress, provides a number of useful case studies which highlight these kinds of outcomes (Harrisson 1977).

Another outcome, which was reported by Litman (1974), is that mediation of the stress of illness or coping can have very different effects. One type of family unit is brought closer together in a corporate attempt to deal with problems, while for others family relationships are made far more difficult than before the onset of the illness.

The impact of chronic illness in terms of psychiatric morbidity among family members has also been documented by a number of writers about a variety of chronic disorders. For example, Allan et al (1974) explored the psychological impact on the individual family members to cystic fibrosis, Sainsbury and Grad (1970) studied the effects of psychiatric illness on the family and a number of recent studies have examined the impact of dementia on family members (Levin et al 1989).

Venters (1981) links better quality of family functioning, as assessed by a composite measure, with two coping strategies. One is endowing the illness with meaning. Rather than living with uncertainty, some families find it positively helpful to interpret the illness and its causation according to a preexisting religious, medical or scientific philosophy and to go on to define the hardships caused by the disease with optimistic explanations. The second coping device was sharing the burden of the illness within and beyond the immediate family so that an equilibrium between family loyalty and social participation provided social support.

Venters considered family adjustment to cystic fibrosis as a process which provided for more positive functioning after the first year, once families had progressed beyond initial confusion and depression. The earlier findings, which typifies familial response as social isolation and a reduction in positive communication between family members, could have been distorted by considering only the early phase of adjustment, before longer-term reorganisation and recovery of family functioning had been established.

Comaroff and Maguire (1981) regard the process of establishing meaning in the case of leukaemia as rather more problematic in the sense of emphasising the greater uncertainties of

this illness. Like cystic fibrosis, leukaemia was once inevitably fatal. Advances in treatment now mean that its most striking feature is the unpredictability of its course and outcome. Thus families are preoccupied by the hope of long-term and perhaps complete remission.

Early in the course of the illness parents react by feeling singled out by an affliction of the type that usually seems 'only to happen to others'. The families of polio patients reacted in the same way (Davis 1963). At this time, too, the uncertain duration and consequences are handled by attempting to construct some norms against which to measure their present state and future prospects. This is achieved by some parents collating all available information in an attempt to postulate timetables and probabilities but, while so doing, maintaining an optimistic definition of their own case for as long as possible. Selective information-seeking and avoidance persists for as long as the illness, its nature changing as the course of the illness progresses. Oscillation between contradictory responses – repugnance, guilt, optimism, pessimism – are a regular feature. Comaroff's and Maguire's (1981) analysis is grounded in the need for parents to complete their inadequate clinical knowledge by transcending the boundaries between what is formally 'known' and 'unknown' about leukaemia.

As well as the more clinical definition of the illness, the moral implications, the explanations of why it happened, were also a recurrent feature of 'meaning'. This was clearly tied to attempts to allocate responsibility for its occurrence. Seeking explanations for cause typically progressed from biological or medical to more ultimate questions of 'Why us?', 'Why now?'. Such questions appear typical of all chronic illnesses. Parents of polio victims were asking the same kinds of questions (Davis 1963). In so doing parents reviewed their own biographies of potential events or factors which might have caused the illness, even to invoking metaphysical explanations: 'It's a punishment for something we've done'. Comaroff and Maguire (1981) suggest that this seeking for meaning is not resolved, unlike Venters who found resolution in the majority of the families. In part, this might be attributable to the different clinical course of leukaemia and cystic fibrosis as understood by the parents, as well as to the stubbornly unknown features of the former to medical science. The aetiology of leukaemia remains a mystery, while treatment efforts are progressing; prognosis is crucially uncertain and there is an ever-present threat of fatal relapse. The uncertainty of prognosis has social implications. It affects social encounters between the family and others who are likely to respond with embarrassment or emotion. Their behaviour can be interpreted by the family as being patronising or sympathetic while they may respond as if the illness was contagious. More crucial are the relationships within the family. While parents may try to conduct as 'normal' a mode of existence as possible, the meaning of the whole domestic context is radically altered. This entails not only the child's perceptions of illness and treatment, but also the parents' relationships with them, which stem from an uncertain future. Situations and cultural constraints often entail efforts to stifle overt acknowledgement of the illness, while at the same time it is responsible for radically altering the meaning of their lives and the future. While most families resist collapse, the disruption of family relations raises searching questions about the meaning of survival.

The implications of severe childhood illness, especially where uncertainty is high, highlight for professional policy the differences between clinical and family values and meanings. The families in these studies of children with different chronic diseases doubted the value of clinical investigations, as well as interpreting their children's state of health and well-being differently from the assessments offered by professionals. Sociological investigations try to encompass the processes by which families respond to having an ill child or the outcomes for families in terms of the quality of family functioning or psychiatric morbidity. What these studies emphasise are the social implications of developments in modern treatment, which often have the effect of exaggerating rather than reducing remaining uncertainties for the families involved. This applies across illness conditions, as well as to features of modern health care like the increased possibilities for survival among babies whose birth weight is very low (McHaffie 1990). The effects of reduced income among families with children who have a chronic illness should not be forgotten.

The effects of chronic illness among adults can be equally devastating, particularly to female members. Robinson (1988) found that women were expected to cope more successfully than men in caring for a spouse with multiple sclerosis. This expectation that women will cope is independent of perceived functional difficulties or whether it is their spouse or themselves who have the disease. In general, Robinson found that women's perceptions of their problems and how to deal with them are more pessimistic than the perceptions of men. There were also gender differences in how marital relationships were perceived. Stress on family relationships, coupled with financial strain, increased the social isolation of family members. The disorganisation of existing family roles and routines is likely for all families caring for a family member with a chronic illness, as well as when life-threatening conditions, such as myocardial infarction, are diagnosed (McEwen & Finlayson 1977, Schott & Badura 1988).

A number of chronic conditions dramatically affect later life, particularly stroke and dementia. One writer, describing his own dysphasia, termed stroke 'a family illness' (Buck 1963). Forster's (1989) powerful novel about a family coping with a grandmother with dementia sums up better than many research studies the nature of dementia as a family illness. Of course, there are also benefits to caring for family members with chronic illnesses which the dominant medical perspective of 'illness as a burden' does not take into account.

Brocklehurst et al (1981) and Anderson (1988, 1992) describe some of the long-term effects of stroke. The psychosocial outcomes of stroke have been well documented (Anderson 1988,

1992, House 1987) and include physical and mental disability, such as immobility and depression, loss of social roles, reduction in social activities, changes to family life, loneliness and social isolation. In their longitudinal study of stroke, Brocklehurst et al (1981) found that three-quarters of the main supporters of stroke victims were women, and of these three-fifths were under the age of 60. During the first year of stroke 14% of the supporters gave up their jobs because of supporting a stroke sufferer and there was a noticeable deterioration in the health of supporters during that period. The major problems arising for the main supporter were related to the patients' behaviour, the need for constant supervision and the supporter's loss of sleep. Families of stroke sufferers were providing considerable support. In over a quarter of cases the individual required help with feeding, dressing and toileting, and a further third for everything except personal care.

Similar findings about the caring role of the family have been found in studies of dementia (Levin et al 1989) and other chronic conditions. In two studies of the terminal year of life (Cartwright et al 1973, Cartwright & Seale 1990) a large proportion of people were found to be as dependent on others for support as found with stroke sufferers. Similar difficulties were experienced by the family supporters, and again they were mainly women. These data reinforce our view that the family is the basic unit in health and medical care. They also help explain why people without families are more likely to end their lives in institutional care (Townsend 1965).

THE FAMILY IN THE CONTEXT OF CARE

As we have seen, when a person is ill it is generally the family that copes. The family will offer remedies and advice; it will take over those roles that the ill person is no longer capable of and it will provide the care necessary until recovery or for long-term support. However, because of traditional gender roles within families, the burden of illness will usually fall on the women of the

family: mothers and daughters. Thus when we talk about care by the family in our everyday lives we are usually talking about care by women. This pattern is reflected in public policy (Secretaries of State for Health et al 1989), and care by women is what is implied by community care (Walker 1982).

Community or family care

Community is one of the unit ideas identified by Nisbet (1967) in his analysis of the sociological tradition. Unfortunately the concept is vague and presents numerous problems in sociological analysis. These difficulties stem partly from the lack of clear definitions as well as from the value-laden nature of the concept. Bell & Newby (1971) prefer a territorial approach to community, which implies a distinct area within which a more or less distinct group of people interact. Others, notably Stacey (1969), use the term to identify a specific pattern of social organisation.

Wilson (1982) argues that it is the value-laden nature of the concept which is more important than problems of definition. 'Community' is an emotive word, which produces images of what is a good life, what kind of life is desirable and what kinds of social arrangements promote intimacy and stability. This vision of life idealises the rural community with intimate personal relationships, constructive methods of social control, the transfer of knowledge between generations and respect for authority and for the status quo. This contrasts dramatically with life in modern urban and inner-city areas.

The concept of *community care* is hazardous to use because of the variety of meanings attached to it. For example, it has been defined as the 'provision of help, support and protection to others by lay members of societies acting in everyday domestic and occupational settings' (Abrams 1978, p. 78). In contrast, it has traditionally been used in Government policy to refer to the care which occurs outside institutional settings, and has most recently been applied to elderly people, people with a mental illness or people with a mental handicap (Walker 1982). This confusion is perhaps best understood by Bayley's (1973) distinction between *care in the community* and *care by the community*. Care in the community refers to the trend of replacing large and often geographically remote institutional facilities with smaller units of residential provision which would, if possible, be familiar to individual residents. This was replaced by the notion that 'community care' referred to the fact that carers or care givers resided in the community, incorporating the notion of the *community* actually doing the caring. Nowadays, the concept of community care by the community dominates the *assumptive world* of policy makers and service providers. (The term 'assumptive world' is used to describe our image or our perception of the environment in which we live (Young 1977).) Following a number of implicit official statements about the nature of community care in the United Kingdom an explicit policy was published for the World Congress on Ageing in 1982:

The primary sources of support and care for elderly people are informal and voluntary. These spring from ties of kinship, friendship and neighbourhood, and they are irreplaceable. It is the task of the public authorities to sustain and where necessary to develop this vast grass roots network, but the responsibility is one for the community as a whole. Care *in* the community must increasingly mean care *by* the community. (DHSS 1982, p. 1)

An examination of the reality of community care reveals that the provision of support and care falls not on the community at large but upon the family. Within the family it is the women who provide the bulk of care (Land 1978, Finch & Groves 1980, Walker 1982, Charlesworth, Wilkin & Durie 1984, Ungerson 1987, Finch 1989, Qureshi & Walker 1989, Finch & Mason 1990, Graham 1991). This observation has been expressed in terms of the double equation: 'in practice community care equals care by the family, and in practice care by the family equals care by women' (Finch & Groves 1980, p. 494) (Fig. 6.2). Even where community care is outside the family, such as in neighbourhood

care, it is women again who provide the majority of support (Abrams et al 1989).

In the United Kingdom there are an estimated 6 million informal care givers looking after frail elderly people, people with learning difficulties and people who have a mental illness (Green 1988). It is estimated that 4 million informal care givers are looking after people with significant disabilities (Martin et al 1988).

Much of the care giving literature has focused on family relationships and gender issues. There is little data about class or ethnic differences. Informal care givers are found at all ages, including children. Most predominantly, however, male care givers tend to be of retirement age and where spouses are the principal care givers of older people they tend, naturally, to be old themselves (Bond 1992).

SUMMARY

This chapter has revealed the cultural context of lay health beliefs and has shown the pervasive influence that the family has in matters of health. While it remains speculative that family relationships may cause psychiatric illness, there is now evidence that they influence the course of schizophrenia.

Child health is in part determined by the behaviour of parents. It is important therefore to discover the social influences on such behaviour. One such influence is the transmission of health culture and intergenerational studies are one way of looking at this. The transmission of health culture, however, has been found to be complex and rely on broader social changes to a greater extent than might have been supposed.

Illness among family members can have devastating negative effects as well as, at times, positive consequences. While families are subjected to social, financial and emotional stress, some also gain in mutual strength and understanding, finding resources previously untapped. While chronic illness, or long-term caring for handicapped or elderly family members, has pronounced effects for the family as a whole, the major consequences are for its female members. The movement to increase care by the commu-

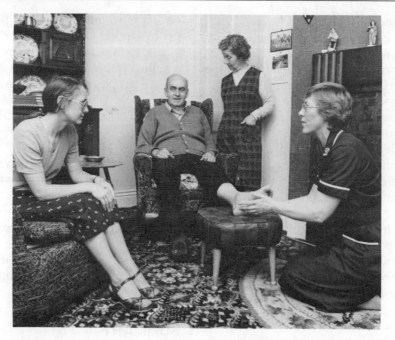

Fig. 6.2   Care in the community means family care, means women's care (courtesy of Rik Walton).

nity, maintaining people who are chronically ill, handicapped or physically or mentally frail within their families, has profound consequences for women – married and unmarried, daughters, mothers and wives. Government and health and social care service policy to expand community care needs to examine and take into account the consequences of such policies for the health and well-being of the family and, in particular, of its female members.

FURTHER READING

Anderson R, Bury M (eds) 1988 Living with chronic illness: the experience of patients and their families. Unwin Hyman, London

Blaxter M, Paterson E 1982 Mothers and daughters: a three-generational study of health attitudes and behaviour. Heinemann, London

Stainton Rogers W 1991 Explaining health and illness: an exploration of diversity. Harvester Wheatsheaf, London

7

Health care organisations

INTRODUCTION

So far in this book we have introduced two universal features of modern societies and discussed their importance in the context of health. First, we identified the concept of social stratification as a cornerstone to understanding the structure of societies, and showed how social stratification could be related to health. We then focused on the family and, in the last chapter, contended that the family is the most important social group within which health is maintained and illness occurs and is resolved. In this chapter we turn to a third universal feature of modern societies, namely organisations, and discuss the relevance of organisation theory for understanding health care organisations.

As with other sociological concerns, the study of organisations can be approached from a variety of perspectives. Silverman (1970), in his influential study of organisations, identifies two broad approaches, each of which comprises a number of perspectives. One approach, generally referred to as *systems theory*, emphasises explanations of behaviour in terms of interaction of systems attempting to satisfy their organisational goals. Systems theory is dominated by structural functionalism and often uses the organic analogy discussed in Chapter 2 to explain the nature of the relationships between different parts of the system. Other perspectives within systems theory do not adopt a sociological frame of reference. Human Relations theory owes most to psychology; Socio-Technical

Systems theory straddles psychology and economics; and Decision-Making theory is grounded in economics and cybernetics as it applies to automatic communication and control.

The other main approach, *action theory*, argues that attention should be focused on the participants in organisations. Each participant might experience and perceive the organisation and its relationship to the wider social world in which they live in different ways. Action theory emphasises the ability of individual participants to create, sustain and change the social environment and nature of organisations.

In the last 20 years the sociology of organisations, like many other areas of sociological concern, has been considerably influenced by the critical theorists. Reed (1992) identifies five current analytical frameworks. In addition to systems theory and action theory he describes three further conceptual frameworks: organisations as structures of power and domination; organisations as symbolic constructions; and organisations as social practices.

The analysis of organisations within a power framework adopts a postMarxist perspective in which organisations are defined as instruments designed to protect and advance the interests of the dominant economic, political and social groups within societies. Thus, the power framework assumes that organisations are created and sustained as viable social units by the wider totality of power structures and control relations in societies, and in which they are embedded.

The analysis of organisations within a symbolic framework reflects the unease with which mainstream approaches ignore the process of organising in everyday life. Organisations are cultural artefacts that are produced, reproduced and transformed through processes of symbolic construction, mediation and interpretation in which all members are routinely engaged. Thus, organisational reality is constructed, internalised, sustained and changed through processes of cultural creation and enactment. The symbolic perspective emphasises the cultural processes that create and sustain a shared sense of organisational membership and identity.

The practice framework tends to provide a synthesis or partial synthesis of the different approaches highlighted above. Thus, organisations are social practices geared to the assembly and integration of other social practices concerned with transforming the conditions under which collective action is made possible.

In this chapter we review these theories of organisation and major concepts like bureaucracy and power. In particular, we show how the functionalists rely on the concept of role, and the idea of organisational goals is expanded in a system theory approach to studying the care of inmates of long-stay institutions. In contrast, action theory relies heavily on the perspectives of those within organisations determining how they operate and we use a study of play leaders in children's wards as an example of this interpretation. We then turn to the negotiated nature of social processes in organisations before exploring the role of power within organisations. Finally, we consider current trends in health care organisations in relation to teamwork and management. We begin this chapter with a discussion of the concept institution, a term which is often used synonymously with organisation.

Institutions

Sociologists use the concept of institution to describe the way we order social life so that we can make sense of each other's actions – *a regulatory pattern* which is programmed by society and imposed on the conduct of individuals. Institutions are experienced as having external reality, objectivity, coerciveness, moral authority and historicity (Berger & Berger 1976).

Externality and objectivity

Institutions have *external reality*; they are not just things we humans imagine as existing. Like rocks, trees or houses, a hospital has a physical presence; or like love or thought, medicine has an abstract presence. In either case, we cannot ignore them when they occur in our daily lives.

They will also have objectivity since in general we all agree that they exist.

Coerciveness

The possession of external reality and objectivity gives an institution *coerciveness* or *coercive power*. We have all experienced the power of the school or the hospital in our everyday lives, perhaps in the way that these institutions get us to wear their distinctive uniforms and arrive and depart at specific times. We would not normally question the power of institutions like the law or medicine for example, to detain a patient under the Mental Health Act, whether or not we agree with the way this power is used. In some instances, however, such as in the case of patients who discharge themselves, people might try to ignore the power of the institution. When this happens the coerciveness of the institution will become explicit. Specific sanctions will be used to bring the defaulting patient into line. Similarly, mechanisms are available to persuade radical members of hospital staff to adhere to hospital customs and practices.

Moral authority

Institutions also have what Weber called *moral authority* – a concept we described in Chapter 3. In other words the institution has *legitimacy*. The institution will have legitimacy when it is generally accepted that the authority of the institution is just and rightfully given. Thus, the psychiatric hospital which prevents patients from discharging themselves has the moral authority as well as the physical ability to do so. Of course, the moral authority will only exist while society agrees that it is the right of the psychiatric hospital to determine which patients should be discharged, or the nursing home to determine which residents should be admitted.

Historicity

Finally, a basic characteristic of institutions is their enduring nature. Most institutions have a history which extends beyond the life careers of the authors and readers of this book. The family and the church have been in existence and are likely to endure for a considerable time, as we saw in Chapter 5, although structures may change.

The sociological use of the term 'institution' has a wider meaning than just physical structures. Similarly, when we talk about health care organisations we shall be concerned not only with the physical structures of hospitals but also with the social organisation of health care and professional occupations. This approach differs from that adopted by many sociologists, particularly the structural-functionalists who have emphasised that organisations are physical entities persisting over time, which are specifically set up to achieve certain aims.

ORGANISATIONS AS SYSTEMS

The structural functionalist perspective on organisations, in common with other systems theories, is based on a number of functions. These are that organisations comprise a set of interdependent parts; organisations have needs which are necessary for their survival; and organisations take actions.

Such assumptions, in the context of health care, appear trivial and common sense. Most health systems, whether they be primary care teams, hospital clinics or whole health districts, can be divided into 'subsystems' by occupational group, speciality, physical location or some other ascriptive category. Thus, the antenatal clinic in one hospital observed and described by McIntyre (1978) would provide an example of an organisation with interdependent parts: consultants, junior medical staff, midwifery staff, clerical staff, pregnant women and their relatives. The stated goals of the antenatal clinic are to screen the total population of pregnant women; to select high- and low-risk groups; and carefully to monitor high-risk groups. This example illustrates a major problem for systems theory. McIntyre's study shows that not all those attending or working in the clinic share the same goals as the medical and midwifery staff running the clinic. Indeed, there may also be disagreements between different doctors or midwives as to the appropriate goals of this particular example of an organisation. Thus, in gaining a sociological understanding of the antenatal clinic we need to recognise that different individuals may hold different goals. System theory ignores this fact.

This kind of criticism of system theory has led to the distinction being made between the *formal organisation*, based on rationality and efficiency, and the *informal organisation*, based on sentiment. Yet if we recognise that formal and informal organisations can coexist, we shall see that the concepts are problematic. The formal organisation is something defined by one set of personnel, in our example the obstetricians, who consciously attempt to impose their definition of the situation throughout the antenatal clinic. However, within the informal organisation the goals of midwives and pregnant women may differ. The aims and interests of midwives and pregnant women will influence their commitment to the rules and routines of the clinic. If their commitment declines, their performance of roles in the organisation may be affected.

The study of roles

A persistent feature of structuralist theories of organisations is the static rather than dynamic nature of the roles occupied by its participants. Our discussion of socialisation in Chapter 5 implies that one of the functions of socialisation is to prepare the individual for different roles in the social system. The concept of role implies not only an expected pattern of behaviour but also that the occupier of the role – what we shall call the *role incumbent* – shows appropriate feelings and values. Patients are expected to comply with doctors' orders, but they are also expected to feel that it is right and proper that doctors issue such instructions. For patients to tell doctors how to treat them or to refuse to accept a doctor's prescription would be regarded as inappropriate behaviour or non-compliance.

Multiple roles

The concept of role has a theatrical analogy (Goffman 1971) in that we are all engaged in acting our various roles. The role is like the part in the play (Brutus) while the way that the individual acts the role is analogous to the performance of the part by a particular actor ('John Gielgud's Brutus'). In real life, as on the stage, we can act more than one role. We act some roles, such as gender roles, throughout our lives while others, such as those of parent, occupational therapist or goalkeeper, will be acquired. We all act *multiple roles* (Fig. 7.1). At the same time as being a doctor a woman can be a feminist, daughter, mother, rate-payer, preacher, car-driver and patient.

Role-set

Merton (1957) coined the term *role-set* to describe the array of roles and expectations that any individual will confront while taking a particular role. The female doctor, while acting as doctor and not in any of her multiple roles, will be interacting with several others playing roles: pharmacist, hospital administrator, nurse, dietician, physiotherapist, patient and patient's

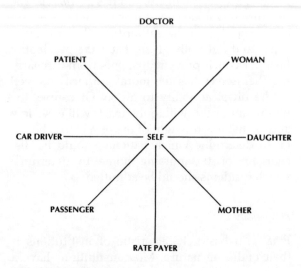

Fig. 7.1 Multiple roles.

relatives (Fig. 7.2). When she acts the role of mother the role-set will include other mothers, son, daughter, daughter's friend, son's teacher. A more complex example of a role-set is illustrated by Runciman (1983) in her study of the work of the ward sister. As a ward sister her own role-set consisted of over 100 role relationships indicating the complexity of the sister's work.

These formal descriptions of multiple roles and role-sets give an impression that roles are uniform and static. Turner (1962) emphasises the important distinction between *role-taking* and *role-making*. The idea of role-taking suggests that

all roles are prescribed and defined by a specific set of rules which all actors comprehend and to which they conform. Military and bureaucratic roles are probably the minority which easily fit this model, since the formal regulation systems of most bureaucracies prevent individual actors from making any modification to the behaviour and decisions prescribed for their roles. They do as 'the system' prescribes with minimum discretion. In contrast, the idea of role-making suggests that actors will usually create and modify roles according to their own interpretation of the role and in response to the way others interpret their own roles in the role-set. This is especially the case when new roles are emerging in organisations – roles such as nurse practitioners or clinical specialists in nursing organisations.

In her analysis of the role of the occupational therapist Fairhurst (1981) shows how, even in a bureaucratic organisation like a District General Hospital, actors are able to make their roles. Fairhurst found that the definition of what constituted occupational therapy advanced by 'official' ideology was not the one shared by the occupational therapists in the hospital studied. They felt unable to take the role of occupational therapist as defined by 'official' ideology. By devising their own strategies, manipulating other people's roles and suspending others' versions of their own roles, they were able to *make* their own version of the role of occupational therapist. Thus, it is useful to see roles as dynamic and something which people themselves develop rather than as static features of people's lives to which they mould their performances. Nevertheless, roles are to some degree constrained by the social environment and there are limits to the behaviour tolerated by others in their expectations of appropriate role behaviour. Bond (1978) observed that some nurses strongly criticised one member of staff who regarded it as within her interpretation of the nurse's role to tell patients with cancer their diagnosis if they asked her. Others regarded this as a medical prerogative and exerted sanctions to persuade their colleague to limit this kind of behaviour.

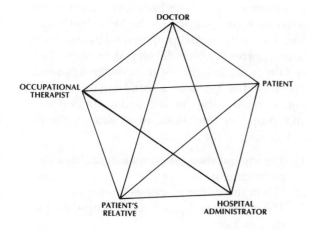

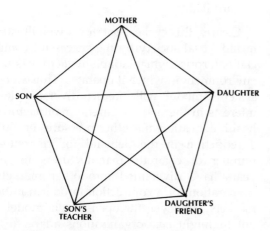

Fig. 7.2   Simplified role sets.

Role conflict

Most of us will act multiple roles throughout our lives, such as doctor and mother, and as a result will experience *interrole conflict*. Holding a perception of the role of doctor which differs from official ideology or of mother which differs from traditional beliefs can lead to *intrarole conflict*.

Interrole conflict means conflict between two simultaneously held roles. A doctor who has to be at work on the afternoon of a child's birthday party experiences *interrole conflict* between the role of doctor and parent. The degree of conflict will reflect strength of attachment to the two roles.

In contrast, parents who disagree with the expectation that a parent should be present at a child's birthday party will experience *intrarole conflict*. Their interpretation of the role of parent conflicts with the dominant view of other similar role incumbents – other parents. In other words, they do not agree with the general consensus of their social group about the patterns of expected behaviour in parents. In contemporary Britain, for example, there are appreciable differences in opinion about the role 'mother' between, on the one hand, the 'feminists' and, on the other hand, the 'traditionalists'. These differences are often expressed in terms of whether mothers should go out to work and the demands made in particular kinds of work. For example, it is often still the case that women with young children are not acceptable as nurses, the prevailing view being that they cannot give sufficient time, energy and commitment to both the job and the family. Are male recruits ever discriminated against in this way? They are probably not. However, they may have problems reconciling the role of man with the role of nurse, since the latter is often regarded as a feminine role.

This approach to role conflict proceeds as if women are forced to choose between two competing sets of expectations, for example, between the 'traditional' and 'modern'. However, in its most general sense, intrarole conflict exists when there is no immediately apparent way of simultaneously coping effectively with two or more expectations of a role. The problem for the individual actor is more fundamental. How should a woman interact with men, some of whom have modern, some traditional, and some mixed, conceptions of the masculine role, and with women who may have the same or different conceptions of the feminine role? To some extent women learn to modify their role in line with the expectations of other men and women who have different conceptions of it. Again, the concept of impression management (see Ch. 3) comes into play.

OPEN SYSTEMS

In Chapter 2 we described how functionalism often uses the analogy of the biological organism. This is the model proposed by the open systems approach which developed in response to certain criticisms against the systems approach. The model emphasises a social organism, existing in relationship to the social environment, and proposes four basic requirements for the functioning of the system:

1. The organisation takes some input from the environment.
2. The organisation processes this input.
3. The organisation produces an output for the environment.
4. The organisation retains sufficient resources from the process of production to allow its survival.

Clearly, this cyclical pattern is well illustrated in industrial society by the successful commercial enterprise which adapts its activities to the environment in which it operates. Thus an open-systems model will predict diversification of interests in the major cigarette manufacturers if health education and other pressures encourage a reduction in the demand for cigarettes. A number of cigarette manufacturers in recent years have diversified into other markets in preparation for a contraction in their traditional markets. However, the open-system model does not highlight *how* organisations adapt to their changing environments.

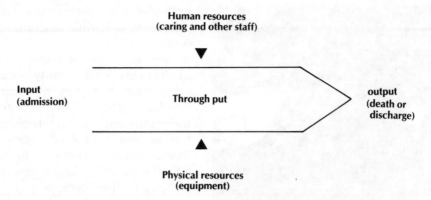

Fig. 7.3   An open system in health care (Miller & Gwynne 1972).

The open-systems model has been used by Miller and Gwynne (1972) in a study of institutions for people who were physically handicapped or chronically sick. The four basic requirements identified above are illustrated by Miller and Gwynne (see Fig. 7.3). The inmates of the institution represent the through-put of the organisation. Caring and other staff are the human resources, and equipment comprises the physical resources. Death or discharge of an inmate represents the output of the system.

This study illustrates some of the difficulties associated with the identification of the organisation's goals and the pursuit of these goals within the framework of a shared set of values. The logical output of this kind of organisation is dead inmates, even though inmates, staff and the outside world find such explicit goals unpalatable. Miller and Gwynne report that the implicit output of dead inmates leads to the development of two contrasting types of value systems, which they refer to as psychological defences.

First, staff, who were committed to preserving life at all costs, were described as providing a humanitarian defence. Thus, although the handicapped inmate may be socially dead, the pressure of humanitarian values attempts to maximise the interval between social death and physiological death. In Chapter 10 we explore the notions of social and physiological death in some detail. Here Miller and Gwynne are using the term 'social death' to describe the implicit rejection by society of the handicapped inmate.

Second, staff who attempted to deny that the handicapped are abnormal, were described as providing a liberal defence. Liberal values aid the handicapped inmate whose capacities should be fostered to their full potential. Physical and social rehabilitation are therefore encouraged.

The type of care provided in the organisation was found to relate to the type of value system present. In institutions where staff were committed to preserving life at all costs the *warehousing* model of care was dominant, while in institutions where staff defined the inmates as normal the *horticultural* model of care persisted.

The warehousing model

In the warehousing model care is provided for the primary task of prolonging physical life. Effective warehousing requires that patients or residents remain dependent and depersonalised, and accepting of their dependency. Any attempts by patients or residents to assert themselves, or to display individual needs other than those previously defined by staff, will be a constraint on the achievement of the primary task. Independence is therefore discouraged. The ideal patient or resident is the one who accepts

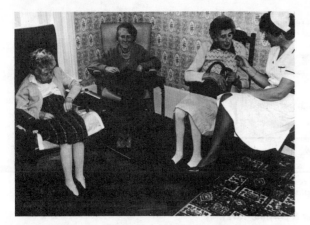

Fig. 7.4 Warehousing may be characterised by the extent to which it is personalised (courtesy of Nursing Standard).

the staff's assessment of his or her needs and the treatment they prescribe and administer.

The warehousing model has been refined by Evers in her study of work organisation in geriatric hospitals (Evers 1981). She describes two kinds of warehousing: *minimal warehousing*, where patients' care is organised entirely on a routinised basis in order to achieve the primary tasks of prolonging life, and *personalised warehousing* (Fig. 7.4), where some attempt is made to provide a personalised service to patients, albeit within a life preservation ideology.

The horticultural model

The horticultural model is a relatively recent development, which is more an aspiration than a reality. Needs for physical care are the constraints in the horticultural model. The primary task of the model is to develop an individual's capacities to the optimum by encouraging independence. This might be achieved through the process of *normalisation*: by organising caring activities around social activities and by providing an environment which approximates to life outside the institution. Privacy, choice and independence should all be respected. The development of small domestic units for people with learning difficulties and experimental NHS nursing homes for long-stay elderly people are

examples of an attempt to encourage the horticultural model while retaining institutional care (Graham 1983).

The limitation of using the open systems model in this kind of study is that it provides no explanation as to *why* different value systems develop within different institutions or *how* these different value systems lead to the contrasting kinds of care regimes described. A desire for explanation led a number of people to adopt a social action approach which, while recognising the structural constraints on action, asks how and why individuals carry on their interactions within that framework.

ACTION THEORY

Action theory has been an influential perspective in the study of health care organisations. The approach is probably exemplified by Goffman's theoretical analysis of the *total institution*.

A number of institutions for the elderly, disabled and young chronic sick exhibit the characteristics of the total institution. The essential feature of the total institution is that, unlike life outside, for inmates there is no separation between the three central spheres of modern life: work, leisure and family. All aspects of life are conducted within the boundaries of the institution and under the control of a single authority. Each phase of daily activities is shared with a large number of other people, all of whom are treated alike and are required to do the same thing together. These activities normally follow a strict routine imposed from above by a system of explicit formal rulings and a body of officials. The routine of daily activities comprises a single rational plan which has been designed to fulfil the official aims of the institution (Goffman 1961).

British studies of long-stay institutions have repeatedly exemplified Goffman's model. The survey by Townsend (1962) of residential institutions and homes for the aged in England and Wales remains, after 25 years, the best description of the ubiquity of the total institution. His case studies of residents in old workhouses, which provided the mainstay of local authority residential services for the old and handicapped, vividly describe the isolation of residents from the outside world, the lack of individual privacy and independence, the routinisation of activities, and the separation between residents and staff. Miller and Gwynne's (1972) study of residential institutions for the physically handicapped and young chronic sick describes a similar situation in some of the organisations they studied. Baker (1983), Evers (1981) and Bond and Bond (1993) in their studies of staff and patients in geriatric hospitals found that the concept of the total institution remains relevant to contemporary British long-stay hospitals.

The characteristics of the total institution identified by Goffman describe a form of organisation in which the prevailing definitions of the situation derive from within the organisation itself. General goals for psychiatric hospitals or prisons may be proposed by society, but the rules as to how these are achieved will generally emerge from within the institution. We draw on Goffman's analysis again in Chapter 8 when we describe how patients are socialised into their new roles as inmates. Members are cleansed of their outside identities by having to undergo a mortifying process during which their personal possessions are almost entirely removed; they may be made to wear a uniform and are recognised by a number, for example when medication is given. They may often react to such treatment by intransigence and withdrawal, both of which are interpreted in some institutions as signs of the disease for which the patient has been institutionalised. After long periods of stay Goffman observed that inmates may generate the adaptations of *colonisation* by establishing an identity within the organisation, which they perceive as being more important than previous identities they experienced in 'normal' society, or *conversion* by appearing to accept the staff's views of them. Both these adaptations are vividly described in his study of *Ways of Making Out in a Mental Hospital* (Goffman 1961), and show how some inmates are able to increase their power and status relative to other inmates, and even sometimes to staff members.

Hall (1977), in his study of the introduction of play leaders into two children's wards, also illustrates the usefulness of action theory. His approach stresses the different perspectives of those involved: the children, the nursing and medical staff, the play leaders and teachers, and the domestic staff. Each participant was shown to construct his or her own definition of the situation which guided his or her actions. Action theory fits Hall's view of disturbances in hospital being caused by threats to the continuity and persistence of individual interpretations of the situation. The recognition of various interest groups at ward level helps us to understand resistance to any kind of innovation. This can be seen as a rational response to threatened disruption of existing social relationships, which carries implications for the rights and obligations attached to socially defined roles. In Hall's study different participants regarded play in different ways, having different conceptions of its value for the care of children in hospital. For the play leaders, play was the *raison d'etre* of their role. Nursing staff saw play as a subsidiary part of their role; they appeared to value the play leaders because, by keeping the children occupied, this allowed them to concentrate on the more technical aspects of their job. For domestic staff, play in the ward, and the greater mobility of children as a result of play, could easily create more work despite any attempts by play leaders to keep their areas tidy. Indeed, the emphasis on play goes against the traditional values of order and cleanliness at all times, to which many cleaners and nurses subscribe. The same may be said of activities in long-stay hospital wards when nurses regard the occupational therapist or 'diversional' therapist in much the same role as play leaders.

POWER IN HEALTH CARE ORGANISATIONS

Any consideration of interactions between members of health care organisations must take account of structural constraints. Structural constraints affect patient and professional alike, albeit in different ways. One such constraint is the bureaucratic setting in which care is usually delivered.

Bureaucracy

Central to any bureaucratic setting is the feeling of *being processed* (Fig. 7.5). This underlying experience is common to all of us when we deal with bureaucracies, whether as students, patients, tax-payers or rail travellers. What is a *bureaucracy*? Few sociologists have attempted a simple definition, and most refer to the basic characteristics of a bureaucracy first delineated by Weber.

Bureaucracies are characterised by a separate organisation with full-time staff – a feature common to all health care organisations. As in the total institution described above, the work of such organisations is segregated from the private lives and activities of staff members, and not infrequently is characterised as impersonal and creating loss of dignity for clients. The work of bureaucracies is usually arranged around fixed areas in which they hold authority legitimised and ordered by specific regulations. The various National Health Services Acts delineate the areas of concern for different health care organisations.

A bureaucracy will assume that each staff member is trained in a rational manner, an assumption often taken for granted by health professionals working in the health service. Part of this training includes the development of an ethos of 'objectivity'. Each client or patient is supposed to be handled according to the rules of the organisation, regardless of the personal feelings of staff and clients. Attempts to be objective encourage the impersonal atmosphere associated with many health service institutions (Smith 1992).

Bureaucracies, in order to accomplish objective activity within a defined area of jurisdiction, are organised in orderly and stable hierarchies. It is this characteristic of health care systems which is particularly important for understanding interactions between health professionals and patients.

At the top of the power hierarchy are senior doctors who achieved their dominant position by virtue of being regarded as having expert knowledge as well as holding sociolegal responsibility for patients (Freidson 1975). This is still the case in the 1990s, at a time when general managers in health care organisations are responsible for the efficient running of the health service. The work of other professional staff is organised by doctors' orders. Thus other staff may be regarded as doctors' agents in dealing with patients. While remedial therapists, social workers and chaplains, like doctors, can lay claim to professional expertise they tend to be 'staff' rather than 'line' personnel and so lack the authority awarded to doctors (Katz 1969). Their subordination to medical authority extends into areas of *nonmedical* expertise, so that doctors can instruct others what to say and what not to say to patients about their illness, functions which have come to be defined as 'medical' (Bond 1978).

Nurses are even more lacking in autonomy. While often acting as the representative of the doctor, they are often reluctant to give care based on their own initiative or to assume personal accountability. Rather, deriving from Florence Nightingale's view of nursing, 'what the nurse did for the patient was a function of what the doctor felt was required for the patient. Even such unskilled tasks as feeding a patient were thus defined as part of the medical regi-

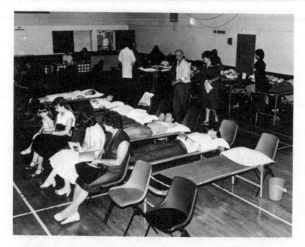

Fig. 7.5 'Being processed' at a blood donation session (courtesy of Nursing Standard).

men. All nursing work flowed from the doctors and thus nursing became a formal part of the doctors' work. Nursing was thus defined as a subordinate part of the technical division of labour surrounding medicine' (Freidson 1975, p. 61). As well as being subject to the orders of doctors, nurses are also subject to the authority of the nursing hierarchy (Fig. 7.6) as well as the general management structure of health care organisations. Although the NHS and Community Care Act of 1990 has effectively removed overall control of nursing staff from the nursing profession, at ward and district level the traditional nursing hierarchy still predominates. More will be said about this aspect of work in Chapter 11.

Nurses and paramedical workers are, therefore, constrained in their relationships with patients by the medical profession as well as by the organisation; but they are still in a position to exert relative power and authority over patients. This aspect of health care organisations is developed in Chapter 9.

Negotiation

Action theory has questioned the use of the rational-bureaucratic model in the study of

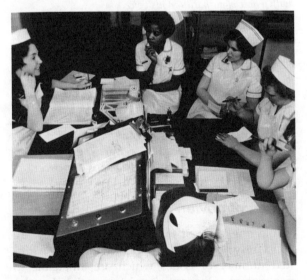

Fig. 7.6 The nursing hierarchy reflected at a ward report (courtesy of Nursing Standard).

health care organisations, arguing that the power structure in any complex organisation is amenable to modification by individual actors. Within any health care organisation there is a variety of personnel: patients, doctors, nurses, therapists, social workers, clerical workers, managers, porters, cleaners, volunteers and many others, all in the same place and ostensibly working towards the primary goal of the organisation, which is to restore and maintain patients' health. These groups bring together different personal backgrounds, different types of training and professional socialisation (a subject we discuss in Chapter 11) and varying amounts of experience. Significantly, as we have seen, they occupy different hierarchical positions in the organisation. Between them they will all hold a multitude of views and perspectives about the restoration and maintenance of health and about dying. Due to these divergent orientations and interests, differences of opinion will regularly emerge in matters of patient care and organisational policy. For example, Bucher and Stelling (1969) found that the different perspectives of the basic science and clinical faculties in the medical schools they studied led to competition for resources and recognition in the curriculum. Even organisations with unusually high levels of consensus between individuals on these issues have the problem of practical implementation of ideas and the assignment of specific tasks. Thus in clinical units there will be competition over resources.

According to the rational-bureaucratic model the organisation turns to its rules and regulations whenever internal problems occur. However, most personnel do not know all of these rules nor how to apply them, and indeed the rules are often neither very extensive nor explicit. Consequently, conflict of interest will not be resolved by the straightforward application of rules, nor even by relying upon the exertion of hierarchical authority within the organisation.

The inadequacy of formal rules and structures to govern activities in organisations sustains an informal structure in which the parties involved maintain social order by *negotiation*. This is done by a continuous process of give and take, diplomacy, bargaining, withholding information and displaying different degrees of cooperativeness (Strauss et al 1963, Strauss 1978). This happens between staff groups as well as between individual staff and individual patients. In Chapter 5 we discussed how individuals are socialised into particular roles, with orderly relationships a function of appropriate role expectations, cooperation and reciprocity. Negotiation is another important process through which social action takes place.

Initially, negotiation was studied in long-term settings. Strauss and colleagues articulated the theory on the basis of their study in two psychiatric hospitals. They found that psychiatrists often disagree among themselves on such matters as diagnosis, ward placement, therapeutic regimes, and prognoses in individual cases. This is, of course, a feature of professional practice which is not unique to psychiatric hospitals or psychiatrists! We have all experienced similar differences of opinion between professionals in all health care organisations and other organisations such as schools, government agencies and commercial enterprises. Such disagreements do, however, create problems for other staff. For example, when a psychiatrist decides to transfer an extremely rumbustious patient from one ward to another, it creates numerous problems for that ward's staff and their manner of dealing with the 'problem' may be to transfer the patient to still another ward behind the psychiatrist's back (Strauss et al 1963).

Within the hierarchical structure of most health care organisations, negotiations between professionals may be extremely subtle. Stein (1978) provides a vivid illustration of the subtleties of negotiation between doctors and nurses in his account of *The doctor-nurse game*. The object of the game is for the nurse to be responsible for making significant recommendations which must nevertheless appear to be initiated by the doctor. To do this the nurse makes recommendations without appearing to be making a recommendation statement. At the same time a physician making a request for a recommendation from a nurse should do so without ostensibly asking for one.

Stein provides the following dialogue to illustrate how the game is played. In this example the medical resident on hospital call is awakened by telephone at 1 a.m. because a patient on a ward, not his own, has not been able to fall asleep. The medical resident answers the telephone:

This is Dr Jones. (*An open and direct communication.*) Dr Jones, this is Miss Smith on 2W. Mrs Brown, who learned today of her father's death, is unable to fall asleep.

(*This message has two levels. Openly, it describes a set of circumstances, a woman who is unable to fall asleep and who that morning received word of her father's death. Less openly, but just as directly, it is a diagnostic and recommendation statement; Mrs Brown is unable to sleep because of her grief, and she should be given a sedative. Dr Jones, accepting the diagnostic statement and replying to the recommendation statement, answers.*)

What sleeping medication has been helpful to Mrs Brown in the past?

(*Dr. Jones, not knowing the patient, is asking for a recommendation from the nurse, who does know the patient, about what sleeping medication should be prescribed. Note, however, his question does not appear to be asking her for a recommendation. Miss Smith replies.* Pentobarbital mg 100 was quite effective the night before last.

(*A disguised recommendation statement. Dr Jones replies with a note of authority in his voice.*)

Pentobarbital mg 100 before bedtime as needed for sleep, got it?

(*Miss Smith ends the conversation with the tone of the grateful supplicant.*)

Yes I have, and thank you very much doctor. (Stein 1978, p. 110)

This example illustrates one way the doctor-nurse game is played. It also illustrates that doctors and nurses hold different types of power.

Types of power

While one view of institutions is that they are constantly negotiated, in practice there are a limited number of issues which are amenable to negotiation. One criticism of negotiated order theory is that it focuses on the minutiae of everyday life in organisations and ignores the wider and deeper aspects of power. The presence of power structures within an organisation puts people in unequal positions before the processes of negotiation even begin. However, as the negotiated order model indicates, most members of an organisation will have some power, albeit rather limited, for some personnel.

One way of looking at social power is to attempt to observe the influence that one person has over another. French and Raven (1968) have identified several types of power by describing the ways in which 'person A could cause person B to do something which was contrary to B's desire'.

Reward power

The power holder may influence behaviour by controlling rewards or resources which are valued by the subject. Hospital cleaners might reward the play leaders for keeping their area tidy by agreeing to the siting of a sand box in the children's wards. Doctors might reward patients for not complaining by discharging them home early. Ward sisters might reward student nurses for extra help by giving them a good report. General practitioners can reward district nurses and health visitors by the amount of space provided for them in the practice premises.

Coercive power

The power holder may influence behaviour by controlling the punishments. A nurse may punish elderly patients for being incontinent by being too busy to attend to them. Any professional can be punished by another professional in cases of professional misconduct by reporting them to the relevant disciplinary body. Such is the strength of 'closing ranks', however, that this is rare.

Coercive and reward power are similar in that the power holder is in a position to manipulate the environment by withholding or threatening to withhold resources considered necessary for the maintenance of a satisfactory environment.

Legitimate power

We have already discussed the concept of legitimacy in relation to social stratification in Chapter 3. Legitimate power is the result of an individual's position within an organisation. It stems from the moral authority of a particular position in the organisation, which allows the role incumbent the right to prescribe particular behaviour. Legitimate power gives the power holder control over invisible assets, particularly information, right to access and right to organise.

Information

Information is power and withholding information is often a very evident form of legitimate power. In Chapter 9 we describe the ways information is controlled in staff-patient interactions. Doctors control information on diagnosis and prognosis, so that other professionals as well as patients are dependent on them for this knowledge. In primary care organisations the general practitioners may control information by, for example, insisting that all patients on a practice list are seen by them before they are referred to other primary care professionals. The general manager may control access to the notes of meetings of the Health Authority.

Right to access

Legitimate power gives the power holder the right of access to a number of individuals and networks. This right to access not only leads to more information, but also the familiarity which often occurs can be used to the advantage of the power holder. The establishment of a general manager in, for example, purchasing authorities would reduce the legitimate power of other members by restricting their right of access to the chairman.

Right to organise

Holding legitimate power gives power holders the right to organise their own work and the right to make decisions. All professionals, to different degrees, are given this kind of power.

Expert power

Expert power is based on the subject's belief that the power holder possesses superior knowledge and ability. As Young's (1961) monograph *The Rise of the Meritocracy* suggests, this form of power is the most acceptable since we all have the opportunity to become experts, even if only in small ways. People also tend not to resent being influenced by experts, except when their power has not been legitimised.

Referent power

This kind of power relates to the prestige of individuals and to some extent relates to the status of a person in society. Thus people who invoke high prestige or charisma are endowed with referent power. The higher status usually attributed to doctors means that they have higher referent power than social workers or nurses. Thus, patients or clients may be more influenced by doctors, because of their status, than by other health professionals.

This approach to the study of power helps to illustrate the variety of influences, interests and conflicts inherent in any organisation before negotiation begins. It also helps to explain why, in social interaction, different actors are able to 'negotiate' different outcomes. Power is a multidimensional concept, so that individuals who have a great deal of legitimate power may have little power on other dimensions and, as a result, are relatively weak in influencing decisions. It may be that these other types of power have a greater influence on people's daily lives than legitimate power.

GENERAL MANAGEMENT AND TEAMWORK

The British National Health Service is a complex organisation employing some 1 000 000 employees representing a variety of skills and professions. It is a unique organisation nationally and internationally. Within the United Kingdom it is the only human service organisation which is available to the whole population and internationally it is the only health care system which is centrally financed and managed. The history of the NHS is also complex and we refer the reader to other authorities for a detailed analysis (Klein 1989, Levitt & Wall 1992).

Since its creation in 1948 the NHS has been subject to increasing rates of change with major structural reorganisation in 1974 and 1983, the introduction of general management in 1984, and in 1991 and 1993 implementation of the NHS and Community Care Act of 1990. Throughout the 1980s the organisation of the NHS was subject to 'fine tuning' (Klein 1989). Perhaps the most significant organisational change has been the switch from an emphasis on *administration* to general *management*. Following the 1974 reorganisation, consensus management dominated the administration of the health service. Doctors, nurses, administrators and treasurers shared in the administration at different levels of the service. Undoubtedly, the traditional power of the medical profession dominated the new management team but the newly created structure also provided enhanced power to nurses which had for so long been the handmaidens of the medical profession (Strong & Robinson 1990). We explore further the importance of this role for nursing in Chapter 11 when discussing professional organisation and professionalism.

The introduction of general management into the NHS in 1984 following the recommendations of Griffiths on the management of the health service (DHSS 1983) saw a dramatic shift of power and influence in the health service at all levels. Under consensus management no single person was in charge. All decisions had to be unanimously agreed to by all members of the consensus teams which assumed collective responsibility for all decisions. Griffiths argued that such a structure was cumbersome and not conducive to good management, particularly where difficult decisions were required to be taken. Griffiths recognised consensus management as slow, yielding lowest common denominator decision-making. The major prob-lem was the lack of clear responsibility at all levels of the NHS, from the central Department of Health to the individual hospitals or service groupings within health authorities.

The implementation of general management into seven district health authorities has been studied using ethnographic methods by Strong and Robinson (1990). They found that the new management approach was based on a wholly new set of principles: on systematic monitoring, on a single line of command, on an integrated structure, on the rules of generalists not spe-cialists, on greater devolution as well as greater central control, on flexible staff and flexible structures, on hybrid staff members who would know something of everyone's job, on micro- as well as macromanagement. After 1984, nurses were not necessarily responsible for manag-ing nurses and any trade or profession could be responsible for the management of the clini-cal trades. Overall nursing continued to have limited influence, although individual nurses who were promoted to general manager roles became individually powerful. In general, doc-tors have lost some influence but where indi-vidual doctors are general managers or management units are based on clinical teams, their power is substantial. How has the intro-duction of general management affected clinical management in health care organisations?

Teamwork and collaboration

It is perhaps assumed that health care organisa-tions are essentially teams of professionals working together to achieve a common goal. We have reported a number of studies in this book which suggest that this official view of health care organisation is not often supported by empirical data. Indeed, a number of writers such as Dingwall (1980) and Reedy (1980) have questioned the usefulness of 'teamwork' as a term which is open to so many interpretations. Reedy (1980) prefers to use the concept of colla-boration to describe those characteristics central to many of the notions of teamwork. Armitage (1983), in writing about primary health care organisations, identifies interprofessional collab-oration as 'the exchange of information between individuals involved in the delivery of primary health care, which has the potential for action in the interests of a common purpose' (Armitage 1983, p. 75). Although this definition focuses on just one aspect of collaboration, namely infor-mation sharing, it is arguably more realistic and useful as something measurable than wool-ly definitions of teamwork.

Table 7.1 A taxonomy of collaboration (From Armitage, 1983)

Stages of collaboration	Definitions
1. Isolation	Members who never meet, talk or write to one another
2. Encounter	Members who encounter or correspond with others but do not interact meaningfully
3. Communication	Members whose encounters or correspondence include the transference of information
4. Collaboration between two agents	Members who act on that information sympathetically; participate in patterns of joint working; subscribe to the same general objectives as others on a one-to-one basis in the same organisation
5. Collaboration throughout an organisation	Organisations in which the work of all members is fully integrated

Armitage goes further than this, in that he identifies a taxonomy of collaboration consisting of five stages (Table 7.1). Although these stages refer only to the level of interaction, it may be possible to use them as signposts to other aspects of interprofessional collaboration. In testing this model Reedy and colleagues found that few primary health care organisations exhibited characteristics of full collaboration (Bond et al 1987, Gregson et al 1991). The measurement of collaboration between district nurses and general practitioners, and health visitors and general practitioners was done by asking respondents to rate their relationship with a colleague from the other profession according to a five-point scale based on the taxonomy of collaboration shown in Table 7.1.

Collaboration in health care organisations is most often an association of unequal partners in which participants are rarely equal in status, prestige or power and, as we have seen, do not necessarily share the same values or goals. As McIntosh and Dingwall (1978) note:

The status of many nurses and health visitors in practice attachments is equivocal. On the one hand they are superficially members of the team, they have direct contact with doctors, and their advice is sought. However, they do suffer a certain subtle, but no less potent, undermining of any aspirations to partnership they may have. If partnerships with doctors exist at all it can best be described as a 'junior partnership' (1978, pp. 130–131).

The British Medical Association's evidence to the Royal Commission on the National Health Service states:

No doctor fails to recognise the necessity of cooperation with the nursing profession and *with other medical workers*. But this does not mean that the doctor should in any way hand over his control of the clinical decisions concerning the treatment of his patient to anyone else or to a group or team. (British Medical Association 1977, p. 303, *our emphasis*)

Although *teams* may exist and *team* conferences are held in hospitals, a clear division of accountability takes place at the consultant level across all medical specialties (Illsley 1980) and, in practice, decisions by doctors continue to be those likely to carry most weight.

Thus although teamwork, or more specifically collaboration, is a dominant ideology of most health care organisations, most doctors will support the view that the doctor should provide leadership. We suspect that a number of other health professionals might also support this ideology; and if there is general support then we must consider how cooperation and consensus work out in practice and its effects on patients. There is growing evidence that in settings where staff perceive greater teamwork, and it is assessed as greater, patient care is more effective (Wilkinson 1991, Knaus et al 1986). However, we need further explanation of the dynamics of relationships between professionals and what processes reduce barriers to real collaboration.

UNDERSTANDING HEALTH CARE ORGANISATIONS

Health care organisations occur in a variety of forms, from a single-handed general practice in rural Sutherland to a large teaching hospital in Central London. However, in this chapter we have suggested that whatever the diversity of size and specific function, health care organisations, like other organisations, exhibit essentially similar characteristics. We have also shown that the physical and social boundaries of organisations do not necessarily coincide. We may have a clear idea about the physical boundary of a hospital, perhaps by the presence of a perimeter fence, but we will have more difficulty in determining its social boundary. Both patients and professionals are part of that particular organisation even though they may not reside within its physical boundaries.

In this chapter we have seen how different sociological perspectives have been used to analyse health care organisations. Systems theory emphasises the formal rules of organisations which guide members' performance of their roles to achieve defined organisational goals. These rules include definitions of organisational goals, definitions of the relative power of members, and rational procedures for identifying methods of achieving organisational goals.

Action theory describes the limitations of this rational-bureaucratic model, emphasising the variability of members' definitions of goals, the way members manipulate the different kinds of power and the variability of methods used to achieve organisational goals.

However, in understanding health care organisations, both perspectives provide useful insights, albeit at different levels of analysis. In attempting to understand the day-to-day routines of an organisation and the processes of conflict and change as they occur at the individual level, action theory and, in particular, negotiated order theory are directly relevant. Together they suggest why different professional ideologies develop and are maintained, why within organisations there is a resistance to innovation and change, but mostly why there is so much variability within and between organisations. Most of these issues are highlighted by our discussion of Hall's study of the introduction of play leaders into two children's wards. Used in this way, action theory illustrates a *microsociological* approach to the study of organisations.

A number of writers, notably Day and Day (1977), have been appreciative, but critical of this microsociological approach. From a *macrosociological* perspective, action theory in general, and the negotiated order theory in particular, fails to explain the ways in which forces external to the organisation do in fact affect the negotiations, relationships, and structures within it. How, for example, are the power relationships which we have identified as being common to most health care organisations contingent on the power relationships of society in general, summarised in our earlier discussion of social stratification (see Ch. 3)? Systems theory too, though to a lesser extent, focuses on the organisation in isolation from the wider social structure. The wider discussion of health care organisations in the context of British society is beyond the scope of this text, although we have indicated in both Chapters 3 and 4 how the social, political and economic structures of society interact to influence health, the maintenance of health and the prevention of illness.

FURTHER READING

Goffman E 1961 Asylums. Essays on the social situation of mental patients and other inmates. Anchor Books, New York

Hall D J 1977 Social relations and innovations: changing the state of play in hospitals. Routledge & Kegan Paul, London

Reed M I 1992 The sociology of organisations: themes, perspectives and prospects. Harvester Wheatsheaf, London

Silverman D 1970 The theory of organisations: a sociological framework. Heinemann, London

Strauss A 1978 Negotiations: varieties, contexts, processes and social order. Jossey-Bass, San Francisco

8

The patient career

INTRODUCTION

Within the life career, most people at one or more times become a patient. Health professionals have little difficulty in recognising what is a 'patient', but we shall show in this chapter that 'patient' can take a number of different meanings. We shall also explore how people become patients, how they adopt the patient role and how they follow a career which is explained by the same kinds of sociological concepts as the life career.

In order to consider patients and their careers, we need first of all to draw on the idea of illness. A great deal is taught to health workers about signs and symptoms which are the diagnostic features of various diseases. Sociologists, however, distinguish between *disease* as a concept, with its origins in medicine, and *illness*, which has a social basis. We say we feel ill, not that we are diseased. Appreciating the social basis of illness is important if we are to understand the behaviour of individuals, patients as well as those with whom they relate, when they are ill, and why different people may behave in very different ways. Why is it that some people with a bad cold retire to bed until it has cleared up while others, with ostensibly the same symptoms, carry on with their work? Why is it that some people who discover a lump in their breast very quickly go to their doctor, while others procrastinate for weeks or months before it is found or they seek help? Sociologists call this *illness behaviour*. We shall examine two contrasting models which have been developed to help explain such differences in behaviour.

WHAT IS A PATIENT?

As members of society, particularly as health care workers, you may think it a little strange and perhaps even trivial that we should ask 'What is a patient?'. How would you answer it? Someone in hospital? Someone receiving medical treatment? Someone attending for a routine chest X-ray or antenatal appointment? Someone suffering pain? These would all be suitable answers, and point to characteristics of some people we would call patients.

When we begin to answer the question in sociological terms the notion of patient becomes less self-evident and, as a result, more useful in analysing the 'patient career' (Fig. 8.1). A recurrent theme has been that sociological enquiry questions many of the taken-for-granted definitions of things, events and actions which occur in our society. We have already noted (in Ch. 5), when discussing definitions of the situation, that people hold different perspectives about social life. It is important, therefore, before proceeding

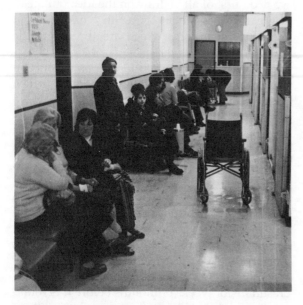

Fig. 8.1 Achieving patient status in a hospital casualty department (courtesy of Nursing Standard).

further that we establish a common sociological notion of 'patient' in relation to some of our taken-for-granted understandings of the term 'patient'.

A patient is someone who receives services from a doctor or other health professional – nurse, dentist, physiotherapist, chiropodist among others. In Britain almost everyone is a patient because, in our system of health care, we register with a general practitioner. Patients are all those currently on a general practitioner's list. This is purely an administrative definition of patient, since all are patients irrespective of whether medical treatment is currently being received or, indeed, has ever been received. In contrast, dentists do not have patient lists. Dentists' patients always receive attention of some description, even if it consists of only an examination to show that there is no need for any other intervention. These administrative definitions and distinctions of what constitutes a general medical practitioner's or a general dental practitioner's patient stems from the different ways that they receive payment for the work that they do. General medical practitioners receive a portion of their income based on the number of people for whom they can be called upon to give treatment, that is, all of those on their list, *whether or not* they receive any treatment. They can supplement this income by carrying out other work on a fee for service basis, for example, carrying out cervical cytology tests on women in the 'at risk' age groups, by providing immunizations, and by attending the birth of a baby in hospital. Dentists, on the other hand, are paid only on the basis of the work that they do, that is, the number of people whom they actually examine or treat.

Someone actually in the process of having medical treatment constitutes a second definition of 'patient'. In the same way, of course, what constitutes treatment is an administrative definition. Social workers, health visitors, nurses, remedial therapists as well as doctors all provide some kind of treatment, although not necessarily medical treatment. Yet social workers call people to whom they provide 'treatment' clients, as do health visitors. Nurses and therapists, like doctors, usually provide 'treatment' to patients, and there is a tendency among nurses who work with people with learning disabilities to call them 'people'.

Medical treatment can only be given by doctors or by people who are under the supervision of a doctor. If we try to define medical treatment we can engage in circular definitions such as 'medical treatment is treatment normally given to patients by doctors'. Such definitions are not necessarily unhelpful, in that they imply that there is a social basis for the administrative definition of what constitutes medical treatment. It is the medical profession with its monopoly of practice which defines the content of medical treatment and regulates who can give it. We return to this subject again briefly in Chapter 11.

Our third taken-for-granted understanding of a patient is someone who bears and suffers pain. Now although many illnesses cause people a certain amount of discomfort, there is no doubt that only a proportion of patients bear or suffer pain. This understanding of the term patient is, therefore, too narrow to be helpful.

How, then, do sociologists explain the labels 'patient' and 'client', applied to different persons by different professionals? In order to understand their explanations we must turn to two important sociological concepts: *labelling* and *deviance*.

LABELLING AND DEVIANCE

The term 'labelling' refers to a social process by which individuals or groups classify the social behaviour of other individuals. In sociology, we are generally interested in understanding the processes by which labelling of particular individuals or groups evolves and the characteristics of the groups which fall within a given label. We include social groups regularly in our conversations – criminals, agnostics, feminists – and we label individuals – old, mad, sexy – in order to classify them. The important thing to note about these examples is that the nouns refer to deviant groups, and the adjectives describe deviant attributes. They imply a shift in some respect or attribute which is away from the normal and valued attributes of the society. In the same way a state of health is the norm and is valued by society while illness is deviance from the norm.

Everyone experiences deviance at some time in their lives and what constitutes deviance varies over time. Attending a funeral without a black tie or turning up to a wedding in a pair of jeans are examples of acts which are considered less deviant today than they were some years ago. In pluralistic societies – societies in which different social groups preserve their own customs and rules – the distinction between deviant and nondeviant behaviour is blurred. In British society it is now quite common and regarded as normal for couples to have sexual relationships outside marriage, yet for many religious groups this remains an immoral arrangement. Thus, for a large proportion of the population this behaviour is not deviant but for others it would be considered a deviant act.

There is general agreement that 'deviance always refers to conduct that is a violation of the rules constructed by a given society or group' (Berger & Berger 1976). Deviance is therefore a matter of social definition. Sociologists have identified two types of deviance: primary and secondary (Lemert 1964).

Primary deviance

Whether a given label will have meaning within a social group will depend on whether that label is permanent and this, in turn, will depend a great deal on whether the person applying the label has the authority to do so. For example, if a man is labelled mentally ill by his spouse or his lawyer this may not be accepted by others in society until a psychiatrist has legitimised this label by diagnosing the behaviour of this individual as clinical depression, or whatever. Legitimisation may not occur until he has been referred to a psychiatrist which reinforces that he is indeed mentally ill.

Another example of primary deviance concerns the person seeking a sick note from the

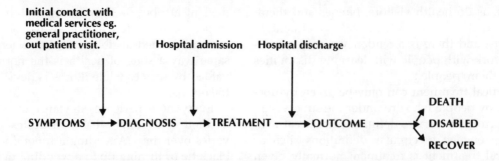

Fig. 8.2 The patient career.

general practitioner. In order that they will receive sickness benefit, or continue receiving their wages or salaries, the Department of Social Security requires that sick people off work for more than one week have their deviant status of being a sick person legitimised by their general practitioner signing the appropriate forms.

Secondary deviance

One of the important features of labelling is the *effect* it has on both the person being labelled and other people around them. We call this secondary deviance, to distinguish it from the attributes which initially triggered the label. Being given a label is likely to affect the way the individual behaves with others. In time, he or she is likely to come to act the role which the new label implies because of the way others have behaved towards her or him, the possessor of the label. For example, if we start to call elderly relatives 'senile' and, perhaps more important, to treat them as if they are senile, it is amazing how quickly they begin to behave in somewhat bizarre ways. This process is sometimes called a 'self-fulfilling prophecy'.

As the above example shows, secondary deviance can have negative effects. This is well illustrated by Goffman (1968) in his book, *Stigma – Notes on the Management of Spoiled Identity*. Goffman shows that certain categories of patient, once labelled, become stigmatised and that the effect of this stigma is to reinforce the deviant behaviour of such patients. This helps to explain why in psychiatric settings patients labelled as 'violent' and responded to in particular ways may exhibit more rather than fewer violent episodes, and why patients in general hospitals labelled as 'demanding' are responded to in such a manner that their 'demanding' behaviour is perpetuated. We return to the concept of stigma again in the next chapter, when we consider how labelling patients influences interaction with them.

We are now in a better position to answer our initial question: What is a patient? We have seen that we use the labelling process to categorise people. Being ill is a form of deviance. People who are ill, and who are diagnosed as ill by doctors, are given the label 'patient'.

Similarly being poor, living in a single-parent household, or experiencing social problems are all forms of deviance. In these cases it is the social worker, among others, who legitimates this status by giving the status of 'client'. As we have tried to show, such labelling processes are essentially arbitrary and are also essentially social.

BECOMING A PATIENT

In describing a life career we introduced the reader to Weber's notion of *ideal type* (Ch. 5). The patient career is a similar ideal type; and it most closely approximates the experience of people entering hospital.

The notion of patient career owes a great deal to the work of Goffman (1961). The value of the concept, as Goffman describes it, is that it has two sides. One concerns the private side of the individual concerning the patient's feelings, image of self and felt identity. The other relates to the patient's public image reflected in her or his status, life-style and relationships with others. Goffman writes of the '*moral career*' of the mental patient, that is, the regular sequences of changes that occur in people's private images of themselves and those changes which affect their public images in the course of becoming psychiatric patients. He describes the moral career of a patient as a series of *status passages* through initial identification of symptoms, diagnosis, treatment and outcome. Although the model described by Goffman is of psychiatric patients, there are close parallels with long-stay patients in nonpsychiatric hospitals and, to a lesser extent, shorter-stay patients. Following Goffman, our ideal type of patient career is shown in Figure 8.2.

The concept of the patient career illustrated in Figure 8.2 is not the average patient career, nor indeed the best, but an ideal type. We consider that this very simple model of progression through symptom identification, diagnosis, treatment and outcome illustrates the variety of patient careers. As with some other aspects of the life career, some patients will pass the career milestones of symptoms, treatment, diagnosis and outcome on a number of occasions. In some instances some of these milestones may be omitted: for some patients symptoms like abdominal pain will be treated without a diagnosis ever being made, while for others symptoms will be identified and the patient will die or recover without a diagnosis being made or treatment being given. Patients with chronic illness will have extremely complex careers.

As patients follow their individual careers they will perceive a change in their public images – in their statuses and roles – and will privately reassess their self-image to match the changing status. For example, the middle-aged man who seeks medical attention because of mild chest pains, may alter his self-image of a youthful squash player to that of invalid if a doctor signs him off work as sick because of heart trouble. As Goffman describes for the psychiatric patient, this process of reassessment will not necessarily take place simultaneously with the person's changing role or status. It may take time and, as in the life career, it happens through a process of socialisation.

Patient socialisation

How does a person with signs and symptoms become a patient? In the context of the hospital, becoming a patient entails behaving differently from how one would behave in other settings. Sometimes it entails removing outdoor clothes and wearing night attire. New patients learn the role and expected status of patients within the particular ward. It may be different from some other wards in which they have spent some time. If they are to obtain information about their condition they must learn who to ask, when to ask and how to ask. Some patients leave behind their adult independence and ask, for example, if they may make a telephone call or take a bath. If they exert their usual degree of independence and take their own medication, on the other hand, they may receive a reprimand from the staff. The role of patient, like other roles in life, has to be learned. This is achieved by talking with other patients and observing how they behave, as well as being explicitly taught and controlled in certain ways by hospital staff. Patients learn very quickly where you can smoke, when it is most appropriate to ask for a bedpan and when are the best times to have a word with sister. In other words, new patients are socialised into their role as patient.

The process of learning the role of patient is well illustrated by Goffman (1961). In his essay,

The Moral Career of a Mental Patient, Goffman is concerned with the processes by which patients reassess their self-image and, in particular, he draws attention to the ways in which patients distinguish between right and wrong ways to behave. Goffman follows the career of psychiatric patients through the process of *institutionalisation*. That is a process by which patients lose autonomy and function completely within and are dependent upon the institution in which they live. When patients become *institutionalised*, when they learn to conform to the rules and routines of the institution, they will lose their 'old' self and obtain a new institutionalised identity. Not only will their public image conform to the institution's routines for eating, sleeping, relaxing, working and bathing, for example, but also the private self-image will conform eventually to this public image.

On entry to hospital some patients refuse to accept that their roles have changed. They may avoid talking with other patients, regarding themselves as different, and they may respond to hospital staff in a manner different from that of other patients, and begin to act more like other patients in patient groups as well as with doctors and nurses. New patients may gradually accompany other patients to the cafeteria to spend some time talking, smoking and drinking tea rather than spending the time alone in the ward or garden. Instead of sitting back and waiting for their names to be called to receive their medication, or waiting for it to be brought to them by a nurse, they join the queue in the ward with other patients at the usual times.

While engaging in this behaviour, however, they may still attempt to withdraw from the patient role in other ways. For example, the businessman waiting for a routine operation or recovering from a heart attack may attempt to continue working while in hospital. In the psychiatric hospital Goffman observed that patients would continue to use nicknames they had earned in 'outside' life and to use the 'cover' address tactfully provided by some psychiatric hospitals, since admitting to being a mental

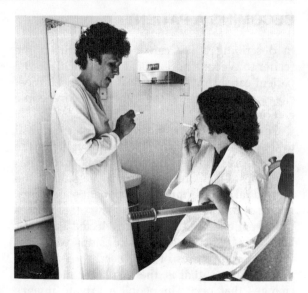

Fig. 8.3   Deviant patients (courtesy of Rik Walton).

patient would be socially stigmatising and contradictory to their own self-image.

In time new patients begin to realise that they are really no different from other patients. Irrespective of other roles in life – plumbers, mothers, fathers, teachers – all act similarly as patients. There is a common core to the patient role – and as with all roles, there are acceptable and less acceptable ways of acting it. The process of adapting or being socialised into the role of patient involves beginning to accept restrictions of freedom and movement, to accept communal living arrangements and to conform to ward routines. These become normal as opposed to alien experiences of the patient's new social status. A good literary example of socialisation into the patient role is described in *Cancer Ward* (Solzhenitsyn 1971). Of course, some patients never learn to act the correct patient role as defined by other patients and also by professionals – they become part of a deviant subculture inside the wider patient culture of the hospital. Anyone who has read or seen *One Flew Over The Cuckoo's Nest* (Kesey 1973) will very readily recognise this (Fig. 8.3).

We have described how patients become socialised into the patient role and, in extreme circumstances, some patients become 'institutionalised'. This presents a problem when attempts are made to rehabilitate long-stay patients from hospitals for the mentally handicapped or mentally ill. These patients need to adopt new private and public images through similar processes; they must unlearn their patient role and associated behaviours and become resocialised into a more adaptive and socially appropriate role in the community.

HEALTH AND ILLNESS

In the context of an ideal type of patient career people become patients because they are ill. Illness and health or wellness are aspects of everyday life, which occur at opposite ends of a continuum. Where people are located on that continuum depends very much on what they themselves perceive as health and illness and what others, particularly doctors, also perceive. Illness, like health (see Ch. 6), is differently defined by different people.

A simple distinction we need to make here is between *illness* and *disease*. Disease refers to a medical concept of pathology, which is indicated by a group of signs and symptoms. The presence or absence of a disease, as indicated by signs and symptoms, is clinically defined by the medical profession. Doctors or their substitutes, using a common body of knowledge, make the decision as to whether or not a person has a disease. In contrast, illness is defined by the person who had the signs and symptoms. It refers primarily to a person's subjective experience of 'health' and 'ill-health' and is indicated by the person's reactions to the symptoms; such reactions include stopping eating, staying off work, going to bed and taking pills. If two or more people are defining the situation in the case of a particular set of signs and symptoms – 'the patient' and 'the doctor' – it follows that some people can feel ill without having a disease, while others will have a disease without feeling ill. We can illustrate this diagrammatically as shown in Figure 8.4.

Sometimes the two definitions of the situation will coincide – when the individual and the medical practitioner agree that the person is well, and when they agree that the person is unwell and has a disease. On other occasions disparities arise. The individual may go to the doctor feeling unwell but the doctor may find no reason for this and, while remedies may be prescribed, the patient is not classified as diseased. The individual may also feel perfectly well but at a routine examination a very high blood pressure may be discovered together with changes in the optic discs, indicating hypertensive disease. Medication is prescribed and the patient is faced with adjusting to a serious chronic condition about which nothing was known.

In this distinction between what Western medicine calls disease and what lay people call illness we have emphasised that different definitions of phenomena – signs and symptoms – can exist within the same culture. Between cultures definitions of what constitutes illness and disease can differ markedly. A commonly cited example is that of a South American tribe where a certain facially disfiguring skin disease is so common that it is those members of the tribe without the disease who are considered 'abnormal' or diseased, and who seek treatment from the local medicine man. We therefore emphasise that definitions of disease and illness are socially determined. In this country there was a time when people sought help from their priest for particular problems rather than from a doctor; this indicates a historical shift in definitions of what constitutes illness and treatment.

ILLNESS BEHAVIOUR

Epidemiological and social research have shown that many people with signs and symptoms do not obtain professional advice and treatment. For example, Dunnell and Cartwright (1972), in their study of medicine-taking, found that fewer than 1-in-5 people who reported symptoms to their interviewers had consulted their general practitioner about them. Hannay (1979), in a study of symptom prevalence, found that two in every three physical symptoms were not

		Medically identified signs and symptoms	
		NO	YES
Signs and symptoms identified by subject and interpreted as 'abnormal'	NO	WELL	WELL BUT DISEASED
	YES	UNWELL	UNWELL AND DISEASED

Fig. 8.4   Relationship between disease and illness

reported to the general practitioner. A number of studies of chronic physical and psychiatric illnesses have shown consistently that for every person with a particular disorder and receiving some kind of treatment from medical services, one or more people exist with the same disorder who are not receiving treatment. Williamson and colleagues (1964), in a seminal work about the unmet medical needs of old people, reported that 58% of their sample had disabilities unknown to the doctor. Brown and Harris (1978) have shown that of 69 women who were suffering from a definitive affective psychiatric disorder in the 3 months prior to being interviewed in their survey, only four had received psychiatric care during the previous year, and almost half were not being treated by a general practitioner. Why is it that some people with particular objectively defined symptoms consult doctors or other health professionals, while others do not? The concept which helps us explain this phenomenon is *illness behaviour*.

Illness behaviour is concerned with those social factors which affect definitions of health and illness and which influence, among other things, the demands people make for medical care. The term was first coined by Mechanic (1962) who defined illness behaviour as 'the way in which symptoms may be differentially per-

ceived, evaluated and acted upon by different kinds of persons'. In other words, illness behaviour is about the social factors which influence the way individuals view signs and symptoms, and the kinds of action engaged in to deal with them. Individuals may recognise signs and symptoms as a medical problem, but they may or may not choose to ignore them, or they may or may not deal with the problem without seeking formal medical care. What are the social factors which influence the use of medical services?

A number of British studies have identified some broad characteristics of people in the four categories shown in Figure 8.4. They have looked at the social characteristics of users of different health services such as general practitioners, outpatient, hospital and antenatal services (Cartwright 1967, McKinlay & McKinlay 1972, 1979, Cartwright et al 1973, Robinson 1973, Cartwright & Anderson 1979). Common social factors were found to be associated with the use of services; for example, age, gender, marital status, social class, religion, employment status and education are all associated with health service utilisation. We know that middle-aged women visit their general practitioner more often than younger women, and more often than younger and middle-aged men (McCormick et al 1990). Working-class people make less use of dental services than their middle-class counterparts (Gray et al 1970) (see Ch. 3).

These studies have shown that the use of medical services is associated with certain social characteristics; in other words, they tell us which kind of person is most likely to use the different services. However, they throw little light on *why* it is that people do or do not use the various medical services. This has implications for policy makers. It is only by establishing these reasons and explaining the differences that policy decisions can be influenced in an attempt to alter the utilisation of services by groups 'at risk' from health problems.

EXPLANATIONS OF ILLNESS BEHAVIOUR

A number of writers have devised conceptual models to help in our understanding of illness behaviour. Many are fairly similar, but we have selected two contrasting models to illustrate not only the complexity of illness behaviour but also the variation in sociological perspectives which have been used to study it. Broadly speaking, these two models are representative of the structuralist and the interactionist approaches in sociology.

A structuralist approach

The first model is taken from a review article by Kasl and Cobb (1966a). The model was developed using the findings from a large number of studies, mainly from the United States, to explain why individuals do or do not go to the doctor with their symptoms. Their model is presented schematically in Figure 8.5.

Kasl and Cobb have listed in the top left-hand corner a number of characteristics of individuals, which have been shown in earlier research to be associated with illness behaviour and with psychological distress, perceptions about the value of seeing a doctor and perceptions about the threat of disease indicated by symptoms. In this scheme it is assumed that if people regard symptoms as a threat and they believe that a visit to the doctor will be of some

benefit, then they are more likely to seek medical aid than those people who, for example, perceive a visit to the doctor to be of little value. The model identifies a number of factors which might affect people's perceptions about the threat of disease and about the value of different actions.

The first factor identified is psychological distress. People react in different ways to symptoms. Many can cause distress, which will mediate a person's way of looking at the threat of disease. For example, two women both find lumps in their breasts. Both might consider that they could be malignant. One may immediately seek medical aid while the other delays, not wishing to confirm whether the lump is indeed malignant. Research has shown that psychological distress in response to symptoms varies according to the characteristics of individuals as listed in the top left of the diagram.

The other mediating factors identified in the model relate to the perceived value of action. The cost to people of seeking medical care in terms of loss of earnings, loss of leisure time, cost of travelling, for example, or the previous

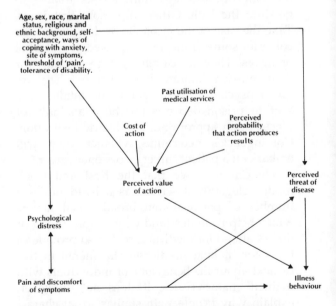

Fig. 8.5 The postulated relationship between symptoms and illness behaviour (Adapted from Kasl & Cobb 1966).

experience of seeking help and the perceived probability that seeking medical aid will have any effect on the symptoms, are all factors which individuals may take into account when deciding whether to take their symptoms to the doctor.

The approach to illness behaviour which Kasl and Cobb's model represents has been used most often to explain the use of services by different social groups in society. However, illness behaviour takes many forms apart from this. To ignore symptoms is a form of illness behaviour just as going to bed without seeking any professional help is equally illness behaviour. The particular form of behaviour engaged in depends on the individual's perception and definition of the situation. A number of writers have identified what Goffman (1961) terms *career contingencies* triggering mechanisms to describe the influences that social factors have on illness behaviour. The person due to start a new job ignores today the symptoms which last week or next week would have kept her or him off work. Some career contingencies are inevitable. For example, the old lady with rheumatism ignores the pains in her legs until she is unable to get into the bath. Others are more fortuitous. Take the case of the alcoholic or drug user who commits some crime in their need for alcohol or drugs. They are caught and go to court for their misdemeanours, but whether they are given psychiatric treatment in hospital or are sent to prison depends on the availability of places in an appropriate psychiatric institution. Contingencies determine whether they will embark on a patient career or prisoner career.

We can now see that the Kasl and Cobb model, elegantly described as it is, identifies a number of personal and broad social factors which help us understand why people attend or do not attend for medical care. It also provides a basis for making predictive statements in this context about the behaviour of individuals with defined characteristics. It does not, however, explain why people with similar social characteristics respond differently to similar signs and symptoms.

An interactionist approach

In contrast Dingwall (1976) provides an interactionist perspective on the study of illness behaviour. Unlike the previous model, which draws on a large number of studies, Dingwall supports his *Illness Action Model* with empirical data from only four substantive studies – on psychoactive drugs (Becker 1967), poliomyelitis (Davis 1963), myocardial infarction (Cowie, 1976) and childbirth (Dick-Read 1958). This does not, in our view, limit the usefulness of his model, which is illustrated in Figure 8.6.

The first thing to note about Dingwall's model is that some of the terminology is different. The title refers to *illness action* rather than *illness behaviour*. What at first reading might appear to be a trivial difference is in fact a crucial distinction between the structuralist and interactionist perspectives. We refer the reader back to Chapter 2, in which we discussed the distinction between *behaviour* and *action*. Behaviour, as we said, implies an automatic reaction to a given stimulus whereas action involves notions of intentions or purpose stemming from within individuals. People, therefore, make choices about if and how they will respond, and the complex array of possible outcomes is included in the model.

Let us now work through this rather complex model which, you will note, has no beginning or end – it forms a loop. We will begin at the left-hand side and explore some of its components.

We immediately come across a second terminological difference from the first model. Instead of talking about signs and symptoms Dingwall refers to disturbance – meaning *disturbance of equilibrium* – as the initiating phenomenon. Three main types of disturbance of equilibrium can be identified. These are symptoms, changes in the individual's lay health knowledge and the identification of signs of disease through routine screening.

Recognising disturbance by symptoms indicates awareness of some abnormal state for this individual. It could refer to symptoms like backache, heartburn or blood loss but the important

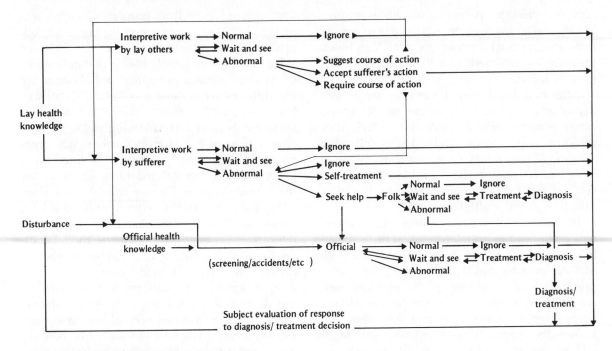

Fig. 8.6   Illness Action Model (Dingwall 1976).

feature is that the individual interprets this as abnormal for him. Therefore the normally office-bound man who has spent the previous day enthusiastically digging his garden only to find that he has a stiff back would feel discomfort but would probably not define his condition as abnormal, and would continue his usual life-style. However, if his discomfort continues for longer than he thinks it should, then there is a disturbance in his equilibrium which will prompt some kind of action.

The onset of symptoms need not be a sudden event. In fact, symptoms may be present for some time, but it is not until the pain becomes so severe that we cannot walk or the headache so intense that we can no longer concentrate that the disturbance of equilibrium is sufficient to influence the course of action.

Whereas symptoms may be a triggering mechanism in many acute illnesses, this will not necessarily be the case for chronic illnesses, where symptoms in the usual sense of the

word are a constant feature of the person's life. What tends to happen is that the ill patient who has a chronic condition, for instance, the man with obstructive airway disease, comes to perceive his morning cough, sputum and breathlessness as normal for him. When this 'normality' is disturbed and there is an exacerbation of bronchitis the individual can follow the pathways through the *Illness Action Model*. He has perceived a disturbance from his own equilibrium.

The second form of disturbance, changes in the individual's lay health knowledge, can come about through watching a television documentary about the dangers of asbestos, for instance, or through reading an article on the harmful outcomes of gross obesity. Disturbance is therefore created by the individual reevaluating the significance of symptoms, which in turn leads to some form of action.

The third type of disturbance comes about after some asymptomatic disease has been discovered through participation in a routine health check. The woman who is discovered to have an abnormal cervical smear or high blood pressure is informed and this leads to some form of action.

After individuals have become aware of their disturbance in equilibrium, the model shows three possible parallel pathways which they could follow. Some individuals following screening or accidents, for example, will already be in contact with medical services, without the sufferer being able to make decisions. Dingwall calls this official health knowledge.

In most situations, however, the disturbance will lead to an interpretation of its meaning by the sufferers within the framework of their own lay health knowledge. This interpretation will be influenced by previous personal experiences of a similar condition, knowledge of others with that condition and knowledge gained through reading newspaper and magazine articles or listening to radio or television documentaries. At the same time, the interpretation of the disturbance by significant others such as a spouse or friend may be sought and this may also influence the actions of the individual.

The result of the interpretation produces in each case three possible outcomes.

One of the recurrent possibilities we see throughout this model is to wait and see what happens. No judgement need be made immediately. It is not unusual in everyday life to delay and wait and see what develops before we act. For example, we tend to wait to see whether a headache develops and persists before resorting to analgesics. Of course, what is important to note is that we all make such judgements differently, using different health knowledge and experiences. In the above example what constitutes a headache for the individual concerned would become a central question. During this waiting time the nature of the disturbance will be reappraised; hence there are arrows in two directions in the model to indicate this.

The other ways of interpreting the disturbance are to define it as normal or as abnormal.

The sufferer, as well as significant others, will engage in forming these conclusions, and folk medicine and official medicine do likewise. What is important to note here is that definitions of what constitutes normality and abnormality can differ between those involved. If the disturbance is defined as normal then it is ignored by everyone. Should early morning sickness occur after a woman has learned she is newly pregnant, then this would be likely to be interpreted by everyone as normal and to be ignored after the episode is over. Each of the interpretations as normal lead straight to the right-hand side of the model. If, on the other hand, a disturbance is interpreted as abnormal, then the model indicates a number of different outcomes for each of the groups which may be involved.

If we focus on the sufferers we see that they can do one of three things: ignore the disturbance, engage in some sort of self-treatment, such as taking an aspirin, or seek help. There are two sources from which help may be sought – from traditional medical services or from *folk* or *alternative medicine*. A good example of folk medicine was the granny midwife, who used to help local women in childbirth. Homoeopathic clinics, osteopaths and those who practice acupuncture are examples of alternative medicine. Individuals providing traditional, folk or alternative medicine will make their own interpretations of the disturbance and act accordingly. If they regard it as abnormal, then diagnosis and treatment will follow. This takes us to the bottom right of the model.

Once an episode of disturbance is complete, and remembering that this may take from minutes to months to accomplish, sufferers will engage in a reevaluation of the disturbance, informed by their evaluation of the diagnosis and treatment decisions. If all is well, the outcome will be a reestablishment of the original equilibrium from which the disturbance was first noted, and the individuals will return to their own normality. Depending on the nature of the disturbance, however, the original equilibrium may never be regained, and sufferers may come to redefine a new equilibrium as normal. The man who had originally thought himself perfectly well, but who suffers a coronary thrombosis necessitating a change in lifestyle and life-long medication, will redefine his equilibrium and this will influence any future episodes of disturbance and their interpretation. Less dramatically, hill walkers who one day cannot reach their favourite summit will redefine their health status and act accordingly. The model, therefore, is circular and demonstrates how past experiences, as they are subjectively interpreted and acted upon, will influence future actions.

Appreciating the subjectivity of interpretation of health, illness and action, and regarding the origin as a definition of disturbance rather than imposing the notion of symptoms which are defined through medical knowledge, provides for a less rigid approach to the study of illness behaviour.

We have discussed these two models at some length and attempted to show that while they provide different interpretations and explanations of illness behaviour, they both demonstrate that illness behaviour can only be understood by looking at it within its social context. To ignore the social realities of an individual's situation is to misunderstand the meaning of an illness to that individual.

Illness is, therefore, both a biological and a social event. It involves changes in both biological function as a result of disease and changes in social function: changes in behaviour and changes in a person's relationship with others. We can now see that people seek medical care and become patients, not because they have a disease, but because of the social response to that disease, as it is defined and dealt with by them. Being ill or being a patient refers not only to a clinical or biological state but also to a social position or role.

THE SICK ROLE

Being a patient implies that you are ill. Parsons (1951) developed the concept of the *sick role* to describe the expectations of people in a society which defines the rights and duties of its members who are sick. Like any of the other social roles we have mentioned adopting the sick role requires cooperation and recognition of that role from all of those around us. The behaviour of sick people and the behaviour of others around them must conform to the particular pattern of expectations that adhere to the sick role.

In his analysis of the sick role, Parsons identified four principal elements. Two of these elements represent the rights and the other two elements the obligations associated with the sick role. The first right that the sick person, that is, the one occupying the sick role, can claim is the exemption from normal activities and responsibilities. Being off work, staying at home in the evenings instead of going out and being relieved of domestic chores are exemptions which some sick people achieve. Sick women often have more difficulty in obtaining these rights, since domestic work might have to be continued whereas employment outside the home would not.

It is clear from our earlier discussions that adoption of the sick role, being ill, will not be directly related to any objective or subjective assessment of symptom severity. The variability of these play some part, but what we have already described as career contingencies interfere with such an apparently straightforward relationship. Claiming the rights of the sick role is also contingency dependent. If there is no one else there to feed the baby, the woman with 'flu will struggle to do it despite feeling extremely ill.

The second right which Parsons identifies that the sick person can expect, is assistance from or dependency on others. Sick leave and other welfare practices are society's recognition of the special status of illness. Similarly, the assistance given by relatives and friends at a time of illness is recognition of the sick role, as is admission to hospital or attendance by nurses at home. While the individuals can lay claim to these rights, they must also meet obligations.

The first of the obligations associated with the sick role is that the incumbent should want to get better and to get out of the sick role as soon as possible. At times we may have come across someone whom we regard as clinging to the sick role for longer than we think is appropriate; the patient appears not to want to get better, wants to linger in bed or in hospital or wants to deter resuming normal activities for a period longer than the time normally regarded as acceptable for a particular condition. They are not meeting their obligations.

At this stage it is necessary to identify one of the difficulties of Parsons' analysis, one which we have already discussed in terms of Dingwall's use of the term normality, that is the difference between acute and chronic illness. When we are ill we all, generally, want to get better. To this extent we should be conforming to the expectations of the sick role. However, for most chronic conditions, by definition, there is no getting better in absolute terms.

The second obligation of the sick role which Parsons identifies is that the sick person should not only try to get better but should do so by acting in an appropriate manner: staying in bed as necessary or seeking medical care when required. Leaving aside the problem of the person with a chronic illness, the major difficulty with this obligation is that there are at least two perspectives as to how to define what is appropriate behaviour. As Dingwall's *Illness Action Model* implies, the sick person, other lay people and the doctor may well hold different views about the relevance or appropriateness of specific treatments. The woman with an arthritic hip may decide to attend a homoeopathic clinic and use their remedies, while her family may know of an osteopath with a very good reputation in dealing with 'hips' and the orthopaedic surgeon representing official medical knowledge may consider that the only effective treatment would be hip replacement. Who is to say what is appropriate?

As an ideal type the *sick role* is particularly useful in providing an insight into the way an individual is expected to behave in the face of acute illness. It is less useful when considering chronic illness or disability. Many writers consider that the concept has been over-used (Mechanic 1978) and to some extent it has become a term used by health professionals to label certain categories of patients. From the perspective of labelling theory, playing or being in the sick role becomes the label we use for groups of patients who are 'normally' ill, i.e. acutely ill. We reserve labels like 'cripple', 'geriatric', or 'alcoholic' for people with chronic illnesses or disabilities. However, as an ideal type, the sick role is useful in helping us understand some characteristics of the patient career.

SUMMARY

In this chapter we have focused on some of the issues which influence how we regard patients, health and illness. The meanings that these terms hold have been explored in some detail to show that they are socially defined and can differ in meaning according to various cultures and subcultures, education, age, gender and social origins. This helps us to understand more clearly the World Health Organization's definition of health which is 'the state of complete physical, mental and social well-being and not merely the absence of disease and infirmity' (WHO 1983, p. 1). Health is not an absolute state of affairs. Rather it is a variable status between different countries, cultures and social groups. This definition is also noteworthy since, as well as physical and mental well-being, health includes a social component. This very broad definition of health clearly implies that it is not the prerogative of medicine to define health, just as we have shown that illness is not medically defined. Being ill and subsequent behaviour depends on how we regard and are influenced by our own particular circumstances.

Equally, how health care professionals regard patients and illness is determined by their own experiences, and to the extent that these differ from those of their patients, so interpretations will differ. Health care professionals deal with illness for much of their working time and come to make assumptions about patients and patient behaviour. They may come to forget that while they regard tests or procedures as routine, they are new and can be frightening to patients, and their beliefs about the reason for a patient's behaviour may be totally alien to the patient's own explanation. Therefore, if health care professionals are to understand their patients – why they discontinue breast feeding within a few weeks, fail to bring children for immunization, wish to discharge themselves from hospital, do not practice their exercises – it is necessary to find out the patient's version of events rather than impose their own views.

In understanding the concept of patient career we note that people coming into hospital have to learn how to become patients, indeed how to become good patients if they want a smooth passage. Simply becoming a patient involves an interactive process between people and their social and physical environments. Understanding how this comes about and some of its implications will be examined in further detail when we consider staff-patient interaction in Chapter 9 and death and dying in Chapter 10.

Another useful way of incorporating patient career into ideas about professional practice is to consider the organisation of care from the patient's perspective rather than from the perspective of a single form of care-giving organisation. Patients may follow extremely complex career pathways, being treated by different doctors, nurses and various kinds of therapists, not only in different hospitals as well as at home but also even in different wards and departments within a single hospital. With conditions like rheumatic disease or cancer, the career can extend over many years and involve many different care givers. By focusing on the patient and the continuous nature of the career rather than on discrete elements within it, this may provide for a more rational and cohesive way of planning and delivering care. This idea is now gaining prominence through care management (Challis & Davies 1986) and having key workers or care managers to coordinate care.

FURTHER READING

Dingwall R 1976 Aspects of illness. Martin Robertson, London

9

Interaction with patients

INTRODUCTION

In this chapter we focus on relationships between patients or clients and health professionals. The investigation of relationships through types and processes of interaction has proven to be a fruitful area for sociological research and reflects the importance attached to this aspect of the work of all health professionals. Ellis (1980) includes nursing as one of the 'interpersonal professions' whose 'primary method is face-to-face interaction and whose repertoire of professional skills would therefore be interpersonal in nature' (Ellis 1988, p. 44).

We begin by discussing some aspects of the basis of relationships between nurses and patients, which leads to a discussion of aspects of professional and client interactions, and how these may be very similar but also vary in relation to time, place and context. Important here are the roles played by participants and we introduce another of Goffman's ideas, namely that *frames* provide structure and meaning for social interaction. Professional client interaction can also be viewed as negotiation, the same process that may be used as one aspect of interactions between different professionals within an organisation (see Chs 7 and 11).

The inevitability of patient classification or typification is then explored in relation to understanding the distinction between 'good' and 'bad' patients and the effects of typification on the way staff frame their interactions with patients. Also relevant to this are definitions of work itself and effects on patient outcomes. Particular attention is given to the way nurses deal with patients classified as neurotic. Finally, an extended example of pain work is used to describe the way professionals, especially nurses, manage interaction with patients.

RELATIONSHIPS BETWEEN CLIENTS AND PROFESSIONALS

The term 'relationship' does nothing more than indicate the relative position of two objects in time and space or in a classification system. When we consider social relationships, we refer to situations in which two or more persons are involved and in which 'in its meaningful context, the action of each takes into account that of the other and is oriented in these terms' (Parsons 1937). This implies that the participants have some understanding of each others' behaviour and act in ways that take this into account. In order to do this, participants have expectations about each other which influence the particular forms actions will take. Sociologists are concerned with the social positions that participants occupy and the roles they act. This concern includes the relative social positions of professional and client.

One of Goffman's contributions has been to provide an analysis of how social actions proceed by conceiving them as ongoing within particular kinds of *frame*. In his book, *Frame Analysis* (1974), Goffman's central concern is with trying to analyse the basis of our social experience. In order to achieve this Goffman suggests that we rely on a number of primary frameworks each of which 'allows its user to locate, perceive, identify and label a seemingly infinite number of complete occurrences defined in its terms' (1974, p. 21). When we attend a doctor's surgery we are likely to behave in a fashion which is framed or structured by those we meet there – the receptionist, the doctor or practice nurse – and our own shared view of the form of this kind of interaction. Frame therefore can be regarded as providing a basic anticipated structure for interactions but, simultaneously, the actors also negotiate and structure the meaning of their

experience – that is, you and your doctor interpret what is going on, interact taking this into account, and achieve a level of intersubjective communication because of the frame in which you are operating. The extent to which frames are shared will influence the perceived smoothness of the meeting. Important here is that a good deal of our activity is reflexive; our understanding of what our activities mean depends on understandings gained from other bits of behaviour, by ourselves and the other actors in the surgery, or the same behaviour under different conditions – in the supermarket and railway station – for which we have established a sense of likely effects. In this way, having frames provides a means of attending to and interpreting social experiences as well as providing a structure and definition for them. Accordingly social behaviour can proceed.

Goffman describes different kinds of framing and ways of moving out of existing primary social frameworks, which provide a background understanding for events. For example, we generally know when a fight is a fight and when fighting is really playing at it. As social products, we are generally adept at constituting what we see in accordance with the framework that officially applies. Goffman uses the example of the right of medical personnel to approach the human naked body and the special efforts taken to infuse procedures with terms and actions which keep sexual readings of the interaction in check. Others have also reported the difficulty of keeping the sexual implications of mouth-to-mouth contact for the purposes of resuscitation out of practice sessions. Lawler (1991) graphically described how nurses go about accomplishing body work. The human body and touching it is but one relevant feature of different kinds of primary frame and we must rely on our interpretative competency to distinguish its particular meaning and act appropriately. Needless to say, each frame we encounter will comprise a host of different features.

Important too is the notion of distinctiveness. We regularly hear phrases like 'the doctor or nurse-patient relationship' or 'client-therapist relationship'. This implies that the special relationship a person has with her or his doctor is different from the special relationship with her or his therapist, which is again different from that with her or his spouse or her or his milkman or the person on the checkout at the supermarket. But is the relationship between nurse X and patient A the same as nurse X and patient B, C, D, E, F, etc. or between nurses W, Y, Z etc. and patient A? Goffman draws a distinction between the *person* or individual participating and the *particular role* that the person realises during the interaction. There is therefore a person-role formula, insofar as there is neither complete freedom between the individual and the role they are in nor complete constraint. To every encounter nurse X will bring self, X, and role, nurse. The components of X and nurse will vary depending upon the frame, one component of which is the patient A, B, or C, etc. and their distinctive person plus role formula.

The particular roles that individuals are permitted to perform, however, say in a nurse-patient encounter, are socially defined and limited. There are questions about role rights and obligations, that is, the right to participate in the application of a particular frame, but also about character rights – the right to participate in that role in a particular way. We have discussed these issues of rights and obligations in Chapter 8 in relation to the patient career.

The nature of relationships between health professionals and patients will have certain aspects in common because of the roles of participants, but they will also vary to some extent because of how the participants characterise that role as well as the personal elements which are added to it. There will also be situational variations, and nurses working in a patient's home or in a residential home will behave differently from the way they do in an acute hospital. However, frames will also vary depending on features like the degree of autonomy of the professional, the awareness contexts pertaining (see Ch. 10) and prevailing ideologies regarding power and position.

The construction of nurse-patient relationships

Armstrong (1983) contends that while the word 'relationship' may have remained unaltered over time, the actual form and nature of the relationship between patients and nurses had undergone a fundamental reformulation since the 1970s in general nursing and rather earlier in psychiatric nursing. His analysis is based on an examination of what has been written about nurse-patient relationships in popular nursing text books which 'attempt to distil the essence of nursing for the benefit of the student' (Armstrong 1983, p. 457).

Contrasting the position in the late 1960s with that portrayed in the early 1980s, the nature of what is implied in nurse-patient relationships changes dramatically. His analysis begins earlier, however, drawing on the writing of Foucault (1973). Foucault's thesis is that traditional perceptions of the patient as a discrete analysable, passive body did not emerge in medicine until the end of the 18th century when various techniques were developed by which to explore the human body. Despite the apparent biological entity which constitutes the body it, like other social phenomena, is socially constructed by virtue of social practices and techniques of analysis. Foucault further identifies the body as having an objective and individual status developed contemporaneously in a variant of institutional settings – schools, prisons, workshops and barracks as well as hospitals – which were emerging at the same time as medical theories of localised pathology. In Nightingale's *Notes on Nursing* (1859) about a century later, emphasis was given to the physical environment in which the patient's body was nursed, together with careful and accurate observation of it. The patient thus became objectified within these physical and physiological realities.

It was not until the 1950s and early 1960s that medical writers began to find patients' personalities, as opposed to their bodies, a factor of importance. This was related to response to treatment, focused on problems of patient compliance with medical directives, and identified doctor-patient communication as problematic (Armstrong 1982). This subsequently gave rise to a considerable literature on the nature of doctor-patient relationships with importance given to work like that of Balint (1956). This work served to establish doctors and patients as 'real' people. This is, rather than both parties being regarded and behaving as objects, they were regarded as having personalities and as subjective and social beings.

There has been a similar change in how nurse-patient relationships are defined and how that definition comes about. Armstrong (1983) uses the analogy of that between supermarket customer and cashier. Both parties have well defined roles, their interaction is usually minimal and neither party expects to have to negotiate differences of meaning or mutual anxieties. Imagine now a large research grant being awarded to investigate the nature of relationship of the customer, cashier and technology. Both parties would have to start examining their relationship so that they could relate their feelings to the research team: the confession of silent thoughts would be encouraged and new problems of misunderstandings would be identified. Gradually our apparently mechanistic relationship – virtually between a bag of shopping and a cash till – becomes problematic in that as the customer comes to look for and respond to the personal meanings of the cashier, so that cashier becomes more than an extension of the till but a 'whole person' in her or his own right. Armstrong writes, 'Until recently the relationship between the patient and nurse was similar in its mechanistic passivity to that between customer and cashier' (1983, p. 458), that is, extremely limited in the identity it provided for its participants. This was associated with forms of organisation of nurse's work which were based on scientific management principles and treated patients as work objects, on which were performed a number of tasks, graded according to the level of nurse required to perform them (Braverman 1974). Nursing auxiliaries did the 'basic care' while students could learn to do dressings and injections, quali-

fied staff did medicines and served meals while sisters accompanied doctors. This form of task allocation, and the division of labour according to a hierarchy of task complexity, is unworthy of a true profession.

The more recent nursing literature indicates that patients have been reconstituted from being passive, with the identities of participants described in such a manner that patients only obeyed and showed respect, and nurses were limited to being biddable and showing appropriate demeanour and manner. In other words, the patient was a biological object and the nurse was part of the machinery of surveillance. The redefinition of the relationship in general nursing now portrays the patient as a subjective rather than an objective being, with nurses responsible for monitoring and evaluating the patient's subjectivity and personal identity, and constructing and sustaining that identity. One such definition from currently popular writers stresses that it is patients' subjective experience that is crucial to the illness experience. They describe how:

The best nursing practitioners... see the patient's story in formal and informal nursing histories, because they know every illness has a story – plans are threatened or thwarted, relationships are disturbed, and symptoms become laden with meaning depending on what is happening in the person's life. Understanding the meaning of the illness can facilitate treatment and cure. Even when no treatment is available, and no cure is possible, understanding the meaning of the illness for that person and for that person's life is a form of healing, in that such understanding can overcome the sense of alienation (or of self-understanding) and loss of social integration that accompany illness. (Benner & Wrubel 1988)

Histories of nursing before 1960 therefore will deal with the patient as object while subsequent histories, for example, Davies (1980) and Dingwall et al (1988) reveal these different interpretations. In this sense, as Armstrong points out, more recent writings on nurse-patient relationships and analysis of nurse-patient interactions are a reflection of current interpretations of the subjectivity of both nurses and patients.

In these formulations of nursing, the emphasis lies in its clinical base. Cited in almost every text is Henderson's (1966) definition of nursing, which emphasises that nursing is about assisting others to do what they would otherwise do for themselves – until they are well or have a peaceful death. Carrying this out requires moving from considering patients as objects within a biomedical framework to a 'holistic' approach enabling patients' active participation in care. The emphasis is on the whole person, not the person as a series of tasks, and a person with psychological and social as well as physical needs. This acknowledges the subjectivity of patients while also recognising the subjectivity of nurses.

Such is the power of this reformulation that it has been provided in introductory nursing textbooks (e.g. Roper, Logan & Tierney 1990) along with the emphasis on rational care planning. The 'nursing process' has found its way into the nursing curriculum, the proposals for Project 2000 (UKCC 1986), writings about new nursing developments (Pearson 1988), the development of nurse practitioner roles (DHSS 1986) and has been disseminated by staff organisations (Clay 1987).

Nurse-patient relationships as partnerships

The educational reforms of nursing (UKCC 1986) include 'new concepts underpinning education and practice' in nursing. These include ideas such as 'enhancing patients' health knowledge and skills, giving patients maximum independence, respect for individual choice and understanding the uniqueness of patients and the diversity of individual needs' (UKCC 1986, p. 34). These have been fashioned into practices involving partnerships between nurses and patients, and promoted in progressive nursing settings like Nursing Development Units. Aligned to the idea of partnership is that of the therapeutic nature of nursing. 'The power of nursing to promote healing lies ... in this therapeutic relationship ... a purposeful, supportive and healing association between

two persons that is *interactive* and holistic...' (Muetzel 1988 pp. 89–90). The close nurse-patient relationship, it is argued, 'not only provides the milieu for expressing therapeutic methods, but has itself the potential to serve therapeutic effect'. This raises the act of doing nursing, rather than nurses doing tasks with, to, or for patients, to a therapy in its own right. Patients' needs can be met through 'meaningful intervention' within a 'holistic framework' which involves nurses in a number of different roles with patients including teacher, practitioner and enabler, and always involving patients as partners in care to enable them to increase their knowledge and improve control of their health. Salvage (1992) analyses the nature of nurse-patient partnerships as it was found in the leading exponent, the Oxford Nursing Development Unit. Partnership ideas are located in preindustrial traditional woman healers and have also been absorbed from the USA culture of one to one private contacts between 'professionals' and clients. They also, however, draw heavily on humanistic psychology, with its emphasis on the discovery of self through relationships. As Salvage notes 'these traditions – medicine and psychotherapy – contain complex assumptions about power relations'. However, as Armstrong (1983) and Silverman (1987) describe in the case of medicine, the treatment of disease now seeks to penetrate the very personality of the patient. The roots of disease lie in disordered life choices, and the mistaken grounds for these choices must be corrected by exploring psychosocial rather than only biophysical aspects of patients' lives. The changes in how patients are conceptualised, as partners in a therapeutic relation with nurses, and as psychosocial subjects, rather than as biological objects, have implications also for relationships within nursing. Only professionals have the knowledge to be involved in therapeutic partnership with patients, and so nursing auxiliaries became care assistants, and their relationships with the nursing staff mirrored the traditional doctor-nurse relationship (see Ch. 11). On the one hand nurses are basing their claims to profession – what Melia (1987) calls the 'professionalising elite' – on their special knowledge while on the other they are seeking to change the nature of the relationship between professionals and patients.

But do patients want to change the quality of their relationships with professionals? As described in the previous chapter, patients have a different set of health knowledge and beliefs. On assuming the sick role they are legitimately relieved of particular responsibilities and, in Parsons' (1951) formulation, will comply with expert prescriptions rather than self-directed actions. Brooking (1986) found patients tended to want to assume a passive role, just as Fitton and Acheson (1979) found that working-class patients in particular, attending general practitioners, wanted their illness fixed up in the same way as a mechanic would fix a car, and did not want to be subject to intrusive personal enquiries. To want to be treated with consideration, worth and kindness, does not mean entering into a quasi-psychotherapeutic relationship. This means laying limits on what has been called 'the emotional labour of nursing' (Smith 1992) to providing relief from pain and easing discomfort as well as promoting healthy lifestyles. It does not mean entering into the different strata of psychotherapeutic relationships, in which the goals and parameters are mutually defined by therapist and client. Further, as Salvage points out, the effectiveness of professional relationships for patients lies in part in the faith they bring to the healing powers and applied knowledge of the professionals. To demystify the relationship and change the professional-patient hierarchical structure by calling it a partnership may actually reduce rather than increase its healing potential.

Relevant here also is nursing defined as women's work. Nursing is synonymous with 'dirty work' because of its attention to bodily products and infections, and women, also regarded as unclean, particularly at times of menstruating, are ideally suited to it (Wolf 1986). Such dirty work, often regarded as 'basic nursing' is devalued and passed down to the most lowly in the nursing hierarchy, the nursing auxiliaries and care assistants to carry out. At the same time, nursing retains overtones of motherhood, further reinforcing the sexual division of labour (Ungerson 1983). This poses further complexities in the nature of relationships between female nurses and male patients, as well as between male nurses and female patients in approaching partnership.

A feature of the nature of the new nursing relationships is 'holism' – the whole is greater than the sum of its parts. However, as Lawler notes, the introduction of personal assessments through 'the nursing process' and ideas about holism have resulted in an increased tendency 'for nurses to pry into an increasing number of things in patients' lives, in order to get a more "holistic" picture of the patient. But greater surveillance (which is what some of these actions are), and more emphasis on measurement and monitoring, neither ensures holism nor a holistic view of the patient. It may lead to more information being collected without necessarily informing and improving practice' (Lawler 1991, p. 216).

From this perspective nursing 'advances' like the nursing process, holistic care, partnerships with patients and, more recently, primary nursing and case management, amount to increasing encroachments on patients rather than equalising relationships. While there are some indications that patients in 'enlightened' nursing units prefer this approach over more traditional nursing (Pearson et al 1992, Bond et al 1989, Bond et al 1991a, 1991b, 1991c), the evidence is far from solid (Thomas & Bond 1991). When Hayward and his colleagues (Hayward 1986) reviewed evidence on implementing 'the nursing process' they could find few examples of success. Rank and file nurses in traditional care of the elderly wards, the specialism in which nursing claims a predominant position over other disciplines and where major efforts have been made (Wright 1990) see it as an administrative chore, with no relevance to patient care (Reed & Bond 1991, Bond & Bond 1993). Buckenham and McGrath (1983) found that nurses support the rhetoric of putting patients first but their primary allegiance is to the health care team, with the main function assisting and supporting the doctor. Other studies have shown that 'getting through the work' (Clarke 1978) is the predominant force and that talking to patients, essential to developing partnerships, is not regarded as 'real work' (Melia 1987, Smith 1992).

These data reveal the different tensions operating to sustain the status quo in nursing relationships while at the same time urging change in the nature of nursing work and its organisation. While promising a new deal for patients through increased partnership, these changes also provide the basis of a professionalising strategy which seeks higher status for nursing's qualified and full-time workforce. Salvage warns against the seductive assumption that 'empowering nurses is the route to empowering patients' (1992, p. 22). We return to professionalising issues again in Chapter 11. Irrespective of the intent regarding the respective roles of nurses and patients, what is sociologically important is that within encounters with patients, nurses need to find ways of sustaining their conduct as *nurses*, and so go through the process of constructing relationships on the basis of taken-for-granted premises about what the roles of nurse and patient imply.

STUDYING RELATIONSHIPS BY STUDYING INTERACTIONS

Despite attention to the idea of relationships Altschul's comment that, 'The concept of relationship remains elusive, even when qualified by such attributes as "personal" or "impersonal" and even more so when terms like "passive, emotionally involved relationship" are used' (1972, p. 9) remains pertinent. Because of this elusiveness, research has tended to focus on the less emotive yet observable *interaction* between clients and professionals.

At one level, generalising about interactions between professionals and patients is not made easy by the extreme diversity of situations in which patients are cared for, the kinds of problems they present, the kinds of knowledge and skills nurses draw upon, and the nature and intent of the relationships formed. One way to investigate interaction is to consider particular types of setting: psychiatric settings (Altschul 1972, McIlwain 1983), intensive care units (Ashworth 1980), general hospital wards (Clark 1983, Faulkner 1980), geriatric wards (Wells 1980, Evers 1981, Reed 1989) and to patients in their own homes (McIntosh 1981). Another is to focus on different client groups, cancer patients (McIntosh 1977, Bond 1978, Wilkinson 1991), antenatal patients (McIntyre 1982), patients in labour (Kirkham 1983), parents of chronically ill children (Comaroff & Maguire 1981), parents of children with Perthe's Disease (Harrisson 1977) and stroke patients at home (Kratz 1978, Anderson 1992), to name but a few. There is also a growing body of work on the analysis of consultations in general practice and in outpatient clinics (e.g. Bloor 1976, Strong 1979a, Silverman 1987).

These studies have variously investigated methods of soliciting information from patients as a basis of making decisions; ideological influences on communication practices; value assumptions as they influence communication and the subsequent treatment of social groups. From these other studies we can draw on some general ideas about interactions with patients and some influences on them. What professionals bring to an interaction will depend in part on the organisational context in which it takes place – whether a general or psychiatric hospital ward, an outpatient clinic or casualty department, a well baby or genitourinary disease clinic. Overriding these are constraints of law, professional ethics, time, space, interprofessional relations and how the profession itself is organised.

Professional-client interactions as negotiated order

In Chapter 7 we developed the idea that institutions are socially created and an important feature of their construction is their negotiated order. This concept is relevant to interaction between professionals and clients as they intersubjectively produce a social order.

Power and control

Central to an analysis of the relationship between client and professional is an appreciation that they bring to the relationship different definitions of the situation, different needs and different aspirations. While these may coincide, the professional and the client may have different ways of achieving them. Both mother and midwife wish to see a successful birth, but the midwife may wish to minimise her patient's discomfort by encouraging the use of drugs for pain relief while the mother may prefer to stay alert throughout her labour without drugs. Somehow they must arrive at a decision about how to proceed. Green et al (1990) found that women rated their experiences of maternity care according to their initial expectations.

Interaction between client and professionals often takes place in institutions, and the earlier discussion of the nature of the institutions provides a broad framework for their interpretation. Riley, in commenting on the structural organisation of maternity hospitals said: 'Institutions which depend on rigidly maintained hierarchy and strict division of labour among their personnel cannot fail to transfer the results in some form to the treatment of patients ... the difficulties of acquiring a theoretical appreciation are as nothing compared with the difficulties of *enacting* flexibility within an inflexibly organised system' (Riley 1977, pp. 69–70). This extreme view of hierarchy and division of labour reflects the structuralist position that professionals have more power than clients, and that all professional groups are likely to be dominated to some degree by doctors. However, as Davies (1983) points out, relationships in hospitals are likely to be as much related to the wider social divisions and ideological positions as the constraints of bureaucracy and profession. Therefore the way that professionals interact with patients will be influenced by their social-class positions and gender as well as ideological views of the relative positions of professional and client.

Nevertheless, one way of analysing a professional-client relationship is in terms of the relative power each brings to it. Freidson (1975) has invested this power in *functional autonomy*, in the independence of the professional from lay evaluation and control. Functional autonomy is imputed as a structural property of a particular class of occupations, namely professions. Those occupying professional positions will inevitably carry out their work with clients from this dominant position. The view of the professional as dominant places the client in a reciprocal subservient position. The professional view in this analysis therefore will prevail because clients and professionals occupy different structural positions.

This is reflected in the different ways that professionals exert control, even to the extent of regulating access to the sick role as discussed in Chapter 8. Professionals exert control in areas as different as deciding which patients should be resuscitated or taken off life-support machines (see Ch. 10), when they should be discharged home (Armitage 1981), to the offering of an aspirin (Fagerhaugh & Strauss 1977) and the provision of a bedpan (Bond & Bond 1993). The amount of autonomy available, however, will depend upon the occupational group to which the professional belongs, doctors being more autonomous than other health professionals, based on their authority position within that group. Moreover, while relationships may be asymmetrical this is not to suggest that patients are devoid of making their voice heard nor are they bound to do as they are bid. As Stimson and Webb (1975) found patients will try to achieve their desired outcomes and try to influence doctors to achieve this through a series of negotiations. While at a disadvantage with respect to knowledge and place with medical territory, they can still decide how much to reveal about themselves. Hall and Stacey (1979) found children adept at controlling staff through asking for attention when staff had to interpret if their need was 'real' or a ruse. While patients can exert some control this is limited by their position in the social order.

Controlling information

One aspect of inequality between clients and professionals is that professionals are regarded as having more knowledge and information, which they are at liberty to withhold from clients. This view is upheld by the many studies which have shown that a major source of dissatisfaction among patients is a feeling of not being kept informed (Cartwright 1964, Reynolds 1978, Royal Commission on the National Health Service 1979, Kirkham 1983). While information may be actively sought by patients, it is the conscious or unconscious control of information by professionals which creates uncertainty and anxiety as well as a feeling among patients that they are ignored. There are many alleged reasons for not keeping patients informed – not least that they would rather not know – which are used to justify staff behaviour.

Professionals regularly act on the basis of *assumptions* held about patients' desire for information, assumptions which can often be quite erroneous (Bond 1978, Madge & Fassam 1982). The effect of information restriction is to deny responsible status with the implication that the patient is incapable of intelligent choice and self-control.

A major concept in information control is the management of patients' *uncertainty*. As Waitzkin and Stoeckle wrote:

A physician's ability to preserve his own power over the patient in the doctor-patient relationship depends largely on his ability to control the patient's uncertainty. (1972 p. 187)

Power therefore rests on the control of uncertainty, which in turn rests on the management of information. Davis (1963) distinguished two types of uncertainty. *Clinical uncertainty* exists when there is real uncertainty about clinical matters and when information of this kind is withheld. However, uncertainty can be projected into a situation where there is no clinical uncertainty in order to manage interactions. This is called *functional uncertainty* and may avoid patients demanding reasons for treatment

or explanation of events as well as, when the news is bad, emotional or disruptive outbursts. In order to maintain information control, staff may resort to a number of linguistic devices and interactional tactics, including structuring interactions and conveying the impression that time is short, so that the patient feels there is no opportunity to ask questions. In turn, patients resort to counter-tactics, including bargaining techniques like appealing against established norms, applying the pressure of a barrage of questions or enlisting the aid of family intermediaries (Roth 1963).

As in any bargaining situation the relative power of participants is important. Patients can increase their power by behaving irresponsibly or threatening to withhold cooperation. However, since health professionals are privy to the information first, it is they who decide how, when and what to tell patients. As well as not telling, they can invoke postponement, selective information giving, and blatant deception. On the whole, paramedical staff concur with medical decisions regarding information. While they may express opinions about the negative effect such practices may have on patients, they usually prefer to avoid conflict with medical colleagues by adopting the same stance (Bond 1978, Wilkinson 1991).

Negotiating information and other aspects of care

Initially, negotiation was studied in long-term care settings (Roth 1963) and was conceived as a series of 'offers and responses' (Scheff 1966). Negotiation also occurs in short term contacts, however. We observed our daughter, when aged 6, who had fallen badly on her shoulder, successfully negotiate that she would not have it examined at the local casualty department unless by a female doctor. The staff on duty reorganised the flow of work so that when it was her turn to be seen, a female casualty officer was allocated and treatment was successfully instituted. She had not been socialised into the patient role occupied by adults and professionals responded to her as a *child* patient and so treated her differently (Dingwall & Murray 1983). Her demands, which in adults likely would have caused them to be categorised as deviants, were met. In adults they probably would have resulted in particular sanctions. For example, Jeffrey's (1979) analysis of 'bad' adult patients in casualty departments showed them to be subjected to delay, inattention, verbal hostility and vigorous restraint. Child patients are treated in a different frame in casualty, just as they are by physiotherapists attempting to carry out particular therapeutic regimes (Davis & Strong 1976).

Negotiation can also take place through a third party. During fieldwork one of us observed a female patient in a radiotherapy ward who staff thought required psychiatric treatment. When this was suggested to her husband he interceded on her behalf, expressing his belief that this would be premature and likely to prompt his wife to discharge herself. In this sense the patient, through her husband, had negotiated her treatment. Through asserting themselves in different ways patients can obtain and retain some measure of control which may be regarded as counteracting that of professionals. Where relationships are harmonious then all parties must be reasonably satisfied with the negotiated order they have created and must feel reasonably in control (Rosenthal et al 1980) or accept their power deficit as legitimate or inevitable. Where either of the parties are dissatisfied then problems in interpersonal relationships will persist.

Of course, as in all walks of life, there are limits to the extent that negotiation can take place, with both staff and patients drawing their own demarcations. Formal policy can limit the extent to which patients may negotiate, for example, a discharge date or a home confinement. While midwives are bound by rules to attend a woman wishing a home confinement there is no similar rule which governs the attendance of a general practitioner, who can refuse to do so. Therefore, in choosing a home confinement, patients may choose to do so without medical cover. In other circumstances they may negotiate that their general practitioner will attend. More informal rules govern length of stay in hospital after surgery, and though patients may wish to go home earlier or later than the routine number of days, whether they can successfully negotiate this will depend on how they are regarded by the nursing staff who may intercede on their behalf, and the medical staff who agree their discharge. In extreme circumstances, of course, where hospital staff refuse to negotiate, patients can discharge themselves. This right of patients has been publicised. The Association for Improvement in the Maternity Services notes:

A mother may discharge herself and her baby from the hospital at any time. An early discharge is sometimes looked upon with disfavour by hospital staff who may require the mother to sign a form stating that she has discharged herself against medical advice. If the mother does not wish to sign this form she is under no obligation to do so. (Beech & Claxton 1980, p. 21)

Yet patients are under strong pressure to sign such documents.

The asymmetrical nature of relationships between professionals and patients is more pronounced in hospital than it is in the patient's own home. McIntosh (1981) observed that district nurses saw themselves very much as guests in patients' homes, which determined to a considerable extent the way in which they managed their interactions and the position from which they could negotiate. For example, guests do not lay down rules and regulations for their hosts whereas the nurse, as professional, has to do so in the course of her duties. Nurses have to learn to exert sufficient control in order to establish their authority in respect of the nursing care of patients but at the same time be enough of the 'guest' to let patients and families feel that they are in control. They also have to establish an appropriate degree of distance. The degree of intimacy which characterises care by family members is the result of sustained relationships which are qualitatively different from those with nursing staff.

Kirkham (1983) observed that patients having home confinements behaved much more assertively than their hospital counterparts. Midwives' relationships with home patients were described as more colleague-like. In the absence of other professional colleagues, the midwives shared what they were doing with their patients, giving them running commentaries about what was happening and announcing their intended actions in advance. This information gave patients the opportunity to refuse procedures which some did, unlike hospital patients. Therefore, the standards by which patients conformed were different at home. Those delivering in hospital had very quickly to learn the standards of the institution, their negotiating position being that much weakened.

Control of work

Control of work involves controlling patients who constitute work. Like all other workers, health professionals try to arrange their work to be conveniently and easily performed. One way of achieving this is to establish a number of *routines* and develop procedures which will encourage patients to accept routine forms of treatment.

One vivid example of routinisation of care is the clerking procedure employed at women's first visit at an antenatal clinic (McIntyre 1978) served by medical staff assisted by midwives. A midwife asks a number of medically predetermined standard questions, sometimes now computerised, and carries out physical checks. The results are entered in the computer or case notes. In this context there is no negotiation about the nature of patients' problems. Any 'problem' identified for the doctor will conform to those predetermined by the questions. Topics not covered by questions will not enter into the realm of what are legitimate problems. If the patients themselves raise any questions then the observed standard response from the midwives is to tell them to speak to the doctor about it. In this routinised fashion large numbers of patients with similar conditions are processed in such a way as to conserve the time of doctors and, to a lesser extent, midwives.

In other settings a variety of routines are identifiable, corresponding to particular patient types. Bond (1978) observes that what nurses tell cancer patients about their treatment and condition is reduced to a number of routine explanations appropriate to the categories defined by the nature of the patient's diagnosis, and type and stage of treatment, more so than individual differences in patients' personal characteristics. By invoking standard routines in many aspects of care nurses are protected 'on the one hand from dealing with the emotional strain of continually working through new interactions with the patient, and on the other from having to negotiate from a position of weakness, with the doctor' (Davies 1977, p. 491).

In using routines, health professionals are also drawing on their habitual knowledge developed over repeated experiences of the same kind of clinical situation. In so doing, the application of routines serves to embody the professionals' relative autonomy because they reflect the purposes of the professional without necessarily taking regard of those of the patient. At the same time routines, because of their structure, serve to deny patients any potential influence (Bloor 1976). However, the extent to which standard routines apply will vary according to the various resources and constraints that clients and professionals feel that the particular setting affords them or imposes upon them.

While routinisation of care goes against an expressed ideology of individualised care, it is regarded as an inevitable aspect of work when a high client-worker ratio is involved (Davies 1976). Routinisation of work goes hand in hand with how patients are classified or, as sociologists would say, *typified*. Routines are developed and applied differentially to the appropriate patient type. These types will be specific to the work problems and situations involved.

Typification

Typification is a process of categorising individuals or events into types. It is a concept particularly associated with phenomenological perspectives. The act of slotting things, events and people into types functions to reduce the complexity of the social world by narrowing the focus of interaction to a small number of recognised types. Available typifications are a major determinant of how subsequent relationships are managed. They take account of the characteristics of the type, more so than those of individuals who constitute the type.

An important feature of typifications is that they are 'plan determined' (Schutz & Luckmann 1974). That is, the practical purposes underlying typification, and the circumstances in which it occurs, will influence the particular patient types constructed. A general case of this arises in the typification of 'good' patients and 'bad' or 'problem' patients. From nurses' descriptions of patients Duff and Hollingshead concluded that: '*problem* patients obstructed work and *no-problem* patients facilitated work' (1968, pp. 221–222). What constitutes obstruction and facilitation of work is, of course, context specific. Murcott (1981) identified cancer specialists' typification of 'bad' patients as those who delayed seeking attention for their condition. This was derived from the particular medical concerns of oncology, where the likelihood of successful treatment diminished the longer a patient delays. In nursing homes, residents with dementia who wander constitute particular problems while those who are 'too able' are equally problematic, especially if they are also assertive (Bond & Bond 1993). In any context it is theoretically possible to determine what kind of patient falls into the problem category.

However, there are different views of how constructing typification takes place (Hargreaves 1977). One way is to compare individual patients against an ideal (Becker 1952). British and North American studies in general hospitals arrive at very similar descriptions of ideal patients (Ujhely 1963, Stockwell 1972, Rosenthal et al 1980):

Ideally, from a nurse's perspective, all patients should be sick when they enter hospital, should follow eagerly and exactly the therapeutic programme set up by the staff, should be pleasant, uncomplaining, fit into the hospital routine, and should leave the hospital 'cured'. Good patients handle their illness well, are cooperative, as cheerful as possible, comply with treatment, provide the staff with all the relevant information, follow the rules, and do not disrupt the ward or demand special privileges and excessive attention.
(Rosenthal et al 1980, p. 27)

In one study, nurses identified two main types of problem patient – 'forgivable' and 'wilful' (Lorber 1975). 'Forgivable' problem patients needed a lot of time and resources from staff, were anxious and complained a great deal. They were, however, severely ill and their behaviour and the problems they created were not viewed as their fault. They were given the attention they demanded, especially if they showed gratitude. Patients categorised as 'wilful' were not seriously ill from the staff's point of view, but acted as if they were. Patients complained, were emotional, uncooperative and were regarded as deliberately deviant, wilfully causing extraordinary trouble. Rosenthal et al (1980) identified similar characteristics which gave rise to the designation 'problem patient'. Some are described as manipulative, demanding or complaining excessively. Some are physically abusive in ways which are bizarre or threatening to staff. Others have unpleasant personalities. Another problem category related to excessive complaints about pain or excessive dependence on medication. Finally, some patients are described as 'career patients'. They sought hospitalisation for its own sake and were not considered to be legitimate patients at all. Included in this category were patients judged not sufficiently ill to warrant hospitalisation or who were inappropriate for a particular ward.

After their thorough review of the literature, Kelly and May (1982) attribute nurses' definition of patients as 'good' and 'bad' to the way in which they either provide or withhold legitimisation of the nurses' role. The role of the caring professional is only viable with reference to an appreciative patient, therefore the good patient confirms the role of the nurse while a bad patient denies that legitimation. This analysis is borne out in the nursing of neurotic patients.

Caudhill reported American nurses' problems in dealing with neurotic patients:

I don't think the nurse has any security. No definite body of knowledge to hang her hat on with neurotics. With psychotics you can read and study what their behaviour means. There are innumerable books on how to handle psychotics but nothing for nurses on neurotics. (1958, p. 184)

Caudhill concluded that:

The nurse was fairly clear about how she was to act toward psychotic patients, but she felt uncomfortable and unsure of herself in her contact with neurotic patients. (1958, p. 336)

John noted a similar phenomenon among British psychiatric nurses:

One frequently heard comments that neurotics were just in to 'dodge responsibility' or 'you don't know how much of the illness is genuine and how much is imaginary' or 'they were too pampered'. This was particularly astonishing in view of the obvious handicaps under which certain patients were placed by their illness, for example, fear of being left alone or even stepping outside their own front door. The attitudes, however, were interesting in the light of the amount of sympathy which was extended to patients with evidence of tangible illness, for example, vomiting. (John 1961, p. 124)

Towell (1976) also found nurses describing patients with nonpsychotic disorders as not being ill and, of course, patients who were not egarded as ill 'thereby lost their claims to receive help' (1976, p. 80). Similarly, Altschul (1972) observed '... the label of neurotic does act as a disincentive to interaction' (1972, p. 80). MacIlwaine (1983) observed that many nurses felt insecure in dealing with psychiatric patients who were not easily cast in the sick role. She judged that nurses were happy *only* with patients who were obviously sick or disturbed, and neurotic patients do not fit what nurses regard as an appropriate sick role.

May and Kelly carried out detailed investigation of the interactional and developmental process of patients being labelled 'problem' and the consequences of their behaviour in terms of the feelings aroused in the psychiatric nurses who had to deal with them. One particular woman had a whole string of diagnoses attached to her over her 20-year patient career. Nurses were confronted with major difficulties in attempting to cope with the extremes of the woman's behaviour, which they attributed in part to her own wilful attention-seeking. The patient's behaviour and attitudes involved a rejection of the help nurses felt uniquely able to provide and the giving of which is central to their activities and a necessary part of their self-esteem and professional image. 'In short (she) denied nurses professional competence and undermined their authority' (May & Kelly 1982, p. 288). This applies particularly to the relevance of legitimacy of nurses therapeutic aspirations. For patients to fail to acknowledge that psychiatric nurses have a therapeutic role restricts them to aperipheral place in the treatment process and underlines their subordinate status positions in the health care hierarchy. The issue of defining problem patients therefore is intimately bound up with nurses' sense of therapeutic competence, professional identity and, with it, their authority. May and Kelly's paper is grounded in empirical observations in a particular psychiatric setting. However, their interpretation is likely to have broader application.

It certainly shows similarities to Jeffrey's (1979) work in casualty departments. Patients labelled 'bad' or 'rubbish' were mostly four kinds: trivial complaints, drunks, overdoses and tramps. Jeffrey argues that they are defined as 'bad' patients because they break one or more of the rules described in Chapter 8 as justifying the sick role:

1. Patients must not be responsible, either for their own illness or for getting better; casualty staff can only be held responsible if, in addition, they are able to treat the illness.

2. Patients should be restricted in their reasonable activities by the illness they report with.

3. Patients should see illness as an undesirable state.

4. Patients should cooperate in trying to get well.

Patients who are 'bad' or deviant, in the sense that they break the rules about the kind of patient who is appropriate for casualty treatment, evoke particular kinds of interactions. Because they may be time-consuming they may be detained until there is sufficient slack time; they are managed in unpleasant and otherwise abusive ways or with superficial politeness subject to post-hoc attacks in departmental gossip. Millman provides a similar example from 'The back-rooms of medicine':

Standing around, waiting for the police to arrive, the resident and the intern make bets on whether the case would be a real emergency or just a teenager who had swallowed too much aspirin. But at least, they assured one another, this time it wouldn't be some old alcoholic who would 'waste' all of their time in the Coronary Care Unit. (Millman 1976, p. 49)

The category into which patients are mentally slotted will influence how subsequent interactions proceed. Evers (1981) compared how nurses worked with patients classified as 'Dear old Gran' and 'Awkward Alice'. The former smiled, conformed to nurses' requests and were grateful. The latter, while physically frail, knew what they wanted and were entitled to, and said as much. The former were given much more and kinder attention than the latter, who came in for quite a rough time.

Attaching even informal labels on patients can have major and minor consequences. Meyer and Mendelson (1961) studied psychiatric referrals in general hospitals. They found those labelled as disruptive, because they refused to submit to hospital routines, were referred to a psychiatrist and so also became labelled as someone with a psychiatric problem. Roth and Eddy (1967) noted that rehabilitation patients typified as abusive and uncooperative were promptly discharged from the ward and subsequently denied retraining. Laryea (1984) observed postnatal care in hospital and found that how midwives categorised mothers in terms of their mothering ability subsequently influenced the extent to which they were regarded as requiring assistance in feeding their babies. This had repercussions for their eventual success in infant feeding as well as the mothers' own perception of their mothering ability.

These examples drawn from different countries and clinical settings demonstrate the fundamental nature of patient typificiation, and the way typifications provide for systematic variation in the manner staff frame their encounters with patients. As such they influence the control of work and have consequences for patient outcomes.

PATIENT-STAFF INTERACTION IN THE MANAGEMENT OF PAIN – A CASE EXAMPLE

An examination of the literature about pain shows that much attention has been devoted to physiological, pharmacological, surgical, clinical and psychological aspects. This reflects the immense importance attached to the management of pain in the work of health professionals. However, there is a marked absence of sociological studies which deal with the organisational aspect of the settings in which pain is managed, or the interactions which take place as part of pain work between patients and their families with hospital staff and among hospital staff themselves. Yet as Stacey and Homans wrote:

The sociology of health and illness is unlikely to be able to go forward if it fails to recognise the impact of suffering upon social relationships ... It is, after all, the existence of human suffering, of the body and the mind, and the desire to avoid it, which have led to the development of elaborate health care systems. Social relations in health and illness may perhaps have a unique quality for this reason. (Stacey & Homans 1978, pp. 297–298)

A notable exception to the dearth of work is a study by Fagerhaugh and Strauss (1977) which deals with sociological aspects of pain management in a number of hospitals in the United States. While this is entirely an American study, using an interactionist perspective, much of the theory it develops is immediately applicable to situations met in British hospitals, although the details are different in some respects. It also raises a number of issues relevant to relationships between staff and patients in a variety of contexts.

Earlier in our discussions of patient-professional relations we touched on some of the features that characterise them. Important among them were power and political differentials. We related these to how patients may negotiate to obtain particular information or manage their treatments. Other tactics include persuasion, appeals to authority, threatening and coercion. These determine which, how, when, where, and by whom things get done, and are as relevant to any other aspect of health care as to the management of pain. However, as we pointed out, any examination of what goes on in hospitals must take account not only of what happens between individuals and groups and the prevailing ideologies of the groups involved but also set these actions within the broader context of the organisation and beyond that, and more generally, the social structure.

Ideology and organisation

Ideologies are ideas and beliefs, which are regarded by those who hold them as true and adequate explanations of phenomena and as furnishing sufficient grounds for them to plan and carry out courses of social action. In Chapter 8 we discussed how the major medical ideology was disease-oriented with its emphasis on an acute-care model characterised by patients with a short-term episode of illness, having treatment and being cured. We argued that this is inappropriate as a guiding principle for long-term and chronic care, and so it also poses problems for the management of chronic pain which comprises a substantial amount of pain work (Kotarba 1983).

Of course, other ideologies cut across the dominant one. The caring which takes place in pain clinics and in some hospitals and hospices, represents a contrasting ideology emphasising patient comfort, and the management of pain in such organisations has developed along lines very different to those in traditional acute hospital wards. As an example of how an organisational setting influences interaction, studies in intensive-care units show interaction between patients and staff to be much more a function of monitoring machines and biological systems (Ashworth 1980) than would interactions in postnatal or elderly-care wards. All hospital wards will have identifiable organisational variables. Here we shall attend primarily to the interactional aspects of pain management – but urge that the organisational and ideological contexts be borne in mind.

Pain work

Pain involves work by both patients and professionals. Pain work, of course, is only one aspect of work. However, interactions involving pain have a number of different dimensions and functions. The *relief* of pain by staff and by patients readily springs to mind as most salient. A few moments reflection gives rise to a number of different dimensions – the handling of *expressions* of pain by patients and response to such expressions, *diagnosing* the meaning of pain, *inflicting* pain in order to carry out procedures, *preventing* and *minimising* pain if possible, and *enduring* pain which involves short or long-term coming to grips with it. It would be possible to draw up profiles for different wards showing how these dimensions are differentially salient.

Of course, for staff and patients to accomplish pain work the cooperation of both parties must be sought. This may be at a simple level, as when the patient is asked to relax a muscle to minimise the pain of an injection or to lie still and not interfere with a painful procedure. The patient may ask for the injection in a particular site and, if the patient's view or definition of the situation coincides with that of the staff member, then there are likely to be no problems. If cooperation is not forthcoming then it may have to be elicited by any of a number of tactics: persuasion, appeal to sense or to authority and, above all, negotiation. In any negotiation, power and authority lie primarily with the staff and their primary aim is not necessarily the alleviation of pain but may be establishing a diagnosis or providing treatments which cause pain, like encouraging coughing after abdominal surgery or debridement of sloughing wounds. Negotiations to carry on can entail who carries out the procedures, when they will be carried out, and even the kind of substances used. We have all met this with children afraid of the sting of lotions applied to a cut knee, or the removal of a splinter with a needle and the kind of negotiation which goes on to allow the action to proceed. It also happens with patients.

In delivery areas of obstetric units there are likely to be a range of cultural, ideological and personal perspectives on birth and its inevitable accompanying pain. The longer labour continues, the more likely it is that discrepant positions between the mother and her attendants will be thrown into relief with regard to pain and its expression. At these times, negotiations take place which can resolve in compromises between the mother experiencing her pain and delivery in the way she chooses and the staff imposing and instituting their views about pain control. Conflicting views can lead to interaction difficulties with each party attempting to assert control over the birth process and negotiated decisions taking place about whether and when the staff can institute pain relief measures.

In any setting there will be various degrees of professional tolerance for lay management of pain and this has achieved particular prominence in the case of birth pain. In other settings it applies to the extent that patients may use their own tried and tested remedies for relief – the trusted hot water bottle, lying in what, to observers, seem to be weird positions, pacing up and down. Again, interaction with negotiation will determine the extent to which patients are permitted to institute their own remedies.

Pain trajectory

One facet of pain work which is important is the expected *pain trajectory*, that is, the course that the pain will take. In specific wards and departments staff will have had repeated experience of pain associated with procedures and conditions and are able to anticipate the normal trajectory for particular conditions. In surgical wards for instance, the trajectories for common operations like herniorrhaphy or hysterectomy are well defined. It is when some unexpected pain trajectory appears, like genuine intractable pain in an acute surgical ward or a patient insisting that normal relief measures are not controlling the pain, that problems become apparent. Staff expectations of the appropriate pain trajectory for a straightforward operation may then fail to recognise the pain of peritonitis.

Hospital wards are not organised, or the staff psychologically prepared, to deal with such events. When patients do not fit either accepted types or the routines established for pain management in a particular ward then they are amongst those likely to become labelled 'uncooperative' or 'difficult' or 'causing a fuss'. This happens in part because of the time and energy demanded by these patients amidst a whole lot of other work requiring sometimes prompt attention. It is also occasioned by the interaction difficulties created for both patient and staff by the patient having to work to legitimise pain and manage his or her expressions of it, while the staff may become frustrated and feel helpless and out of control in the face of unpredictable pain. It is not a matter of either patients or staff being at fault, but such occasions can give rise to mutual blame and recrimination. This will create a downward and often irretrievable spiral in the quality of relationships.

Other patient trajectories

Of course, the pain trajectory is only one of a number of trajectories relevant to patients.

Illness, medical care and social trajectories are features of the patient career and biography. We know, for instance, that different cultural groups have different ways of expressing pain (Zborowski 1969) and that different people control their pain in very different ways (Copp 1974). Patients with long-standing pain will have worked out a drug regime which is tolerable and controls the pain; yet when they come into hospital staff can take over the relief work and an effect of drugs or allergens will be ignored to their cost. Patients' negative experience of hospitals, which could have involved misdiagnosis, iatrogenic trauma, or their complaints being rejected, will create specific interaction problems on their next admission. Patients who have repeated admissions will be able to compare different hospital and individual personnel in terms of what they regard as competence in pain control and its corollary, incompetence resulting in unnecessary pain. An examination of patients' written notes typically reveals that little of what could be available about patient biographies is related to pain and its management.

Professionals' interpretation of pain

Professionals are charged with deciding *is* the patient in pain *and* is he or she suffering? Edwards (1984) considered the distinction between pain which is located in a specific bodily area and spiritual pain which is nonlocalised and has no specific bodily place. Bodily pain can of course give rise to mental or spiritual pain, but spiritual pain often exists alone due to loneliness, knowledge of terminal illness or what are usually referred to as psychiatric conditions. Edwards' view is that by far the greater emphasis has been given to the alleviation of bodily pain.

The imperative to assist the patient gain relief from the unnecessary mental pains arising from his illness should be at least as strong as, if not stronger than, the imperative to assist in the relief of unnecessary bodily pain. Yet, it is precisely in this area that there seems to be the greatest patient neglect ...

for it happens that a patient's suffering is dismissed as 'psychological', 'imaginary' or 'unreal' when it is thought not to be bodily localised in nature. ... Those who believe that pains of soul are somehow unreal also find it easy to convince themselves that the ethics of pain management does not apply to that kind of suffering. (Edwards 1984, p. 516)

How professionals interpret pain therefore will be affected by their orientation towards bodily or physiological pain and spiritual pain, what they regard as appropriate work, and by how they interpret different indicators or cues provided by the patient.

If professionals accept an obligation to help relieve the unnecessary pains of patients then it falls to them to be able to determine with reasonable accuracy not only *that* the other is suffering but also the kind of pain and its intensity and duration. However, only the person who is feeling pain can directly perceive it. This information has to be relayed to others. It can be done verbally, but onlookers expect to see signs of pain: pallor, clenched fists, perspiring, wincing or groaning. For pain to be attributed, these signs are particularly important when a pain trajectory is not normal for the ward or condition. Patients are sometimes accused of reporting more pain than they have, pain when they have none, and this is more so when they have acquired a reputation. In pain work assessing pain and legitimising pain are associated processes. Pain assessment has a number of dimensions. Listen for them when you are in any ward. You are likely to hear questions like: Does she really have pain? Is it as bad as she is making out? Is it getting worse? Is the pain real or psychological? What is causing this pain?

Staff base their assessment on their ability to read the signs, the patient's expression and other evidence of pain. This will be influenced by the staff's experience and it is not unknown for an inexperienced midwifery student to dismiss a patient's backache, in the absence of other signs, only to discover she is well advanced in labour. Patients sometimes have to work in order to have their pain accepted.

They need to be aware of the social rules that apply in a particular setting and what they need to do. It is no use waiting and tolerating, expecting to be asked about pain in a setting where the staff wait for patients to report it before they act.

Davitz and Davitz (1981) found cultural differences among nurses' perceptions of pain and suffering. Of 12 countries studied, English nurses were ranked ninth in their inferences of psychological distress and inferred the least amount of physical pain. They report that English nurses working in the United States find difficulty in adjusting to the apparently low tolerance of their patients, which is in striking comparison to the British 'stiff upper lip'. Nurses' own inferences of pain and suffering are their learned behavioural responses of their culture or subculture. However, these are modified by perceptions of patients' characteristics. In general, lower-class patients were regarded as experiencing a greater degree of physical pain than middle-class patients. While patients' age made no difference to nurses' perceived physical pain, children were viewed as experiencing less psychological suffering than patients in other age groups. Nurses, therefore, interpret from an adult perspective, making children's work to establish their suffering that much more difficult.

Patients' ethnic origin also influenced nurses' perceptions. Jews were consistently rated as having greater physical pain regardless of age, diagnosis and social class, with the ratings moving down through Spanish, Negro, Mediterranean to Anglo-Saxon and Oriental at lowest (Davitz & Davitz 1981). While such cultural differences exist both in influencing nurses' responses and in how patients are perceived, other patient characteristics are also influential. Patients who are believed to be responsible for their own conditions, like a drunk driver or those in Jeffrey's (1979) 'rubbish' category, are treated differently. Conditions difficult to diagnose precisely also raise doubts for some staff about the reality of the pain being reported. All of these mean extra work for patients to legitimise that they have pain and its severity.

Legitimising pain

In different contexts pain is perceived as having different degrees of legitimacy. In particular, Fagerhaugh and Strauss found that both physiotherapists and nurses tended to discount the severity of patient's low back pain and this created a breakdown in cooperation over pain work. This rejection of patients' expressions of pain occurs because of professionals' interpretation of behaviour:

Physiotherapist: 'You can tell by the way she moved around the room; if you are in a lot of pain you just can't do that. She acts as though it were a hotel rather than a hospital room.' (Fagerhaugh & Strauss 1977, p. 120)

Tactics can then be adopted to deal with this appraisal. One tactic is to disregard complaints of pain, telling patients they are doing well, on the assumption that if there is no real pain then, providing one waits long enough, patients will stop 'complaining' or reduce claims to pain. Patients who send out wrong behavioural cues or employ unfavourable tactics come to be negatively stereotyped, which makes the job of convincing staff about the meaning of the pain all the harder. In time, patients may just give up trying to persuade staff of the legitimacy of their pain.

Most often patients do not need to legitimise their pain. However, when they do, they need to find ways of telling staff and convincing them. They may show obvious outward signs like crying, banging, complaining regularly, growing more urgent in their requests for relief or becoming angry. If they are convincing then attempts at relief will be instituted. However, if staff are not convinced, then they are likely to become labelled as over-demanding and dishonest about their assertions. In order to assess the 'real' nature of pain staff may resort to more extreme tactics like giving placebos instead of analgesics or observing patients' behaviour without them knowing. The interactional difficulties this creates can then become extreme.

Petrie demonstrated that there are natural variations between individuals in susceptibility to pain. Therefore as well as social differences, there are also physiological differences, giving rise to three groups of people – 'The reducer, the augmenter, and the moderator' (Petrie 1967, p. 1). By definition 'The reducer tends subjectively to *decrease* what is perceived; the augmenter to increase what is perceived; and the moderator neither to reduce nor to augment what is perceived' (Petrie 1967, pp. 1–2). These three types, and particularly the reducers who tend to be regarded as stoics, and the augmenters, create interactional difficulties. Stoical patients may be experiencing severe pain yet do not show signs of it. To offer relief, staff must find methods of establishing and managing their pain without making patients feel loss of face or that they are giving in. On the other hand, augmenters may be subject to various forms of staff abuse which not only challenge their claims concerning their own suffering or need for help but also more widely their moral standing in the ward and broader community.

Balancing

The control of pain involves the balancing of priorities. We have all met this ourselves. We have to decide whether to endure a headache, which may be short-lived, or resort to aspirins which will relieve it although we dislike taking medication. There are equally simple choices to be made by patients – like whether to endure a minor pain of a procedure which will increase the chance of a better diagnosis. There are also more complex and difficult decisions like whether to undergo neurosurgery which will almost certainly yield pain relief but can also produce blindness or other sensory deficits.

Staff as well as patients are involved in a balancing process. For them it may involve the knowledge of producing addiction versus providing reliable pain relief for nonterminal patients. Patients and staff will become involved in interactions which regard balancing from their different perspectives as the focus, and which then create contests over control. Hospital patients temporarily cede to staff members considerable control over some, although not all, aspects of their lives, behaviour and bodies. There is not always agreement about how much control has been handed over – how much right the staff have to continue with therapy despite the pain it may cause, whether as well as managing and taking decisions about some aspects of medical therapy, the staff may control pain medication in its entirety. It is for reasons of *not* wishing to hand over control that some patients choose to have their babies at home and most would like to die at home in order to be sure of maintaining their essential rights and in their own style.

In every situation there are a number of choices or options and these will be different for different people. Whether to have surgery to relieve pain which will also severely restrict mobility has very different consequences for the patient than for other family members. Extending the time between drug administrations to fit in with a routine drug round has different implications for nurses and for patients. Differential judgments in balancing pain work can have personal, cultural and social roots and also depend on the position of the individual in the organisation – patient, relative, nurse, nursing auxiliary, doctor or physiotherapist. When decisions have to be made each will weigh somewhat different considerations, or the same ones in a different balance. In addition, balancing will be profoundly affected by the information available. Patients cannot weigh potential addiction in the balance if they do not know of its possibility; nursing staff will note addiction possibilities but may not realise the patient's terminal condition and so it is of little relevance.

Patients and staff may disagree over choices and disagreements can be implicit or explicit. They may lead to controversy and disagreement between patient and staff as well as between staff members themselves. Unforeseen yet profound consequences can emerge with mutual antagonism: staff withdraw from patients and patients reject staff – even to self-discharge and attempted suicide.

The interactional consequences of the care of patients with pain are relevant for both patients and staff. For patients, this involves not only the amount of suffering and relief they experience but overlaps their feelings about hospitals and their staff, their own self-concept, family relationships and the way they manage their lives. For staff, depending on how they have managed pain, there may be a growth in professional stature brought about by a job well done or a blow to personal identity when incompetence has caused or failed to reduce pain. The experience of intense involvement with a patient with pain can hold major personal significance.

SUMMARY

In this chapter we have dealt with some of the important determining features of relationships between patients and nurses. These apply to some extent to relationships between any group of clients and professionals but, as we have pointed out, a major influence in relationships between health and patients or clients is their standing in relation to medicine.

We described how changes have occurred in the discourse of nursing with regard to how patients and their relationships have been portrayed. 'Professionalising' nurses are promoting exclusivity with patients, through primary nursing. The concept of the 'named-nurse' has been adopted by the state and introduced into the Patient's Charter (Department of Health 1991). This is in keeping with the changes described in Chapter 7, related to the introduction of new management principles and the changing ideology of health services into a market economy. This means that some people 'deliver' health care while others 'receive' it, patients are referred to as 'consumers' or 'customers' and others are the 'providers'. Consumers should act *rationally* according to market principles.

From nursing's perspective one aspect of these new rational ideals is patients wanting to become partners in care but, as we have described, this partnership is anything but straightforward. It encroaches on the whole meaning of nursing work and the division of health labour. It needs to take account of the perspectives of all parties to the relationship, and patients do not necessarily want it. As yet, empirical work on 'the new nursing' with its emphasis on deeper, therapeutic nurse-patient relationships is limited, and prospects for radical change are associated as much with priorities for staffing the service and adjustments to the 'grade mix' in nursing as they are with ideological shifts in the nature of professional relationships. Rank and file nurses are more likely to negotiate some aspects of patient care with them, but the limits of any negotiation are related to a host of social factors, not least the relatively powerless position of patients. As we saw, patients are not entirely without power, however, but how they are treated will relate to social contextual factors and to how they are defined by staff irrespective of their personal qualities. Individualising patient care has to contend with the social functions of its routinisation.

Our major example of professional-patient interaction concerned the management of pain. While pain is a unique experience for every patient it is such an ubiquitous aspect of health professionals' work that it tends to be taken for granted, a routine aspect of work. On occasions, it becomes a major problem for staff to manage. It is when nonroutine measures come into operation that profound interpersonal consequences can emerge. However, even in *routine* pain management, we have shown that issues of power and control are all important together with other features like patient typification, negotiation, persuasion and legitimation which arise in interaction. Careful sociological analysis of relationships between clients and professionals assists us to understand how interaction proceeds and why at times this may become difficult for everyone. By learning to place particular interactions in work and organisation contexts we see there is nothing *abnormal* in regarding patients as difficult or unpopular – it is a perfectly rational response to attempting to get through the work. By drawing awareness to these problems it may be possible to increase professionals' understanding of them, to discuss them and come to terms with some of them. To do so will certainly mean attending to the organisational structure in which care is given as well as to the behaviour of the individual practitioners. As we saw, this is clearly the case in the management of patients with nonroutine pain.

We take up some of the issues of interpersonal aspects of care again in the next chapter.

FURTHER READING

Kelly M P, May D 1982 Good and bad patients: a review of the literature and a theoretical critique. Journal of Advanced Nursing 7: 147–156

Salvage J 1992 The new nursing : empowering patients or empowering nurses? In: Robinson J, Gray A, Elkan R (eds) Policy issues in nursing. Open University Press, Buckingham

Silverman D 1987 Communication and medical practice. Sage, London

Smith P 1992 The emotional labour of nursing. Macmillan, Basingstoke

10

Dying, death and bereavement

INTRODUCTION

Sociology is concerned with human existence and has always had an interest in the boundaries of that existence, birth and death. Until the 1950s the interest in death was submerged and in 1976 Vovelle published an article arguing that the recent attention given to the subject was due to the displacement of a deeply seated taboo on the subject which had lain hidden in the shadows of the Western psyche since some time in the 19th century. This relative banishing of death is associated with the idea of death as an isolated event, privatised and described by Elias (1985) as essentially lonely, a process linked with the rise of individualisation. Other writers have considered death as bureaucratised, medicalised and hospitalised to such an extent that it has been dehumanised (Benoliel 1978, De Vries 1981, Hinton 1972, Kubler-Ross 1970). Prior (1989) argues that death has not simply emerged in some mystical process of evolution but has undergone a series of transformations which impact on the ways that we understand, respond to and organise death in society.

Of particular interest here is the development of interest in death from that of the disciplines of demography, where death is one feature on which populations are built; pathology, which recognises death as a feasible starting point for the study of health; and sociology and anthropology which had discovered in death, like birth, something which reinforced and reflected the nature of the social world.

Demographic studies, however, did not deal with death but reduced this phenomenon to mortality and rates of mortality associated with different social groups, like those we have described in Chapter 3 in relation to social class. This concern with registering and mapping patterns of births and deaths was regarded by Foucault (1979) as a biopolitics of the population. The collection of such statistical information served a technology of life with con-sequences requiring that we meet the various apparatus of surveillance which are focused on our bodies: registration of deaths as of births and marriages, examination and physical control. There has been increasing sophistication in how mortality has been expressed through finer and finer divisions like infant, perinatal, sex- and age-specific, and cause-specific mortality. The ways that mortality rates have been calculated have also increased in sophistication, but none of these allude to the meaning of death. Rather attention to deaths as mortality indices is a reflection of attention to social 'things' from a scientific perspective in which there is a search for the laws of population growth and decline. So defined, the revelation of meanings has no place (Weber 1948b, p. 142).

The interest in death by pathologists is part of the development of modern medicine in which understanding the causal sequence linking death and disease was made possible by making visible human organs and tissues. Like demographers the pathologists also treated their objects of study as things whose essential nature could be understood and revealed according to the laws of human biology. The pathological view of mortality, like that of the demographers, had social consequences on the organisation of death: it justified the postmortem as a method of inquiry; it generated the need for a mortuary as a site of investigation; it structured the language of causation which is used on death certificates; and it justified an understanding of death and disease in terms of anatomical subsystems. In short, it elevated the human body to a central place in the network of objects that could explain and account for death (Prior 1989).

SOCIOLOGICAL PERSPECTIVES ON DEATH

Both the demographers and the pathologists operated their analysis of deaths from the basis of *positivist* science (see Ch. 12), searching for laws which would explain the structure and function of living organisms, the laws which would define the nature of population growth, the growth of healthy tissue and the development of disease. In this sociologists were no different. Indeed, Durkheim makes plain in his preface to *Suicide* that his aim was to study this specific form of death according to the canons of science and on the 'basic principle that "social facts" must be studied as things' (Durkheim 1952, p. 37). This approach to the study of death reflects the sociological interest of the time with its enduring and overriding interest in causation. For much of this century the study of death was the study of suicide and the approach taken was the study of social causation. We take the development of studies of suicide as a case example in Chapter 12 and leave that topic here. Enough to say at this point that suicide was considered as a social fact and from the perspective of its social functions (Hertz 1905, 1960) rather than the meaning of this category of death and dying for the individuals concerned.

Since the late 1950s there have been shifts in the sociological study of death. First, there have been shifts from an objective and scientific language which speaks of mortality, disease and causation to one which is concerned with attitudes, sentiments and awareness. Second, there has been a refocus of interest from the study of mortality to the examination of the meanings and sensibilities of those involved in the process of death and dying: people who are bereaved, professionals involved in managing death and dying and those who die. Just as the earlier 'scientific' study of mortality gave rise to recording and measuring institutions like the registration of deaths, mortuary practices and the Coroner's office, there have also been developments arising from the refocus of interest. The human side of death and attention to the quality of dying, awareness and experiences of death and bereavement have given rise to the hospice movement, bereavement counselling and voluntary organisations like Cruise.

The movement over the past 30 years has also turned attention away from atypical deaths like suicides, to the routine conditions in which these experiences occur and the social relations which surround them. While birth and death are at the extremes of the life cycle, they offer an opportunity for consideration of how these events are similar not only as significant biological status passages or 'existence transitions' but also in a number of ways that are sociologically significant (De Vries 1981). These include the social construction of birth and death, the modern experience of birth and death, the role of the family in existence transitions, the control of information about the process, the role of medicine, collective social concerns with birth and death, and the social rituals and social distribution of sentiments surrounding these events. It is by considering together such seemingly disparate events as birth and death that sociologists develop middle-level theories to explain social phenomena of the kind listed above. In this chapter, however, our focus is death.

Most people personally encounter death rarely, but we cannot avoid it secondhand if we engage with the media. As we reported in Tables 3.4–3.6, childhood and infant deaths have decreased over this century and life expectancy has dramatically increased, as shown in Figure 10.1. Expectancies about dying have changed and 'premature death' has come to be associated with dying not only before the allotted biblical three score years and ten but also before our expected biological life span.

Death is one of the great certainties of life, and in professional life personal encounters with

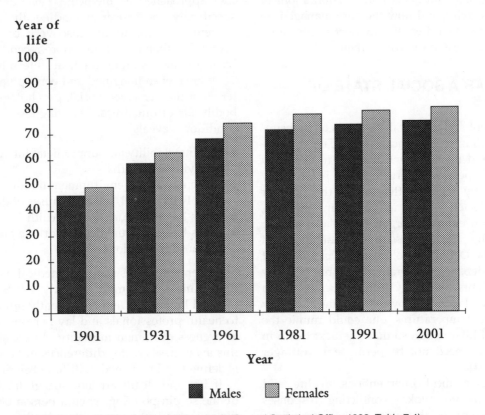

Fig. 10.1 Expectation of years of life at birth (Central Statistical Office 1992, Table 7.4).

death cannot be avoided in the same way as by many people in society. Our conceptions of death, and its relationship to life, are generated through the culturally specific forms or institutions through which we manage death. While particular deaths have significance for us as individuals, in C. Wright Mills' (1970) terms death is also a *public issue*. A situational analysis of dying – the role one plays, the expectations of others, the organisation of social space and relations, the management of self-integrity and composure – all influence the quality of dying and experiences of those involved. In some settings like intensive care units, hospices and nursing homes, death is a more frequent experience and hence features differently in the organisation of work than in maternity or ENT wards. However, how death is organised is influenced not only by its frequency but by the way in which it is framed. The organisational and interpersonal dynamics of particular settings strongly influence both the definitions of death and dying and how they are managed, to create radically different experiences for those who work, live and die within them.

DYING AS A SOCIAL STATE OF AFFAIRS

Death is not and never can be characterised simply according to biological 'facts'. The comprehension and management of death in everyday practice is socially constructed. This is forcefully exhibited by regular attention in the popular press to such issues as abortion, stillbirth, research on embryos, organ transplant, genetic engineering, use of life-support machines and euthanasia. Definitions of death are clouded not only by debate over brain death but also by developments like the Cyronics Society which believed that at death, by maintaining the body in subzero temperatures, one could mimic the process of hibernation so that 'the next death in your family need not be permanent' (Ettinger 1965, p. 194).

Making medical interventions in life and death situations evokes conflicting responses from different social groups as these situations are themselves equivocal and ambiguous. Tech-

nological advances relocated definitions of death away from the respiratory system to the brain and opened out the debate to include the value of life and the essence of human qualities of those kept alive by machine.

While society as a whole has become increasingly medicalised (Strong 1979b), and medicine carries the powers once attributed to magic or religion, writers like Illich (1975) and Sontag (1983, 1990) shed light on the myth of medical infallibility, challenged by illness like cancer. In 1991 a quarter of all deaths in the United Kingdom were due to some kind of cancer (CSO 1992) and projected cancer deaths at 2031 are almost 343 000. These deaths challenge not only medical skill but also the conceptual frameworks by which medicine works. The invasiveness and unpredictability of cancer is not yet encompassed within current medical frameworks and it is noteworthy that many alternative approaches to medicine have developed specifically for cancer, including the hospice movement. Prior to the discovery of streptomycin, TB, then cancer and more recently AIDS, have resisted simple medical interpretations. They have been imagined and conceptualised in terms of the perceived social, psychological and bodily ills of our times. The diagnoses of these conditions reveals:

- the inevitability and unpredictability of individual's deaths
- the cultural and environmental rather than purely biological/medical causes of death
- class-based inequalities in wealth
- class-based inequalities in working and domestic conditions.

In remaining resistant to medical interventions cancer, and more recently AIDS, reveal medical limitations and consistently bring home to health professionals and lay persons alike an awareness of human mortality. As we shall see this awareness creates differences in how dying is defined and managed in different settings.

If life and death are not straightforward to define so pin-pointing when a person begins to die and a patient becomes 'terminal' are equally socially constructed.

The dying trajectory

Recognising dying is not the same kind of activity as noticing a haemorrhage or tachycardia. There are relatively precise definitions for these physiological events. Not so for dying. Neither is dying a diagnosis and should patients ask what is the matter, they are unlikely to be told that they are dying. Rather they would be given a symptom, a disease label or a euphemism for it, if it was too difficult or considered not in the patients' interest to know the truth. Dying is a *predictive* term, indicating the likelihood that someone will die within a socially defined time perspective. This time perspective has been called the *dying trajectory* by Glaser and Strauss (1968). They describe it in this way:

When the dying patient's hospital career begins – when he is admitted to the hospital and a specific service – the staff in solo and in concert make initial definitions of the patient's trajectory. They expect him to linger, to die quickly or to approach death at some pace between the extremes. They establish some degree of certainty about his impending death – for example, they may judge that there is 'nothing more to do' for the patient. They forecast that he will never leave the hospital again, or that he will leave and perhaps be admitted several times before his death. They may anticipate that he will have periods of relative health as well as severe physical hardship during the course of his illness. They predict the potential modes of his dying and how he will fare during the last days and hours of his life. (Glaser & Strauss 1968, p. 30)

Dying trajectories have two characteristics. They have 'shape', in the sense of the dying trajectory plunging straight down as with a road

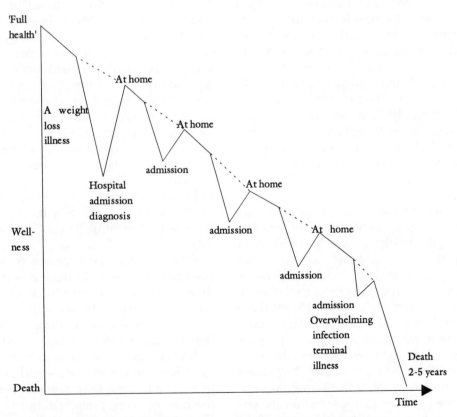

Fig. 10.2   A typical dying trajectory of patients with AIDS (Adapted from Nursing Standard 1990 5(6) : 5).

accident fatality, or showing ups and downs which would be typical of most chronic illness until the final descent. Figure 10.2 depicts a typical illness trajectory of patients with HIV infection taken from records of patients treated in Glasgow. As with all aggregated data, this curve is relatively smooth and removes the particular process for individual patients. The curve also demonstrates duration. All trajectories are plotted against time. Health professionals recognise particular physiological benchmarks which they relate to the progress towards death.

Dying as a social construction

In his important ethnographic studies of deathand dying in two hospitals in the United States, Sudnow discusses 'death and dying as social states of affairs'. He went beyond the taken-for-granted meaning that health professionals hold regarding dying to conclude that the idea of dying 'appears to be a distinctly social one, for its central relevance is provided for by the fact that [it] establishes a way of attending to a person as a predictive of characterization, [it] places a frame of interpretation around a person' (Sudnow 1967, p. 68–69). Sometimes this prediction is well agreed. A great deal of attention had gone into developing prognostic indicators but even so there is a tendency to be optimistic about remaining life (Parkes 1972).

This tendency, and whether patients are labelled as dying, is associated with whether those doing the labelling will be involved in the eventual death. Sudnow observed that there was a greater tendency to label patients as dying when they would create organisational, interactional or professional problems for those assigning the labels. Patients in hospital in objectively the same state and with the same prognosis are defined as dying if they remain to be cared for over the duration of their last illness or if they involve the staff in making arrangements for their transfer to a hospital for the terminally ill. In both cases hospital staff will be involved in a variety of activities. Patients dis-

charged home are far less likely to fall within the 'dying' category since their discharge absolves staff from death related work. Definitions of dying by hospital staff therefore depend on the patient's death impinging on their work. Arguably, the same happens in home care – the patient comes to be defined as dying by professionals when this process directly involves the primary health care team or indirectly involves them in making alternative arrangements for care.

A second important feature of who is defined as dying is the person's social value. Characteristics included in how we define social value are age and status. If a prognosis of 2 or 3 years is given to a 30-year-old, it has different social relevance from the same prognosis given to an 80-year-old. The patients are in very different positions in their life careers. The younger patient is still very early in the work career, may have a young family, an active leisure and sports life and, in the normal run of things, could look forward to a long, happy and fruitful life ahead. This is not so for older people who are already oriented toward forthcoming death. The family is increasingly independent, references to the future are curtailed and the life career is regarded more in retrospect than in prospect (Cumming & Henry 1961). The death of an old person requires less drastic revision of others' life plans than when a young adult is dying. Blackburn (1989) and Seale (1991a) both note the difficulty in determining or 'diagnosing' dying in elderly patients, particularly those with dementing illness (Brechling & Kuhn 1989).

Social significance is also defined by status positions in society. Sudnow observed tremendous efforts to keep alive those who were 'special cases' – particular individuals whose lives were considered especially worthy of saving. On the other hand, those deemed socially unworthy – drunks, suicide attempts and other types of morally improper persons – had far less attention given to them to sustain life. Particularly in the case of those brought into the Emergency Unit as possible 'Dead on Arrival', the social status of the patient as much as their physiological status influenced subsequent events. Depending on the category into which patients were slotted, they were treated in organisationally routine ways. When patients did not fit neatly into prevalent classifications – atypical deaths like that of a child or a young adult or on the other hand a morally imperfect citizen – then disruption of routinised meanings, activities and consequences was observed. The types of disruption depended on the social status and worth of the individual involved.

The process of becoming a dying person influences and is influenced by orientations toward the future rather than the past or present. Activities of families and hospital staff become organised around expectations of death. To be dying places a framework of interpretations around the individual which influences social activities.

Categories of death

When we hear of a death we may classify it in different ways – untimely, a waste of a life, a happy release from suffering. In sociological and anthropological literature there have been a number of consistent categorisations of death. The most common of these are social and physical death; 'good' and 'bad' deaths and natural and unnatural deaths.

Sociologically, Sudnow (1967) distinguishes *clinical* and *biological* death from *social* death. Social death is when the individual is treated as a corpse but is still socially alive. More rarely the opposite happens, when someone has biologically died and is treated as if they are alive, for example, by being spoken to. Staff may adjust patients to look *as if* they are alive or busy themselves doing other things to avoid having to carry out 'last offices', a task not relished in most settings and observed by James (1986) to be a cursory affair in hospital wards compared with a hospice.

More regularly, the patient is treated as socially dead while still alive in biological terms. Examples of social death include seeking permission to carry out postmortem examinations before the person has actually died. Patients can also be said to be socially dead when the doctor passes by and no longer pays attention to them on the ward round. They are no longer of interest in respect of further diagnosis or treatment. Nurses treat patients as socially dead when they pack up their belongings for removal prior to the patient's clinical death. Physiotherapists do so when they cease attempts at treatment while relatives, by stopping visiting, terminate social life.

Observation of the management of dying patients demonstrates the definition of patients' states. At one time, in Nightingale-type wards, when patients were moved to the bed adjacent to the door this was an indication that they were dying. One of our grandmothers was admitted to hospital as an obstetric emergency. She was placed in a small room immediately beside the front door of the hospital. This was a cue to the family that she was not expected to survive. She did survive, however, and was subsequently admitted to a ward. In effect she had been treated as a corpse until, despite the expectation of dying, she lived and was subsequently afforded patient status. This is an example of movement between life and death, with social life reinstated.

Hockey (1990) similarly describes the movement of elderly people in residential homes who become incontinent, unable to walk or 'confused in their minds' to rooms in the 'frail' corridor. The very name alludes to 'their own death-evoking physical and mental deterioration' taking place within the homes' implicit task of channelling deteriorating elderly people towards their deaths. As they became more nearly the corpses, which is the unspoken end product of all social care homes and nursing homes, they were separated and placed in an alcove convenient for staff attention rather than joining the more able residents in the main lounges. Surprisingly James (1986) also observed people in a hospice attached to a hospital also moved into a single room as death approached. The distancing and separation of dying people in institutional care is a microcosm of the less obvious but powerfully pervasive death-distancing strategies in our society at large.

Closer still to death, behavioural changes of staff toward the patient can be observed. As observation of biological life signs show a decline and death approaches, attention shifts from caring for the patient's possible discomforts and carrying out regular physical treatments to defining biological events. Traditional practices of suctioning, mouth care and repositioning the patient diminish while observation of pulse volume and respiration depth and rhythm become important. Routine drug therapy may be omitted.

A contemporary form of the social/physical death distinction resides in the somatic versus brain death classification where sociability is seen as residing in human consciousness and the absence of such consciousness is equivalent to death (Glaser & Strauss 1965).

Most societies hold views on the nature of good deaths and bad deaths.

A 'good' death in anthropological literature is one ... which suggests some degree of mastery over the arbitrariness of the biological occurrence. By contrast, in nearly all our examples, those deaths which most clearly demonstrate the absence of control are those which are represented as 'bad' deaths and which do not result in regeneration. (Bloch & Parry 1982, p. 15)

A timely death in which ritual can be properly attended to, and power and influence can be appropriately redistributed, remains the preferred mode of death (Glaser & Strauss 1968). Staff themselves categorise deaths as 'good' or 'bad'. Wright (1981) comments on a formal reviewing system of all recent deaths by hospice staff. Deaths are evaluated on a 10-point scale. In this case staff have formally defined what they regard as the characteristics of a 'good' death. High on the list is dying free from pain and with 'dignity'. Less formal accounts of what constitutes 'good' or 'proper' deaths are likely to be along similar dimensions, although they will be context specific. A 'good' death in a special care baby unit will not be the same as that in an adult intensive-care unit or in a geriatric ward.

Wright found difficult deaths characterised by ineffective pain control and feelings of inadequate interpersonal relations with the patient concerned. A major contribution to a 'bad' death in the context of the hospice was the occurrence of an atypical trajectory. These may be deaths judged as abnormally quick or lingering and which, as a consequence, influence the feelings the staff have about the adequacy and appropriateness of the care given. Also patient behaviour during dying, defined by the staff as inappropriate as judged against standards of proper conduct, can render a death 'bad'. Wright (1981) cites the case of a male patient, known to be adulterous and known to grab the nurses in an affectionate way, who was labelled uncooperative.

Glaser and Strauss (1965) note two kinds of obligations which staff expect to be met by dying patients who are aware of their terminal status. First, patients should not act to bring about or hasten their own deaths, for example, by attempting suicide. Second, patients have certain positive obligations to meet standards of courageous and decent behaviour. Their partial list includes:

The patient should maintain relative composure and cheerfulness. At the very least he should face death with dignity. He should not cut himself off from the world, turning his back upon the living; instead he should continue to be a good family member, and be 'nice' to other patients. He should cooperate with staff members who care for him, and if possible should avoid distressing or embarrassing them. (Glaser & Strauss 1965, p. 86)

It is much easier for staff to appreciate those who exit with courage and grace, not merely because they create fewer scenes and cause less emotional stress but because they evoke feelings of professional usefulness. It is far less easy to endow deaths with positive evaluation when patients behave improperly, from the staff's perspective, even though it is possible to sympathise with their terrible situations.

A distinction is also drawn between natural and unnatural deaths. The legal manual for coroners contains the statement:

All deaths can in a sense be regarded as natural. This is true in a philosophical sense in that it is part of man's lot to die. It is also true in a medical sense in that in all cases death is brought about by one or other of man's organs. In order, therefore, to distinguish between one sort of death and another it is necessary to consider not only the terminal cause of death but the cause which was the real cause of death. (Jervis 1957, p. 83)

This provides a major classification of death in which the presence of disease marks a natural death in the absence of human agency. Deaths which at one time were attributed to 'the hand of God' in the absence of human agency are now often filled by the concept of 'accident'. Deaths attributed to accident place them in the context of unintentional events whereas deaths which are intentional include suicides, homicides, infanticides and acts of war.

An example of shifts in the natural/unnatural classification are sudden infant deaths. These were once classified as unnatural but in recent times they have been reclassified as natural deaths, despite the fact that they remain unexplained and cannot be accounted for (Knowelden et al 1985). This late recognition of naturalness is primarily due to the medicalisation of these, like other deaths. A syndrome, sudden infant death syndrome (SIDS) was first recognised in the United Kingdom in the 1950s but not officially reported on until 1965 (see OPCS 1982). Sudden infant death provides a model for understanding the way in which deaths are classified as natural or unnatural. Any death which is regarded as unnatural would be reallocated to the natural realm should it be attributed to a disease factor. The increasing demand of clinical medicine to expel humanistic labels and use disease categories means that it is unlikely that old age, hunger or poverty would be cited as causes of death. Social actions and social structures are suppressed in explanations of death. As Prior noted in Belfast, an initial somatised explanation of death due to a plastic bullet was 'Bruising and Oedema of Brain associated with Fractures of the Skull'. This was reclassified after the victim's family brought legal action which challenged the relegation of the socially relevant cause of death to somatic conditions. The death was subsequently redefined as 'Died as a result of injuries received after having been struck by a plastic bullet, and

we believe her to have been an innocent victim' (Prior 1989, p. 65).

Place of death

Examination of the data presented in Table 10.1 show that more people die in hospital or other institutions than in their own home. From national samples of people in the last year of life, Table 10.1 shows the dramatic change between 1969 and 1987 (Cartwright 1991a). A quarter of those dying had spent no time in hospital in the last year of their lives and least likely to be admitted were those over the age of 85 years (Cartwright 1991b). However, almost a quarter of adults who died spent at least part of the last year of their lives in a nursing home or social-care home (Cartwright 1991c). People from rural areas are more likely to die at home and Doyle (1980) indicates that nearer 70% of urban deaths occur in hospital. This is despite the fact that most people would prefer to die at home (Parkes 1985). Townsend et al (1990) also found among terminal-cancer patients who had a preference for place of death that only 20% wanted to die in hospital. Whilst their own home was the preferred place of death for 94% of people who died there, 69% of people who died in hospital had previously stated a preference to die elsewhere. Hospitals with their ethos of cure are therefore the most likely yet least popular place of death. Why this is the case is understood by examining the development of the hospice movement.

The first hospice to emerge in the United Kingdom since the medieval period was St Joseph's Hospice in the East End of London in 1902. However, it was in 1967 that the hospice movement was given impetus with the establishment of St Christopher's Hospice by Cicely Saunders. The need for such a development was directly related to the failure of hospitals and medicine to provide for 'good' deaths. Since then there has been a proliferation of services, extending the inpatient hospice concept to home and day care and symptom-control teams (Fig. 10.3). Hospice type inpatient facilities are also proliferating and being provided directly

Table 10.1   Place of death in 1969 and 1987

Place of death	1969	1987
	(%)	(%)
Hospital	46	50
Hospice	–	4
Other institution	5	14
Own home	42	24
Elsewhere	7	8
Number of deaths	785	639

Source: Cartwright A 1991a Changes in life and care in the year before death, 1969-1987. Journal of Public Health Medicine 13:81–87, Table 2

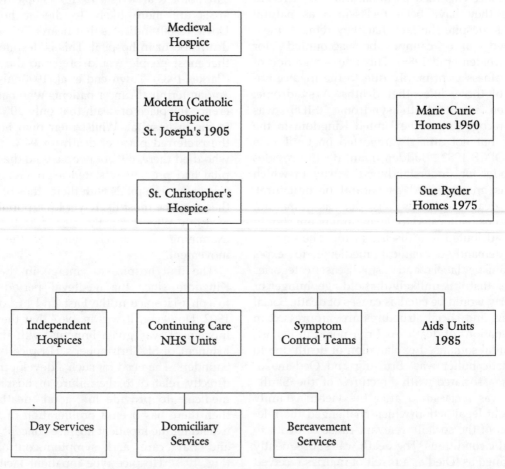

Fig. 10.3 The development of hospice care and other services for the terminally ill.

within the NHS as well as by their purchase of care from hospices in the voluntary sector. Table 10.2 shows 145 different inpatient facilities classified as hospices.

Hospices were set up to provide better deaths. However, initially they maintained the separation of people who were dying by placing them in a special institution devoted to death work. However, this was death work different to that provided in hospitals where Glaser and Strauss (1965) characterised deaths as involving impersonal routines and strict control over emotional expression and openness about death. Research-based criticism of hospital deaths has continued while hospice staff themselves find justification for their expertise in telling stories about hospital failures (Wright 1981, James 1986).

Hospices pioneered what they claimed was a different approach to dying. This is characterised by emphasis on palliative medical therapies rather than curative ones, and on careful attention to the relief of symptoms associated with advancing disease. Of particular concern is the relief of pain which is reported by 84% of patients dying of cancer (Cartwright 1991a). In hospices the aim is to provide pain relief in such a way that patients are not rendered unconscious (Wright 1981, Saunders & Baines 1983). The other major innovation in hospice care was to provide for emotional care, respect and dignity in accord with the patients' state of awareness about the illness.

Awareness of death

The patients in Sudnow's (1967) study were like those in most acute care settings in this country. They were expensive acute facilities and patients stayed there for the minimum number of days. His focus therefore was on sudden and quick deaths rather than the lingering deaths often found in hospices. Awareness of dying was not an issue for many of the deaths observed. Neither is awareness for patients an issue when they are comatose or with babies or young children. However, awareness becomes an issue when deaths are lingering and patients remain alert. Lingering and unpleasant deaths are still commonly linked with cancer, and despite the progress in symptom control Seale (1991a) reports that 60% of cancer patients suffering pain reported it to be very distressing. However, the duration of the period of distressing symptoms was shorter than for patients dying from other causes like stroke or respiratory disease, while the intensity of the distress was greater. Nevertheless, the dying period for most patients is such that awareness of prognosis is an issue and 68% of hospital deaths are expected as well as more than 60% of deaths in the community (Seale 1991b).

Table 10.2   Estalished UK hospice inpatient units

Type of unit	Number of units
Independent free standing units	114
Macmillan continuing care units	12
Macmillan mini-units	7
NHS continuing care units	14
Sue Ryder homes	10
Marie Curie Memorial Foundation	11
Total	145

Source: Griffin T 1991 Dying with dignity. Office of Health Economics, London

How patients become aware that they are dying and how hospital staff manage patients' awareness was the focus of work carried out by Glaser and Strauss (1965). In this study the definition of dying was not regarded as problematic. What was important was how staff managed their social interactions with dying patients, in such a way as to attempt to exert control over how much patients were aware of their condition and how much patients could express of their awareness. Sudnow described how patients were treated – the handling of bodies, administering the flow of incoming and outgoing patients, doing diagnoses, prognoses, teaching and so on – in such a way as to fit the institutionalised daily ward routines, 'routines built up to afford mass treatment on an efficiency basis'. Glaser and Strauss observed what happened within interpersonal interactions with dying patients and how they differed according to the awareness context in which they took place.

Glaser and Strauss found that the kinds of interactions which occurred between dying patients and hospital personnel could be explained in terms of what each party knew of the patients' prognosis at any particular time. What was important was knowledge of certainty of death – that the patient would die, and time of death – when death would be likely to occur or when this question would be resolved. Patients can be placed in any of the four categories, as demonstrated in Table 10.3. These categories represent a movement from living to dead and each is essentially a different point in a status passage. Patients move through these statuses; they are transitional points along two continua.

Let us consider an example. A man falls into category 4 before he is ill. He loses a considerable amount of weight, has problems in eating and retaining his food and develops abdominal pain. He consults his general practitioner who refers him straight away to surgeon. It is decided to carry out some tests and exploratory surgery. The man now shifts into category 3; there is not yet certainty about the nature of his illness or whether he will die but we know when the question will be resolved. In theatre a stomach cancer is found. At this point he moves into category 2; that is he will die because of his pathology but we are left with uncertainty about when he will die. He can continue to exist in category 2 until the point comes when time of death is clear. In this sense dying is a status passage although variations in the timing of the schedule, its onset and transitions between stages can vary enormously. This variability, which is beyond our control, caused Glaser and Strauss to call dying *a nonscheduled status passage*.

An important part of this status passage is the legitimate determination of when patients are in passage and changing status. It is regarded as doctors' work to make definitions of the time scale involved, to announce such definitions at appropriate times to professional colleagues, relatives, perhaps even to patients, and to coordinate the passage.

The prerogative to disclose information about diagnosis and prognosis remains with doctors, particularly hospital doctors (Seale 1991b). While nurses may be more able and likely to

Table 10.3 Certainty and time of death

			Time of death		
Certainty of death	Yes	1.	Certain death at known time	2.	Certain death at unknown time
	No	3.	Uncertain death but known time when the question will be resolved	4.	Uncertain death at unknown time when the question will be resolved

answer patients' questions than they used to be (Bond 1983, Field 1989, James 1986, Wilkinson 1991) this is still dependent on having discussed it with the doctor first, or the doctors giving the information and nurses talking it over with the patients afterwards. Nurses, therefore, are no more likely to be involved in 'breaking the news' but are more likely to be open once this has occurred. How much patients are informed also depends on the disclosure norms of the ward. What is disclosed will relate to a prevailing culture. The hospice movement has changed the likelihood of disclosure of diagnosis to patients with cancer, so that patients nowadays are much more likely to have been given diagnostic information about their illness than they were 20 years ago (McIntosh 1977, Cartwright et al 1973, Seale 1991b); as is shown in Table 10.4. While Parkes (1984) and Gilhooley et al (1988) found no difference between hospital and hospice patients in the proportions who knew their diagnosis and prognosis, only one third were judged as knowing their prognosis, rather less than that reported by Seale. Hockey (1990) observed that only patients who knew that they were terminal were admitted to one hospice. There is a difference, however, between knowing that the illness is fatal and *when* death will occur. Maintaining the ignorance of many of those thought not to be aware of their approaching death, and the way in which the others have become aware, involve social processes.

Awareness contexts

Interaction between individuals takes place in what Glaser and Strauss term *awareness contexts* – what each knows about the identity of the other and his or her own identity in the eyes of the other. Four awareness contexts are identified:

1. *Closed awareness* in which the patient in question does not recognise impending death although everyone else does.
2. *Suspicion awareness* in which the patient suspects what the others know and he or she attempts to confirm her or his suspicions.
3. *Mutual pretence awareness* in which both patient and others define the patient as dying but each pretends the other does not know.
4. *Open awareness* in which both staff and patients define the patient as dying, are openly aware that each holds this definition and act relatively openly in response to this knowledge.

The tactics used by professional staff in their interactions with patients are determined, in part, by their expectations of certainty and timing of the patient's death. How they talk with patients, the time spent with them and how the ward atmosphere is controlled are related to expectations of the patient's death and also the patient's state of awareness, as well as the disclosure norms of the setting.

If the patient is not defined as dying then there is no particular reason to avoid discussion of death, apart from the fact that it is still a relatively undesirable topic and could potentially lead into discussing other patients. If the patient is dying, however, this can create many more problems. The nature of these problems is in part determined by the awareness context in which the interaction is taking place.

The different awareness contexts pose different kinds of problems. With closed awareness, the problem is essentially one of maintaining the patient in that state. Staff are in the position of having to construct an account of the patient's future biography that he or she will accept. As an example, a young man in category 1 was moved to a single room. He was thought not to be aware of his impending death. The reason given for his move was that he had developed an infection, which explained why he felt so ill, and which necessitated barrier nursing. Fiction was enhanced by the use of gowns and masks and much handwashing. The staff attempted to maintain a closed awareness context for as long as possible to avoid the more difficult problems they assumed would follow from a change to

Table 10.4 Dying person's knowledge of condition*

	Deaths from cancer		Deaths from other causes		All deaths	
	1969	1987	1969	1987	1969	1987
What was wrong	%	%	%	%	%	%
Knew	29	73	57	60	49	65
Did not know	49	16	27	28	34	24
Uncertain/other comments	22	11	16	12	17	11
Number of deaths	204	158	478	285	682	443
Likely to die	%	%	%	%	%	%
Knew certainly	16	44	18	22	18	30
Knew probably	21	20	20	20	20	20
Probably not	8	8	10	9	9	8
Definitely not	39	14	31	30	33	24
Unable to say	16	14	21	19	20	18
Number of deaths	213	159	478	283	691	442

* Excludes sudden or unexpected deaths of those under 65 years of age. Data obtained from relatives and close friends

Source: Seale C 1991b Communication and awareness about death: a study of random sample of dying people. Social Science and Medicine 32; 943–952, Table 1

another context. For the same reason, delaying tactics are engaged in when patients are to be transferred from a general hospital to a hospital or home for terminally-ill people. To divulge this would certainly create suspicions which some patients would then attempt to confirm. The resulting interactional problems are largely avoided when patients are genuinely unaware.

In suspicious awareness one difficulty staff face is whether patients are really suspicious or may even know. You may hear staff discussing whether or not a patient knows that he or she is terminal, and what kinds of cues are being omitted which give rise to the staff's suspicion that

the patient is suspicious. If it is recognised that patients suspect that they are dying then tactics have to be adopted to avoid disclosure of information which would reduce patients' levels of uncertainty. It is unlikely that certainty about dying would be increased intentionally by professionals other than, on rare occasions, by doctors and then in response to a patient's obvious efforts to find out.

It is possible to maintain uncertainty in many ways – verbally by referring to the future, being brisk and cheerful within normal limits, by chatting about anything and everything and so preventing opportunities for 'difficult' conversations to arise. It is also possible to avoid patients except to carry out 'essential' care, to linger for as little time as possible and then to avoid creating intimacy by involving others. In short, by behaving as if the patient is not dying and acting in such a way that there is no time to talk, patients respect this right that 'other work' is more important. Should the patient ask directly, and they rarely do, then some stock response may be at hand 'I don't know, I'm not the doctor' or 'Only God can answer that' or, more simply, carry on as if the question had never been asked.

Field (1989) found in surgical wards that it was students and auxiliaries who had most contact with patients, although the behaviour of staff in his study and that by Wilkinson (1991) show how important ward sisters are in determining the nature of interaction. Where there is a culture of nondisclosure students very quickly learn how to control patients. They observe the common tactics available in the different settings in which they work and how to have their rights honoured. Learning is more by observation and imitation of their seniors than formal teaching. Professionals can claim the right not to respond to a difficult question by just staying silent – in effect, saying I will not answer that, I do not need to.

Mutual pretence awareness is perhaps the most common context in hospitals. The staff know the position and know that the patient *must* know although the patient does not openly acknowledge this to them and neither do the staff. There are two rationales for this pretence from the perspective of hospital staff. First, it is argued that this is the best thing for the patient, and that no good would come of open discussion because both the patient and staff would become upset by it. Second, not to have to confront the patient with the subject allows for better forms of care to be carried out.

Glaser and Strauss comment that for mutual pretence to be sustained there is extensive use of props. This extends from continuing to carry out particular forms of care not only associated with keeping the patient comfortable, by maintaining adequate hydration and clean and intact skin, but also extending to maintaining elaborate drug therapy for no therapeutic benefit in a physical sense. Routines like recording temperature and writing up fluid balance charts are continued. As Sudnow (1967) observed, when nurses see death approach they may omit some of their routines; in other words some of the props are dispensed with. However, by this time the patient would not be in a state to notice. So long as the patient is sufficiently alert to know what is going on, then the props must be sustained if mutual pretence is to continue.

Avoidance of dangerous topics is important. If the patient chooses to refer to the future *as if* it will be then staff will go along with this just as they will allow him to totter to the toilet unaided in a brave show of pretence. While the aim is to focus on safe topics which suggest that life is going on as usual, if there is a slip then *both* parties will minimise and conceal it, each actively sustaining the status quo. Otherwise mutual pretence would change to an open awareness context.

Open awareness reduced some of the interactional problems just described but other complexities take their place. Two important types of difficulty are associated with time of dying and the nature of dying. While patients may know that they are dying, they may not know when. They may or may not wish to confirm this. Patients may also have definite ideas about how they wish to die and these ideas may or may not be in accordance with those of their families or the professionals charged with their care. Their main concern may be freedom from pain irrespective of drug dosage while the staff may remain concerned about frequency and levels of narcotics being administered. They may wish to die at home while their family fears having them home because they cannot cope. Being able to discuss these things can create all manner of problems.

This can be exacerbated by expectations held by professionals of how patients *should* behave. If nurses consider the maintenance of appropriate fluid intake important whereas a patient has decided not to drink or eat any more then the patient will resist attempts at persuasion. Patients who are afraid of dying may want some one by them almost constantly whereas nurses have other demands on their time and some cannot tolerate spending long periods with dying patients. Some patients themselves attempt to act as if dead before they die – 'turning their face to the wall' by refusing to talk and hiding themselves below their sheets. Open awareness is acceptable only so long as the patient shows courage and grace, does not create scenes and does not make emotional demands. Patients who die gracefully are often long remembered by staff.

For community nurses things are likely to be different. Hunt (1990) found that all of the nurses who formed a symptom-control team espoused a philosophy of 'honesty'. They adopted a uniform strategy to find out what patients had been told which comprised regular stages:

- *Preamble* setting the stage to elicit information from patients and giving them the opportunity to express the gravity of their conditions.
- *Confrontation* in which patients were encouraged to face up to the fact of having cancer and that there were no cures at this stage of the illness.
- *Diffusion* when there was information passed on offering interventions which could not cure, but which could ameliorate the symptoms.

Almost three quarters of community nurses who, with families, provide the bulk of terminal care at home find this aspect of their work more stressful than caring for other patients (Seale 1992). Compared with the nurses in the symptom control team, only 49% of this national sample of community nurses considered that they knew what the patient had been told of the prognosis at the first visit. However, Hunt's symptom-control-team study based on tape recorded interactions shows that the nurses worked on information provided by patients and did not rely on what may or may not have been told by any number of other health professionals or found out in other ways about their condition.

PROFESSIONAL COMPOSURE AND EMOTIONAL LABOUR

As Hockey noted after comparing dying in old peoples' homes and in a hospice, 'controlled caring and caring control must be continually maintained – lest they be transformed into uncontrolled, unmanageable caring or careless, callous control' (Hockey 1990, p. 196). In the old peoples' homes there was much greater control over all aspects of life mediated through the asymmetrical distribution of power between staff and residents and a greater separation of life from death. In the independent hospice there was far less separation, more autonomy for patients with control related to symptoms, and Christian care offering unconditional support to patients and staff. In a hospice established within the boundaries of an NHS hospital, however, James (1986) found that in many respects the autonomy of patients was similar to that in the host hospital.

Familiar professional, social and gender-based hierarchies were maintained within both hospices, albeit 'carefully submerged within the much-discussed and highly-valued concept of the "caring team" ' (Hockey 1990, p. 194). We will deal with issues of profession and gender in Chapter 11. What is important here is that the work of providing care in direct contact with patients who are dying is primarily women's work – with few exceptions matrons, sisters, nurses, auxiliaries, cleaners, clerical workers and volunteers are women while medical directors and doctors, administrators, chaplains and chefs are predominantly men. Is it mere coincidence that the founder of the modern hospice movement was a woman doctor – who had also trained as nurse and social worker?

The care provided to dying patients can be considered as relating to their physical needs and symptom relief, the latter particularly included within the province of medicine, and psychosocial care, usually encompassed within the province of nurses and their assistants. Writing in the United States, Mor (1987) notes that 'hospice is primarily a nursing intervention'. We may contrast this with hospitals which are medical in their orientation and where 'comfort work' and 'sentimental work', which includes composure work to enable patients to maintain their self control, are secondary to the main purpose of efficient medical care (Strauss et al 1985). However, carrying out the sentimental tasks enables the nonsentimental medically driven work to be completed. De Swann (1990) analyses the way the affect is managed in cancer wards and comes to the same conclusion as Strauss et al that time constraints mean that what is in short supply is attention. While attention in the form of physical comfort and medical care can be obtained, other forms of attention, like information, may be less forthcoming as we described above. However, turning to affective attention or emotional support through comfort, sympathy, listening, encouragement and understanding 'no division of tasks has been defined and the needs appear accordingly limitless' (de Swann 1990, p. 40). In hospitals, appeals for attention are construed as complaints and patients 'somatise' them by turning them into symptoms which justify staff attention. Nurses are well aware that it is not a physical need that is being communicated, as the following quotation from a 19-year-old in the hospice studied by James demonstrates:

Possibly because I feel very young, very inexperienced, and how dare I go up to these people who are in great mental and physical suffering and offer my easy platitudes. Sometimes it's easier to give them an injection, take away the pain. You remember Mr Toon? The time he was buzz, buzz, buzz, calling for us. And it was never really very much he wanted. It worked as well to come and just stand by his bed, and just hold his hand. Often he'd just grab your hand, someone to hold on to. Walking in the valley of the shadow of death. It's not just the physical act of dying, it's all the mental anguish that goes round it. That's what this place is trying to treat. There are so many instances of people being scared, patients being scared. Crying out for someone to help them. I feel very inadequate. (James 1989, p. 21)

The extent to which patients and staff are able to express the kind of mental anguish described above depends on the 'sentimental order' of the ward or hospice. *Sentimental order* is a construct derived from the collective expression of attitudes and mood and the forms of behaviour used to manage different kinds of work pressures. One aspect of the sentimental order of wards is the death ratio – the proportion of patients who will die. The socially determined appropriate level of involvement with patients depends on the death ratio, with higher levels of involvement permitted where there is a low death ratio.

While it may be possible to gauge the level of involvement deemed appropriate for a particular ward, over involvement by individual members of staff can happen by virtue of particular relationships with patients. They may have cared for them in an earlier hospital admission, patients may resemble a close relative or friend, the illness may be like that of a family member, it may be easy to identify with patients' age or other social attributes. Close involvement is far less problematic when death is uncertain than when death and time of death become progressively defined. On the other hand, an inappropriately low level of involvement can also create problems. Distance with the patient may have been established because death was expected and, for some reason, dying has become protracted and time of death less certain.

Composure is also influenced by the extent to which staff feel negligent, either about particular features of care or about standards of professional conduct. Saving a patient is a high achievement and failure to save can seriously threaten composure when death becomes inevitable. When a patient moves into the 'nothing more to be done phase' and, while time of death is unknown, a major goal of care is comfort. Providing good quality comfort care can counterbalance previous feelings of negligence. However, it is not always possible to achieve this goal. Then, as at other times, a major composure strategy is to forget the patient – out of sight out of mind – but this is incompatible with giving good comfort care involving regular and sometimes prolonged contact. Thus composure is threatened.

Furthermore, expression of emotions in hospital wards (Bond 1978) as well as in some hospices (James 1986) is fraught withcontradictions. De Swann observed that while it is not official and public medical opinion, in a cancer ward the prevailing unrefuted, half-concealed and pseudomedical idea was that patients should be strong and was best served by controlling emotions and not complaining. Emotional expression and dealing with other people's feelings as emotional labour does not fit with standard ideas about what should occur in the workplace. While modern nursing advocates attention to caring as a central concern (McFarlane 1976, Leininger & Watson 1990) there is no place for it in managerial methods of determining staffing requirements (Jenkins-Clarke 1992). While the caring component of nursing is professionally recognised (Salvage 1992), 'emotional labour is subject to the circumstances in which it is carried out. It does not exist on its own but it requires a form of organisation which allows for spontaneity, flexibility and space to initiate and respond to need for attention' (James 1989, p. 37). While hospices give credence to the demand for emotional care, 'if blocks of time cannot be made available on demand, together with the more routine moments of personal intimacy, emotional labour is lost amongst the apparently more pressing demands. Emotional labour cannot, therefore, be slotted in as an extra within a job, the job has to be flexible enough to accommodate emotional labour. The predominance of the working routine, of the physical labour over emotional labour, shows that even at hospices, particularly at times of pressure when it is the physical work which has primacy' (James 1989, p. 35).

These findings suggest that both the professional composure and the legitimacy of emotional labour in hospices are likely to offer experiences of dying which are different to those in hospital. Yet the data we have from studies in the United Kingdom (reviewed by Seale 1989) as well as from the United States (Kane et al 1984, 1986, Mor 1987), show that as hospice-type care becomes better known, hospitals have adopted some of their practices. At the same time, the more integrated are hospices with conventional hospital systems, the more like hospitals are they in their organisation, relations between staff and care work norms.

BEREAVEMENT

Death is an event which marks the discontinuity between living and not living. Those who experience the death of a loved one are bereaved, and bereavement can be identified as an event with both personal and social elements. All societies are used to death and have developed laws, customs and conventions as well as beliefs for dealing with it. By contrast, the individual who is bereaved is characteristically unprepared for it. Bereavement is the experience of disruptive change, characterised by loss of what has previously existed. In the context of death, the loss of a person also usually involves a radical disruption in the pattern of familiar social relationships. The discontinuity, occasioned by the loss, is an example of disruptive social change and the process of adjusting to it involves grief and mourning.

Bereavement is only one example of disruptive social change. There are other changes characterised by loss – amputation of a limb or breast, loss of a job, moving house and slum clearance programmes (Parkes 1986, Marris 1986; see also Ch. 4). Similarly, people who have lived in institutions for many years and who are then moved to community residences also suffer loss – of valued relationships, of the security of familiar routines and locales (Booth et al 1990). While it is important for health professionals to appreciate the consequences for individuals of being bereaved, there are two components to consider. Grief, which is the subjective experience and involves psychological and physiological response patterns; and mourning, behaviour influenced by customs and mores, through which grief is expressed (Averill 1968).

The ways in which normal felt grief is expressed vary according to cultures and, as far as Durkheim is concerned:

Mourning is not the spontaneous expression of individual emotions.... Mourning is not a natural movement of private feelings wounded by cruel loss; it is a duty imposed by the group. One weeps, not simply because one is sad, but because one is forced to weep. (Durkheim 1964c, first published in French in 1912, p. 397)

However, the intensity of publicly expressed grief and the form that it takes are socially patterned. Marris describes the English traditions of mourning and how they symbolise grief:

Traditionally, full mourning in England would begin with the shuttering of the house, and the hanging of black crepe, while the dead person was laid out in his or her old home. The funeral procession itself was decked with as much pomp as the family could afford, or its sense of good taste suggested. Thereafter, the nearest relatives wore black for several months, and then half mourning for a while, gradually adding quiet colours to their dress. They lived in retirement, avoiding public pleasures or any show of gaiety until their mourning was over. Cheerful events in the family, such as a marriage, were postponed a while: and a widow or widower could not decently consider proposals for remarriage until the mourning had run its term. But the term was limited by convention, and the social pressure which would condemn too hastily a return to normal life also reproved an overprolonged indulgence in grief. At first, the family might visit the grave often, laying fresh flowers there; in time they would go less and less, but a visit on the anniversary of the death might become a perennial ritual of remembrance. Such customs symbolise the stages of grief: at first the household withdraws, shutting out life; then, by the ceremony of the funeral, it emphasises its concern for the dead; then, through the months of mourning, it gradually comes to terms with its loss. And when the period of mourning is over, it can take up the thread of life without guilt, because the customs of society make this its duty. At the same time, the observance of these rituals sustained a relationship with the dead: it was done for their sake, as much as for the world. Conventional Christianity allowed the bereaved to imagine that the dead looked down from Heaven, saw the flowers on the grave, and appreciated them. Thus the relationship was not broken abruptly, but attenuated through all the acts that turned the harshness of death into the gentler sorrow of laying to rest. Yet these acts also acknowledged death – they related to one who had died, not a pretence to the living person. (Marris 1986, pp. 29–30)

No matter the society, the rites of mourning interpret a conflict between the acknowledgement of death and the continuity of life. Changes in social behaviour in Britain – the absence of public expression of mourning by dispensing with black, the growing interest in secular rather than religious funerals, increase in cremation over burial, high remarriage rates among the younger widowed – all stress the living rather than the dead.

While these social phenomena are relevant to social expressions of grief, our understanding of grief is based to a large extent within the context of normalising psychology. Freud in 1917 wrote an essay distinguishing between mourning as normal and pathological melancholia, and so began the trend to medicalisation of grief. This trend was furthered by Lindemann (1944) who was the first to establish a 'symptomatology of grief' and its subsequent management. Like Freud, he distinguished between normal and morbid forms of grief. These were assessed according to the intensity and duration of the symptoms, and treated according to the principles of clinical medicine. The medicalisation of grief was continued by Engel (1961) in a paper entitled 'Is grief a disease?' which compared grief to pathogenic bacteria. Through subsequent decades Parkes (1965, 1972) characterised 'pathological' forms of grief as a mental disorder. With other writers responses to grief were described as stages over a timescale. Kubler-Ross (1970) analyses this into five stages: denial and isolation, anger, bargaining, depression and acceptance. Kavanaugh (1972) lists seven stages: shock, disorganisation, volatile emotions, loss, loneliness, relief and reestablishment. Backer et al (1982) describe three stages: yearning, anger and guilt.

While these writers focused on the subjective experience of grief, Marris (1958) and Gorer (1965) turned their attention to the social structuring of bereavement, and related the expression and intensity of grief to social factors like the nature of the relationships involved. The loss of infants or very elderly people, for example, is less disruptive than the loss of children or economically active adults. While there are also social variations in how grief is expressed, Rosenblatt et al (1976) compared different anthropological studies and concluded that these rituals contained certain common elements associated with *rites de passage* as found in all life transitions. It was Gorer's (1965) thesis that abandoning these customs was an expression of the denial of death in Western culture. This leads people to adopt roles in society in such a way that they express their grief by seeking help from doctors so that the 'patient' is confirmed in the sick role. The prescription of drugs to block the feelings of grief serves only to delay or distort its expression rather than promote working through it. Bowling and Cartwright (1982) found a tendency for general practitioners who had little contact with widows before they were bereaved to prescribe them tranquillisers, sedatives or antidepressants. They were regarded in turn as less caring by the widows. The quality of social relationship with professionals in the period around the bereavement appears to influence grief resolution. Ransford and Smith (1991) found that surviving spouses showed greater grief resolution when the death had been associated with hospice rather than hospital care. The anticipatory guidance given to relatives by staff before the death, associated with expression of anticipatory anxiety, opportunities for continued interaction and communication with the dying person and the chance to make restitution for failure in the relationship by contributing to the care of the dying person are all indicated as influencing subsequent adjustment to bereavement (Parkes 1985). These are most likely to be found in the networks of care which surround the family as well as the patient in hospices. The importance of the quality of social relationships is further enhanced by prospective studies of bereaved widows and widowers (Raphael 1977) who found the poorest health outcomes after bereavement were among those who perceived their family as 'unhelpful'. Poorer outcomes are also found when multiple losses are involved and when the quality of the relationship with the dead person was ambivalent (Parkes 1985) or the

marriage was unhappy (Bowling & Cartwright 1982).

Thus, despite attention to social influences on grief:

It was psychology which ... dominated the study of grief and bereavement during the 20th century, and, overall, the problem of grief, like death before it, became medicalised and individualised and subsequently fell under the control of medical personnel. Thus, the priest was ousted from the aftermath of death in favour of the doctor and grief was treated (in all senses of the word) as a private and segmented emotion. (Prior 1989, p. 137)

However, as Parkes accepts, 'how a person mourns is determined, to some extent, by the way he is expected to mourn. But the mourner also determines, to some extent, the way others will react to his mourning'(Parkes 1985, p. 12). Durkheim (1964c) takes a stronger line, however, in arguing that the intensity of grief is dependent on socially constructed formulae. For this reason its public manifestations are socially variable, and the social location of the deceased person in terms of social characteristics like age, class, status, and other forms of valuing, have a great deal to do with how grief is expressed. Grief is distributed according to social principles and how grief is experienced is in some measure reflected in its public expression. Prior goes as far as to say that 'all public expressions of grief act as a mirror in which private feelings are reflected, and as the public expressions wax and wane so does the social base of the sentiments behind them' (Prior 1989, p. 141).

Prior's analysis is based on an analysis of death notices in newspapers in Northern Ireland. Only one of these notices is informative in announcing the death and providing information about the burial or cremation. All of the others are expressions of sorrow or support and acknowledgment of social bonds. By analysing the characteristics of the deceased Prior found different distributions in the number of death notices as shown in Table 10.5. This table shows that factors of gender, occupational groupings, marital status and age make a significant impact on the public expression of grief through notices. Also important was mode of death, with deaths due to violence stimulating most notices.

Evident within the notices were different amounts of privacy in the mourning. The starkest notices, shunning ceremony and restricting the grieving process to the immediate family, were distinctive of professional workers, while among the working classes grief was placed on public display. This public display was dominated by notices from the kinship group, with much rarer expressions from neighbours or friends, except when violence had been involved. Grief is the province of the family circle unless it has implications for the wider community. Thus, most deaths are privatised within the kinship group and this is especially so with Protestant deaths. Irish Catholic deaths take place within a culture which is more public and the community is urged to take part in the grieving process by attending ceremonies. The death notices of Catholics were also much more likely to contain religious references and to portray death from the particular stance of seeking intercession to permit entry of the deceased into Heaven. In Northern Ireland the sectarian social arrangements dividing communities along reli-gious lines were also given expression and reinforced through the particular newspapers in which they were placed and the announcements of the different cemeteries in which the bodies would lie. The publication of death notices then serves as an expression of the social distribution of grief while it also serves as a mechanism whereby kinship, community and political groups can reaffirm and reassert their solidarity.

As we described earlier in this chapter in relation to the social determinants of sentiment around dying, there are social continuities in the distribution of sentiments after death. Those excluded from death notices also have particular characteristics. Those whose physical disabilities or social behaviour preclude full participation in social life – very old people who suffer from dementia, people with learning disabilities, elderly single women of no known occupation, or single men whose occupations were socially isolating, such as the lighthouse keeper or merchant seaman. Many of these are found some considerable time after they have taken place and reflect Marris's claim that grief depends on the degree of disruption experienced by the severance of social relationships. Clearly falling into this group too are the outsiders who

Table 10.5   Mean number of death notices per death in a 10% sample of deaths in Belfast, 1981

Demographic variable	Number of deaths	Mean number of notices
Occupation		
Nonmanual	106	4.03
Manual	270	8.59
Gender		
Male	176	8.29
Female	200	6.44
Age		
1–59 years	65	12.37
≥ 60 years	311	6.25
Marital status		
Married	159	9.16
Unmarried	190	5.79

Source: Prior L 1989 The social organisation of death. MacMillan, Basingstoke & London, p. 114

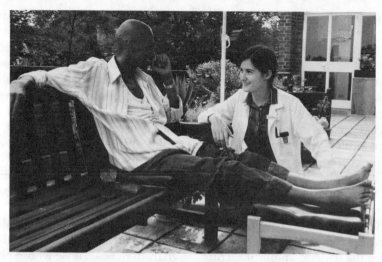

Fig. 10.4   Medical staff learn jow to managed open communications with dying patients at St Christopher's Hospice (courtesy of Derek Bayes).

were not admitted into the society in which they died.

The second major group are those who have never been admitted to the full flux of social life because they died before they were old enough to do so – stillborn babies and neonatal deaths as well as the deaths of infants who were handicapped from birth.

MISCARRIAGE, STILLBIRTH AND PERINATAL LOSS

Legal definitions of what constitutes miscarriage have changed over the years and from one country to another. In the United Kingdom, the legal definition of stillbirth is related to the number of weeks of gestation, marking the probability of a viable live birth. Where there are sophisticated obstetric and paediatric services, the possibility of survival is increasing for lower-birth-weight and lower-gestation-age babies. It is now possible for babies born as early as 23 or 24 weeks with sufficient weight to survive. This means the gestational age at which a birth is defined as a stillbirth rather than as a miscarriage or abortion, has been successively lowered. The mother of an infant born at 24 weeks before the 1980s

would have thought of herself as having a miscarriage. Nowadays, it is possible for a mother to emerge from the trauma of a preterm delivery at this stage in pregnancy with a live and healthy baby. An intrauterine death at this age is now more likely to be considered as a stillbirth.

Women's reactions to miscarriage vary according to the length of pregnancy, previous experiences with pregnancies and the emotional investment in this particular pregnancy (Oakley et al 1990). A common-sense view is that the earlier a pregnancy fails, the 'less' the loss, the 'less intense' the grief. This logic would mean that having a miscarriage would entail less grief than having a stillbirth, which would be less than having a live baby who died. This simple scale to measure appropriate feeling takes no account of the meaning of the pregnancy or birth to the individual but recognises the different legal definitions of the birth products. All live births require a birth certificate and both must be given some form of burial or cremation. Miscarriages, on the other hand, may be treated as the same as gynaecological scrapings and either incinerated or macerated and flushed away. Lovell (1983) examined the consequences of the ambiguities about the status of fetuses and the outcomes of pregnancies which did not result in a live birth. Quoting from some correspondence in *The Lancet* in 1981, she shows that since weeks of gestation are inexact, some probable stillbirths and neonatal deaths are recorded as miscarriages to save the expenses of a funeral and with the assumption of reduced distress to the parents. However, her findings and those from Oakley et al (1990) on miscarriage challenge this view. Mothers differ and often it is those whose babies have lived, even fleetingly, who got over the tragedy better. Those who actually saw their dead babies had a positive view of the experience and they know what subsequently happened to them. Those who had what were classified as miscarriages did not see them, nor did they know what had happened to them:

I think the worst thing about it for me was the fact that your grief is 'intangible' – no name for the baby, never seeing it, no grave to put a flower on, just the horrible thought of it being slung in an incinerator or worse, when you wanted it so much. (Quoted in Oakley et al 1990, p. 106)

To be able to give a baby an identity is associated with having a person over whom to grieve. However, under certain conditions, being able to construct an identity for the baby was interfered with. For women who miscarry staff refer to the 'pregnancy' or the 'fetus' but not the baby. Having a damaged or imperfect baby inhibited staff from showing it to parents. More than three quarters of women who had a termination of pregnancy for fetal malformation experience acute grief reactions but only 1-in-6 received a domiciliary visit from a health professional afterwards (Lloyd & Laurence 1985). It is as if babies who do not look right are morally as well as physically imperfect. Since well-formed babies are described in terms of their 'perfectness', mothers of deformed babies felt guilty and doubted their own self-worth. For those who have a termination rather than a stillbirth, response appears more severe. These babies were defined to them by hospital staff primarily in terms of their abnormality and physical appearance rather than their social meaning.

In contrast, perfectly formed babies, beautiful babies who die, are by implication a tragic loss. Rather than being unfit to be seen, unfit to be loved, unfit to live and so not worthy of mourning, babies defined as beautiful fall into the social stereotype 'beautiful is good'. Mothers whose babies were normal in appearance were not discouraged from seeing them in the same way as were mothers of deformed babies. While professionals may believe that the sight of a deformed baby would be distressing, arguably fantasies about the baby are more frightening than reality. Even seeing part of a deformed baby is better than nothing but without a record deformities may be exaggerated. Nowadays, photographs are often provided as a positive reminder (Lewis 1976). When one of a twin pregnancy is lost, a photograph of an ultrasonic scan is a potent and precious proof that there were two babies.

Loss of a baby also produces loss of anticipated roles as mothers and fathers. Through the course of pregnancy prospective parents are gradually socialised into parenting as preparations proceed, women wear special clothes, give up work and buy baby clothes and equipment. After a stillbirth this is all lost, and women said that they felt as if they caused embarrassment to the hospital staff because they had no baby and had failed to produce what every one had wanted. No longer can the parent of a stillbirth be addressed as 'Mum' and 'Dad'. Lovell (1983) noted women were addressed as 'Mother' from the beginning of antenatal care. In a short space of time, in her assumptive worlds a woman can become a 'mother' and then not a mother and, as well as losing her anticipated new role, she loses the anticipated new baby as well.

Women in maternity units who are no longer pregnant and do not have a new baby may also be stripped quickly of their status as patients. Maternity units are geared to the production of live babies and nonmothers present problems since they do not have babies to wash, feed, change or coo over. They have no legitimate role and Lovell observed that at times women without babies were isolated from the others and would be avoided by staff to the extent of omit-

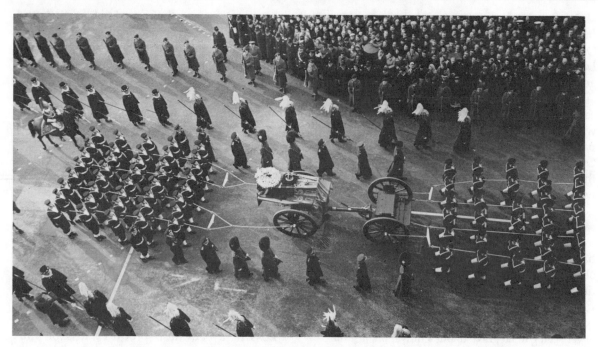

Fig. 10.5   The symbolism of a state funeral (courtesy of BBC Hulton Picture Library).

ting routine care. They may also be sent home with indecent haste. Women felt a 'strong sense of dismissal'. This was particularly the case when they felt that the loss could have been avoided.

While women will have mixed response to miscarriage, stillbirth and neonatal deaths, how they respond is associated with the personal meaning of what was anticipated and the emotional investment in the pregnancy. However, there are societal reactions to losses that will serve to mediate personal responses. The goal of midwifery is to produce healthy mothers and babies. Feelings of failure occur around many hospital deaths, and still birth is no different. This means that women can be handled in such a way that the failure felt by the staff and unacceptability of the failed outcome, are extended to them. Trite comments such as 'See you next year' implying another and more successful attempt – in which case the patient would be more acceptable, are hurtful. Similarly, when one of a pair of twins has died, to

hear 'At least you have one healthy baby' causes pain and resentment since no parent can be expected to find comfort at the death of one child in the survival of its healthy sibling. Ejection from hospital into the community does not mean a more comforting environment, since lay and professional attitudes mirror each other – the life and death of a baby are treated as if the latter cancels the former, and renders the lost baby 'invisible'. Only for the would-be parents may there be an enduring sense of loss:

'You keep thinking of what he/she would be doing as the months and years go by.'

'We are low just now because had our first child been born she would be 11 this week, which means she would be commencing secondary education next term.' (Quoted in Oakley et al 1990, p. 108)

SUMMARY

In this chapter we have reached the end of the life career, which in some cases had hardly begun before it was ended in physical and social terms. The impact of being involved when someone is dying and of bereavement for those who provide professional care and for those who are bereaved have been described. As in other aspects of health and illness, gaining a sociological perspective on everyday events provides us with different insights in their construction and processes. The major advantage of gaining a sociological understanding of dying, death and bereavement is to assist in making these events more bearable to those involved – be they health professionals or lay people, for health professionals are also bereaved in their personal and private lives. Meeting death in the wards for the first time is a powerful experience for students (Quint 1967, Field 1989) and if badly handled may cause them to leave (Birch 1975). To have patients die contravenes the ideological basis of providing health care in our society which focuses on 'saving' patients and restoring them to health. Only in hospices and the growing number of palliative-care and symptom-control teams are these ideals adjusted to trying to achieve 'good' deaths. But these too are professionally defined.

We have alluded to a number of studies which highlight the difficulties experienced by professionals when coping with the final drama of life. Just as lay people try to deny death or at least avoid it, the feelings of failure of staff intrude on professional demeanour and at times this leads to insensitivities in behaviour which have negative effects. Feelings of failure do not fade with experience. Oakley et al (1990) found some doctors were very distressed when they were responsible for the care of miscarrying women. They may then avoid them, and midwives do likewise. Gaining an understanding of this may not lessen feelings of failure but understanding the consequences of its expression may go some way towards changing it. As we have described, the social context in which bereavement occurs and the perceived involvement and caring of staff as well as family members have effects on felt grief and the expression of grief of those who have been bereaved. Whether people can express their grief, and the social structuring of bereavement, can be understood by reading

texts like that by Oakley et al (1990) relating to miscarriage and by Oswin (1991) relating to people with learning disabilities who have been bereaved.

We are mortal, but many deaths are premature and avoidable. It is these deaths that create most distress, particularly when they are sudden, painful and when whole communities are involved. Large-scale disasters create major social and psychological traumas for communities, and health professionals are often those involved first at the scene and subsequently in offering support. To do so effectively means understanding the social significance of the loss as well as the prevailing mores surrounding and defining this particular status passage. While it is tempting to lay down benchmarks against which response to bereavement and appropriate expressions of grief can be marked as normal or pathological, the meaning of death to the individuals concerned, over and against any wider social significance of the death, needs to be considered. But as we have described, how individuals respond to bereavement is socially variable, and the social location of the dead person in our assumptive world has much to do with how grief is felt. How it is expressed is socially derived. In multicultural Britain, these differences will be even wider than those we described using Belfast as a case example. Equally, how dying is handled will vary according to the culture of the institution in which it is managed – hospital, hospice or residential home – or the person's own home where most people would prefer to die.

Death, like birth, creates ties with the unknown. Both require cultural constructions which serve to explain human existence as part of the wider metaphysical realm, and the transition between one state of being and another. How society deals with births and deaths is central to its prevailing beliefs and practices; in particular, how we treat those who are dependent on others is indicative of wider social values. Medicine and technological developments have given immense comforts and gifts, as well as opened up opportunities for the perpetration of atrocities. Medical control has been increased through the changing technologies of transplant surgery, genetic engineering and artificial reproduction. The social consequences of these new technologies have yet to be understood, but they are potent illustrations of how health care professionals are responsible for creating and influencing the quality of birth and death experiences. These events also have been increasingly institutionalised, and as such 'have been stripped of the long established traditions and support systems built up over centuries to help families through these highly meaningful transitions' (Klaus & Kennell 1976). Not surprisingly there are opposing movements to reduce medical control and increase individual control over birth and deaths.

FURTHER READING

Field D 1989 Nursing the dying. Tavistock/Routledge, London

Glaser B G, Strauss A 1965 Awareness of dying. Aldine, Chicago

Kearl M C 1989 Endings: a sociology of death and dying. Oxford University Press, Oxford

Oakley A, McPherson A, Roberts H 1990 Miscarriage. Penguin, Harmondsworth

Prior L 1989 The social organisation of death. The Macmillan Press, Basingstoke

11

The professional career

In this chapter we deal with the concept of career in its more traditional sense of occupational or professional career. The idea of profession is approached by considering it in relation to occupation and the division of labour as it influences nursing. The development of professionalism is traced, indicating the dynamic nature of the concept by describing changes in how profession is considered from Nightingale to the present day. The socialisation of students into professional nursing roles is related to the varying conceptions of profession, while secondary socialisation deals with nurses becoming health visitors.

These are interrelated themes. Gaining any understanding of the current nursing occupation, its divisions and educational status, requires it to be grounded in both the historical and the current social and political interests that have shaped and influenced developments. Important among these social structural influences are gender, ethnicity and class, as well as state-legitimised credentials in the development of the hierarchically structured division of labour in health care. In Chapter 7 we have already described some of the changes which have taken place in the organisation of health care. In this chapter our attention is focused on the paid workers who provide health care in contrast to the army of unpaid workers who operate in the domestic sphere.

PROFESSIONS AND OCCUPATIONS

As with other sociological constructs, there is a tradition of debate about the meaning and sociological value of the term *profession* and whether it may be distinguished from other kinds of *occupation*.

Sociological definitions are more specific and empirically grounded than are common sense definitions and a useful way of thinking about professions is to consider their similarities and differences from other kinds of occupation. Certainly, the Registrar General's and other measures of social class use the idea of profession to classify a broad range of occupations and some of those, and the distinctions between different classification systems, were described in Chapter 3. What these particulars may be are not necessarily fixed in time or context, however, and in Chapter 3 recent changes were described. Another way to consider professions is to list traits. One example of the trait approach is quoted by Becker:

Professional activity was basically *intellectual*, carrying with it great personal responsibility; it was *learned*, being based on great knowledge and not merely routine; it was *practical* rather than academic or theoretic; its techniques could be taught, this being the basic of professional education; it was strongly organised *internally*; and it was motivated by altruism, the professionals viewing themselves as working for some aspects of the good of society. (Becker 1971, p. 88)

Freidson (1983) has argued against definition as a list of traits and proposes that there are two distinct ways that profession is used. The first is an occupation that has assumed a dominant position in the division of labour so that it gains control over determining the substance of its own work. It is also autonomous or self-directing and is able to sustain this special status by the extraordinary trustworthiness of its members. The training which professionals have, typically in higher education as well as in practice settings, provides them with specialised knowledge, ethicality and claims to social importance which enable them to have a special kind of control over and market rights for clients.

Johnson (1972) also stressed that the key to professions lies in particular institutionalised client control. Clients lack the specialist and esoteric knowledge of the professional, lack the sources of power of the professional and are relatively helpless. This enables the professional to dominate in relationships with clients as well as achieve work autonomy.

These knowledge based 'disciplinary techniques' (Foucault 1980), however, are the outcome of wider social and political processes. This is especially the view put forward by Johnson, who regards the client/professional relationship as rooted in the characteristics of the societies in which it is found. Thus professions develop in relation to the dominant existing class structure. Indeed, Johnson (1977) expounds the traditional Marxist view of professionals as 'fulfilling the global functions of capitalism' by legitimising the existing class structure while claiming moral neutrality in this respect.

Others have also taken a macrolevel approach to professions. Parry and Parry (1976) argue that doctors in the 19th century, through the control of the professional organisations, were able to gain social advantage. As the class system was emerging in industrial capitalism, so the new breed of doctors and their wives were part of the development of new status groups. Class is only one form of social stratification and Stacey (1988) draws attention to the importance of gender as well as class status in the development of professions. Europe has been male dominated for centuries, following from the patriarchal structure of domestic kinship relations. The public domain, as it developed as separate from the domestic domain, replicated domestic marital relationships. In the 19th century, the public domain was almost exclusively male and women, particularly middle-class women, were increasingly domesticised. Men ensured that the occupations which succeeded in their claims to professional status were male occupations.

The achievement of professional status in medicine was associated with achieving regulation but only after many attempts. The 1858

Medical Act established the General Council of Medical Education and Registration, known as the General Medical Council. This was charged with regulating the medical profession on behalf of the State, overseeing medical education and maintaining a register of qualified medical practitioners. This means that only registered practitioners can call themselves qualified medical practitioners. The Act enabled a distinction to be made between the qualified and the unqualified, to restrict entry and manage the labour supply of qualified doctors. During the 19th century medicine became secure, stable and rewarding, doctors enjoyed 'a steadily increasing degree of control over their work, their patients and their careers'. They were 'emerging as a profession' (Waddington 1984, p. 205).

Semi-professions

Others in the division of labour also lay claim to professional status. Etzioni (1969) called occupations with less autonomy over their work or control over education and a subordinate position in the occupational division of labour, the *semi-professions*. Freidson (1975) uses a similar concept – the *para-professions*. These are occupations organised around a dominant profession and are reflected in the ways professions describe themselves, for example, 'professions allied to medicine', in the names of their formal organisations 'The Council for the Professions Supplementary to Medicine' and official classifications such as 'paramedical groups'. Freidson contends that the close proximity of these occupations, which include nursing, to the truly professional groups encourages them to take on professional attributes and make claims to be professions. Their challenge to medical *hegemony*, the domination of one social group over others, will be addressed in a later section.

PROFESSIONALISM AND NURSING IN THE NIGHTINGALE ERA

The above brief introduction to the notion of profession and the instance of the profession of medicine, presents a backcloth to the development of nursing since the two occupational groups are closely related. British nursing had its antecedents in the handywoman class, which Abel-Smith (1960) regards as no more than a specialised form of charring. In the 19th century workhouses the work was performed by able-bodied paupers, and elsewhere women from the respectable working class were recruited to do a job without training or high status, poorly paid and with poor work conditions.

After 1840 nurse training was introduced in circumstances associated with the success of pioneers, of whom Florence Nightingale is the most well known. Two aspects of this success are noteworthy. First the upper-middle class background of Nightingale was totally different from the handywomen nurses. As well as being well educated, she was financially independent and able to cultivate favour both among politicians and the governors of the powerful voluntary hospitals. Also at this time the British State was involved in the first modern industrial war, in the Crimea, and as a result became the first unified and large scale consumer of nursing services. This was in contrast to the former practice of nursing services being provided within the home environment. Hospitals were regarded by all social groups as institutions of last resort. The Crimean War was used by Nightingale to demonstrate the value of organised nursing services in the 'national interest'. It was with the development of hospitals that nursing took on a recognised occupational role rather than a community, domestic role.

Gender and patriarchy

An initial organising principle was gender – nurses were female. This reflects the origins in domestic service and the Nightingale training course was specifically suitable for 'daughters of small farmers who have been used to household work and well-educated domestic servants' (Nightingale quoted in Abel-Smith 1960, pp. 21–22). The positive emphasis on the female gender was associated with trained subservience to the male, and specifically male medical, authority. Understanding this relationship requires an understanding of the relationship between professionalisation and patriarchy which has been taken up by feminist writers like Garmarnikow (1978) and by mainstream sociologists like Hearn (1982).

'Patriarchy can be defined as an autonomous system of social relations between men and women in which men are dominant' (Garmarnikow 1978, p. 99). Rather than being biologically or naturally determined, patriarchy designates social relationships between men and women. As we discovered in Chapter 5, the feminist critique of the family examines male exploitation of women with husbands owning and controlling wives' unpaid labour. All professions throughout history have been male dominated. This analogy with the family is extended by describing the position of patients like that of children. As we saw in Chapter 9, as with children in the family, patients come lower down the hierarchy of social relations in health care. Nightingale entrusted nursing with two main functions – hygiene or 'nursing the room' and assisting the doctor. Both can only be practised *after* medical intervention, particularly making a diagnosis. This maintains both a subordinate position to medicine and the division of labour between the two occupations. This was reinforced by the alleged scientific nature of medicine, and the nature of interprofessional relations reducing the nurse to a nonscientific aide whose authority derived from her relation to medicine. Thus nursing became an occupation *primarily defined by its responsibility for executing medical orders and directives*. As Gamarnikow observes, however, it was believed that the healing process was dependent not only on obedience *per se* but also, more importantly, on the harmonious relations between the two occupations. Any power struggle was to be suppressed. This has its modern counterpart in analysis of 'the Doctor-Nurse Game' (Stein 1978, Stein et al 1990) described in Chapter 7, whose cardinal rule is avoidance of open disagreement, particularly where nurses wish to offer and doctors ask for recommendations about patient care.

A middle-class occupation

Nursing became an occupation specifically attractive to middle-class women who had to earn a living. It became a paid job rather than another form of voluntary female Victorian charity. Nursing reformers of the Nightingale era were therefore successful in creating paid jobs for women by, at the same time, not threatening medical control over health care. Nursing was women's work – a good nurse is the same as a good woman. It was *character* that mattered, character linked with the moral attributes and qualities of femininity. Nursing reforms were associated with a training that cultivated feminine character, thereby increasing the difference between men and women. Later came an emphasis on learning tasks to be accomplished – tasks associated with motherhood and other features of running a home. 'Good woman' still equated with good nurse, reemphasising hygiene. It is in hygiene that any scientific claims of nursing are rooted. Future debates addressed issues of whose province was hygiene because of its close links with menial work. Items other than the personal sanitary aspects of patient care were hived off to maids and orderlies, and nursing kept for itself those aspects of care more directly related to medical intervention.

The lady nurses and matrons were the power holders in nursing, they developed an authority structure in hospitals which reproduced a Victorian class and domestic structure (Carpenter 1977). The care functions of hospitals were carried out by the lower class of female workers but under the moral leadership of upper-class women. Even in psychiatric hospitals, where there were large numbers of male attendants, women without psychiatric training could be in charge. There was reinforced a structure encompassing harsh discipline, total commitment and low pay (Carpenter 1978).

While nurses evolved a sphere of autonomy, they remained subordinate to the medical and male division of labour. As Runciman noted in the Records and Rules of the Lady Superintendent of the Royal Infirmary of Edinburgh in 1881: 'No nurse shall be dismissed without the circumstances of the case having been previously referred to the Physician or Surgeon to whose ward she is attached' (1983, p. 22). Matron was head of the female side of the hospital and this situation, while holding certain economic advantages for the health service, could not be called managerial. As Carpenter (1978) reports, the prime practice of nursing organisation and authoritarian tendencies, crystalised in the voluntary hospitals, was to create and sustain vocationalism.

Occupational closure

Nurses were recruited on the basis of the minimum of educational attainment and the maximum of moral stature. Through the notion of vocationalism nursing came to be perceived in a unique way that emphasised its claims to exclusivity. While offering paid employment, it was not undertaken purely for commercial motives nor as spiritual outlet, yet it was sanctioned by the Church for the working out of one's social and feminine conscience. The reforms and training instituted major themes in the discourse of nursing – gender, subservience, vocation, discipline and morality (Chua & Clegg 1990). There were also three main structural consequences which can be interpreted in the context of Weberian ideas of *occupational closure*. Closure involves a general principle by which social groups try to maintain exclusive power over resources, limiting access to them. This involves using all of the characteristics Weber associated with status differences. In the context of 19th century nursing these were that:

1. The newly trained nurses and matrons were invariably unmarried women – there was a prejudice against married women, staff lived on the premises and the mystique of vocation required renouncing husband and bodily temptations. Until the 1900s the voluntary hospitals refused to admit men for training in case they might 'usurp the functions of the doctor' (Select Committee on Registration 1905, p. 4, quoted in Chua & Clegg 1990).

2. Most of the trained nurses were relatively young. Matrons could be appointed to the voluntary and workhouse hospitals from the middle and higher social classes in their mid-20s.

3. Nursing became an acceptable occupation for women of higher social classes who could afford fees to train. They sought to restrict entry to daughters of similar birth who would go on to from an elite cadre of sisters and matrons who controlled the major voluntary hospitals and workhouses in London and the other important centres. A significant number also returned to nurse their own class privately in their homes.

Like the doctors, and in keeping with other aspirant groups like midwives and teachers, the lady nurses at the turn of the century sought state-sanctioned professional closure by petitioning for nursing to become registered. Being registered is significant in demarcating an occupation's boundaries, by separating those who are 'insiders' from those who are 'outsiders'. There were several reasons for nursing wanting to accomplish this – untrained people working in a private capacity being passed off as nurses, no standardisation in what constituted training, support from the powerful London doctors who believed there would be an increase in good nurses for their wealthy patients both at home and in hospital, while at the same time women were agitating for greater recognition and the vote. The absence of closure on the title 'nurse' also threatened the self-image of a group of lady nurses led by Ethel Bedford Fenwick. She sought to extend the Nightingale concept of 'the trained nurse'. It is important to note that there still has not been closure on who is entitled to use the term nurse. Leaders of nursing still regularly use the term 'auxiliary nurse' for those who have minimal training and are not registered.

Nursing up to the Second World War

Nightingale opposed registration and the whole movement to establish examinable competence as the basis for registration and the award of the title 'nurse'. Opposition also came from small hospitals which feared that they would not be recognised as training establishments, as well as from some doctors who feared that registered nurses would encroach their territory. However, the lady nurses campaigned successfully for a central body that would scrutinise nurse training courses provided by hospitals and establish a national examination. At the same time, exclusivity in restricting would-be nurses to those of higher social classes was maintained not only by demanding certain educational standards but also by erecting financial barriers and charging for tuition and taking examinations. It was not until the First World War, and again a national emergency, that 3 years training and examinable and certified competence through registration gained acceptance, and a statutory register was created in 1919. In part, the creation of registration and gaining the vote were a measure of the public debt to women in general and nurses in particular who had 'nursed the wounded, manned munition factories and replaced men in a variety of essential jobs' during the war (Abel-Smith 1960, p. 92). Examinable competence and long years of training became the dominant themes of nursing discourse in the early part of the 20th century (Chua & Clegg 1990, pp. 147–148). The voluntary hospitals were able to insist on probationers having secondary education and there continued an unspoken prejudice against married women. At the same time salaries were kept low so as not to attract unsuitable kinds of women. Men were excluded except in the asylums and a survey conducted by the Athlone Committee in 1937 found male nurses comprised 0.5% in the voluntary hospitals, 4.3% in municipal hospitals and 44.8% in mental hospitals (Ministry of Health and Board of Education 1939). Men in nursing did not share the same class origins as the lady nurses.

While the 19th century nurse was typically a mature woman and the lady nurses at the end of the century began training in their 20s, the age of entry to training was successively lowered until 18 years was the norm. The Nightingale elite had relied on the cultural notions of gender, subservience, discipline and quasi-religious morality and these were gradually replaced by examinable competence, vocationism, gender and youth (Chua & Clegg 1990).

While there was a drive towards occupational and professional unity among trained nurses, there were also inevitably territorial disputes over control. Splits were created by having nurses who were trained and untrained, as well as other more subtle distinctions around married nurses, male nurses, nurses in the voluntary hospitals and the larger training institutions and those in smaller local-authority workhouses for chronically-sick people. These divisions gave rise to an element that was fundamentally contradictory to the nursing elite's notion of professionalism – the incipient identification with the trade union movement. The College of Nursing explicitly rejected the notion of links with the working classes and industrial labour by rejecting trade unionism, the idea of striking and even the concept of overtime as paid work. Nevertheless, during the 1930s trade unions like the National Association of Local Government Officers, the National Association of County Officers, the National Union of Public Employees and the Transport and General Workers Union all actively recruited nurses. This was particularly so in the psychiatric and mental handicap spheres and trade union activity was critical to their emergence as distinct occupational groupings (Carpenter 1980, Dingwall et al 1988). The College of Nursing clearly saw the unions as a threat and opposed them as well as their campaigning for improved conditions by state regulation of the working hours of nurses and funding of nursing services. Despite the College's resistance, something had to be done about conditions. An interim report of the Athlone Committee proposed taking the elitist voluntary hospitals into state control and thereby funding increases in nursing salaries as well as reducing working hours and increasing supporting domestic staff. These proposals were not acted upon until yet another war convinced the Government of their necessity.

Nursing after 1945

After the Second World War there was a continued shortage of trained nurse labour. In part, this was due to the education requirements set by the General Nursing Council which retained exclusivity for those who received their credentials through registration. However, the result was that, because of the trained nurse shortage, to maintain the labour force meant the introduction of new grades. The enrolled nurse, a grade which was also credentialed but at a lower level, was legalised in the 1943 Nurses Bill. Nursing auxiliaries who had no formal training were also accepted as assistants to perform unskilled tasks, while the trained nurse did the most skilled work and the enrolled nurses with lesser entry requirements and a shorter period of preparation were somewhere in-between. Nurses who were trained maintained their position over the enrolled nurses by the delegation of certain tasks while maintaining claims to professional expertise and skills. However, there is no precise definition of what constitutes such skills. They were imputed by the superior and longer education, a permitted set of tasks which other nursing staff were denied, the supervision of nurse learners and promotion potential. Symbolic differences reaffirm the manufactured differences in skill – uniforms and badges, calling learners 'pupils' rather than students who had to satisfy 'assessors' rather than 'examiners'.

While nurses renegotiated their position, the state established the Woods Committee to comprehensively review the nursing services as a requirement of the National Health Service Act of 1946. The Committee (Ministry of Health 1947) made some far-reaching recommendations as a means of increasing the number of trained nurses. It proposed that all nurse training should be of 2 years duration, that the enrolled grade be abolished and that students be given 'full student status'. This would entail removing students from the hospital workforce, relieving them of routine domestic duties, treating them as students and offering an education dictated by their leaning needs rather than service needs. In addition, the proposal was that they would be financed by regional nurse training boards, thus taking them out of the control of the hospitals and the matrons. These proposals were not accepted in full. Although nurse training committees were established the other proposals had to bide their time.

BUREAUCRACY, MANAGERIALISM AND KNOWLEDGE-CREATION

The establishment of the National Health Service, with the creation of hospital groups and new governing bodies, weakened the power of the matrons compared with the group secretary and medical superintendents who operated at the level of the governing body. At the same time, there was a continued nursing shortage. Increasing numbers were recruited from Ireland and the Commonwealth, while nurses were treated as an expendable and easily replaceable workforce, continuing the long-standing myth that there was an endless supply of 'ladies' to fill the qualified-nurse role. The continuing shortages led to yet another report, the Platt Report (Ministry of Health & Department of Health for Scotland 1961) which recommended better pay and working conditions for learners and, again, separation of training from the hospital base. Again these proposals were rejected as likely to 'bring the wrong sort of girl into nursing' while there was dissatisfaction at the loss of decision-making authority among the matrons in the service. This did little for nurse education, regularly the loser to service pressures (Davies 1980), but produced a wide-ranging review of the administrative inadequacies of the hospital structure. The Salmon Report of 1966 (Ministry of Health 1966) on hospital services and the corresponding Mayston Report (1969) on local-authority community-nursing services produced a watershed in introducing bureaucracy and managerialism into nursing. Management structures appropriate to industry were directly transposed into nursing and, for the first time, nurse managers were brought directly into the senior levels of decision-making. At the top of a hierarchical nursing structure, chief nursing officers, along with top level doctors, administrators, treasurers and works officers, were charged with managing the service. The NHS was a complex organisation:

Because of this complexity, organisation in a single hierarchy controlled by a chief executive is not appropriate. The appropriate structure is based on a unified management within hierarchically organised professions, on representative systems within the nonhierarchically organised medical and dental professions and on coordination *between* the professions. Coordination between professions at all levels will be achieved by multidisciplinary teams through which the managers and representatives of the relevant professions can jointly make decisions. The teams will be consensus bodies, that is, decisions will need the agreement of each of the team. (DHSS 1972, paras. 1:24–1:25)

For nurses, the structure placed them at the most senior management level, at least in theory at the same level as the other players, and in control of a nursing hierarchy managed separately from other occupational groups. Indeed, the NHS was described as 'rather like a feudal society in which independent authority is exercised by a number of groups' (Day & Klein 1983). However, this consensus arrangement was not a success in management effectiveness terms and was ill-adapted to the financial and political climate of the 1980s.

Reforms of the eighties

In 1983, Roy Griffiths, deputy Chairman and managing Director of Sainsbury's the retail chain, with a small team, set out proposals for a radical internal reorganisation of the NHS (DHSS 1983). The time was ripe for an idea which had been proposed for the health services management on several previous occasions – the introduction of general managers to run units within the NHS. There were units at different levels beginning with Regions in England, below which were Districts (called Areas in Scotland and Wales and Health Boards in Northern Ireland) and these were units which would comprise hospitals or groups of hospitals, community services or geographically organised groups of services, each with a general manager in overall charge. The proposals met with vigorous resistance from the professions, including nursing, but to no avail. At the root of

the problem were the growing demands of the health service for resources and their concentration in the acute sector services. The commitment of the Government to cut public spending while retaining the NHS, demanded that resources should be used more efficiently (Ham 1985). The need was to change the administrative culture to a managerial one with someone to give direction and to be held accountable for NHS performance. Summing up, Griffiths wrote:

In short, if Florence Nightingale were carrying her lamp through the corridors of the NHS today, she would almost certainly be searching for the people in charge. (DHSS 1983, para. 5)

General management and nursing

Salmon and Griffiths brought some fundamental changes to the gender theme. Until the 1940s, male nurses were confined to a separate register. Even in the psychiatric sector, which had large numbers of male workers, the education and administrative power rested with female nurses with the chief male nurse's power limited to the male wards. The effect of the increased managerialism in the NHS was to increase the number of management posts which were attractive to men and relatively unattractive to women ward sisters. This was associated in part with the absence of patient contact and caring, 'the quintessential discursive basis for nursing femininity' (Chua & Clegg 1990). Women who are married are likely to take time out for child rearing, to face the disadvantages of part-time work and, even if in full-time employment, are less able to be geographically mobile to climb the management ladder because of family commitments. As a result half of senior nurse managers are male while they constitute less than 10% of the nursing labour force (Gaze 1987).

Nurse education

While managerialism has changed the power base, there have also been changes in the rhetoric of nursing professionalism. Nursing legitimised the position of the lady nurses through the ideal of vocational service, an ideal which initially served to exclude the handywomen from professional ranks. The professional version of nursing then sought exclusivity in its high moral ideals vested in the status of the lady nurses. Over the years this claim to profession has declined, and with it the symbols of vocationalism. Claims to professional status favour entrance based on educational credentials which have increased in importance as nursing jostles in the marketplace for girls with appropriate qualifications amidst competing opportunities. The need for nursing recruits amid changes in the demographic base, which again threatens the supply of sufficient entrants to nursing at the same time as there is emphasis on efficiency and value for money, continues to provide for tensions between professionalism and managerialism.

While nursing leaders in the past (Abel-Smith 1960) and the not-so-distant past have campaigned for an all qualified workforce, there have always been significant numbers of unqualified nursing staff. The adoption of the proposals in Project 2000 (UKCC 1986) has ensured that nursing has attained the educational reforms which have given entrants student status and removed them as a cheap form of labour. At the same time, the registered/enrolled nurse division has gone with the introduction of a mandatory 3-year course, of which the first 2 years are common, with specialisation of the different parts of the register in the 3rd year. These different parts of a single register have replaced the different registers which previously existed for nurses in the general, psychiatric, mental handicap and children's nursing fields. To compensate for the loss of student labour unregistered assistants are introduced, under the control of the registered nurse. However, in keeping with the national drive towards gaining formal credentials, National Vocational Qualifications have been introduced for this occupational group (DHSS 1987), thereby maintaining a hierarchy within nursing staff.

The shift of nurse education into the higher education sector, the process of specialisation in nursing through both initial and continuing education courses and the development of certified specialist practitioners who can act as consultants to other nurses, makes nursing more like the professional education of doctors. The registered nurse is recognised as a professional 'knowledgeable doer', with a practical career which requires a high level of decision-making and analytical skills, and also as a member of a progressive and well-established profession.

The development of 'professional caring'

The education theme as the basis of profession is further amplified by the development of over 20 degree courses in nursing in the past 30 years. This provides a basis for developing claims for the scientific basis for professional knowledge through research, and the development of 'theories of nursing', as well as the dissemination of professional values. Disciplines with university status also have a potent resource with which to press for wider prestige and honour.

Claims for professional status are also being made through the adoption of a managerial decision-making approach to patient care. The international dissemination of the 'nursing process' was described by the World Health Organization as:

The rational application of relevant knowledge and technology to nursing intervention and the subsequent development of the body of knowledge and technology in nursing. (WHO 1976, p. 1)

The problem-solving stages of the nursing process have been used as the basis for the curriculum (Rhodes 1980) while this is overlaid with ideas about 'total patient care', 'primary nursing' (Pearson 1988) and the 'named nurse' (DH 1991). The importance of these developments for claims to profession lie in:

An image of individualistic care that is scientifically grounded and carefully researched. Such care is delivered by an educated, rational, 'health professional' who has studied personnel management, psychology and sociology in addition to physiology and anatomy. Today's nurse is not a 'skilled auxiliary of the doctor' but a manager. (Chua & Clegg 1990)

By this means, current claims to profession through managerialism, and aligned with the notion of private practice in the relationship between individual nurse and patient, are precisely in line with the Griffiths rhetoric of efficient resource management. Perhaps it is for this reason that the Government was so willing to accept the idea of the 'named nurse' in its Patients' Charter. While proponents of primary nursing and the named nurse pose threats to health service managers because of their demands for increased qualified nurse labour to carry out 'professional' care, at the same time, the managerial emphasis also provides a means of holding nurses accountable and disciplining them should they be found wanting (Dingwall et al 1988 p. 220), as well as challenging professional values in seeking 'value for money' by employing more unqualified, hence cheaper, labour.

THE DIVISION OF LABOUR IN HEALTH CARE

Nursing is one occupation in a division of labour whose boundaries are in a constant state of negotiation. At the outset of the NHS there were three important groups: doctors, nurses and administrators, with the doctors predominant. Advances in knowledge and technology have increased the division of health labour to create a host of technical and other professions allied to medicine. At the creation of the NHS Bevan said:

It is obvious that the [health] auxiliaries must remain under the supervision and tutelage of the general medical profession. Only in that way can we ensure that the craft is kept in proper order. (Quoted in Armstrong 1976, p. 157)

While this view is reminiscent of the rhetoric considered essential to bring doctors into the NHS, at the same time, the division of health

labour was enhanced by the state providing for formal regulation of professional groups like physiotherapists, occupational therapists and chiropodists like the nurses before them, through registration. As described above, the power of nursing was also enhanced by their inclusion in the highest management tiers, and when general managers were introduced after Griffiths they were open to competition, not only from all professionals and NHS administrators but also from managers from outside the NHS as well. As Table 11.1 shows there was initially a preponderance of former administrators in general management posts, and Whitehall was no longer willing to leave things to the doctors.

Several writers (Armstrong 1976, Alaszewski 1977, Baer 1981) consider that since the 1950s all of the professions, like nursing, have become more self-conscious and attempted both to extend their knowledge base and to exert control over their work. In so doing, they have attempted to encroach on new territory and so engage in 'professional mobility'. However, in an analysis of the relations between medicine and other occupational groups, Larkin (1983) modified the notion of medical dominance by distinguishing between overriding power and immediate responsibility. Recognition of the skills of paramedical workers does not necessarily imply a change in medical hegemony. It is possible to redraw the boundaries without changing the relative positions of the different occupational groups. Larkin distinguishes those occupations whose power is constructed around control of a few tasks from those which are agents of the division of work itself. Medicine falls into the latter while the paramedical professions belong to the former. They may negotiate the boundaries of their competence, but they cannot define them. They may seek, and have obtained an occupational monopoly in their sphere of competence, by negotiating role boundaries with the more powerful medical staff, but they did not challenge medical dominance.

Similarly, nurses may wish to extend their roles and carry out tasks which were previously

Table 11.1   Former jobs of new General Managers in 1986

NHS General Managers	Regional Health Authorities	District Health Authorities	Units (hospitals)
Former NHS administrators	9	132	364
Doctors	1	15	110
Nurses	1	4	7
From outside the NHS including the private sector	3	38	54
Vacancies		2	13
Total	14	191	611

Source: Owens P, Glennerster H 1990 Nursing in conflict. Macmillan, London, Table 5.1, reprinted from The Economist, 4.10.86

within the province of medicine. McFarlane (1980) argued that such extensions, even when competence is assessed, are in danger of taking nursing away from its caring and hence unique professional base, to carrying out medically delegated tasks within a medical model of care. This poses problems for nursing in its attempts to escape the 'handmaiden' image and assert its independence from medicine while medicine retains final responsibility. While nurses may find ways of influencing decisions, by negotiating over clinical matters and being involved as a member of the 'team', such teams remain medically dominated. This applies even to health visitors who, unlike other nurses, have direct access to patients (Dingwall 1980). Recently, there have been important changes in nurses' powers: to prescribe a limited range of products; in palliative care teams to change drug dosage; and to effect patient discharge from hospitals. These developments are not in any essential way associated with, or a result of, an overall decline in medical dominance. Nursing remains within the medical division of labour and accepts medicine as the senior partner, while also being squeezed by the application of business principles by general managers (Hart 1991).

Challenge from below

Within nursing, there is continued challenge to the claims it lays to professional status from the brigade of unqualified workers who work with nurses. While there have been recent attempts to professionalise and redraw the boundaries of nursing to exclude nursing auxiliaries from tasks which are deemed the province of nurses because they involve direct patient contact (Pearson 1988), the stress on value for money in the health service as an element of current management interest is pushing the boundaries in the opposite direction. Thus, successive reports associated with the NHS Management Executive call for a reduction in the qualified workforce in settings like outpatient departments (NHS Management Executive 1990) and in the community. Great interest was expressed in a long-stay ward established without any qualified staff, apart from visiting as requested to do 'technical' procedures (Dopson 1990).

With the removal of students from the labour force comes the introduction of the new breed of nurse support worker which is intended to replace the nursing auxiliary grade. The credit accumulation schemes established by the

National Council for Vocational Qualifications provides for a new system of credentials which will enable those without formal educational qualifications to amass sufficient credits to enter formal nurse training through this route. The closure nursing brought about by demanding a particular level of academic attainment from entrants will be challenged by this new open entry system as a channel of recruitment.

This has been well recognised by the Royal College of Nursing which has perennially dithered over what to do about nursing auxiliaries who had no training to speak of, and now dithers over nurse support workers who have credentials. While the College balloted their members in 1992 to ask their opinion about their admission to membership, with an associate status rather than full entitlement, there was not sufficient support to take this forward. With a desire to increase its membership and reduce the power of the Trade Union Congress affiliated health service unions, the College maintains a second purpose of increasing the distance between nurses and their assistants. History replays itself as the demand for nursing labour and controlled expenditure ensures that the support worker replaces the enrolled nurse as a challenge to professional closure:

With great reluctance, nursing was obliged to accept the SEN in order to have some influence over the growth of assistant nurses and to regulate their competition with SRN [RN] grades. (Dingwall et al 1988, p. 229)

We shall observe whether the same process happens with support workers for, as Baly observes:

The purists may fulminate, and legislation may change the legal position of the nurse, whether she is village nurse, ordinary probationer, or enrolled nurse, it seems that nursing will always need some kind of two-tier system. Either there are not enough wholly trained people to undertake all the tasks, or there is not enough money to pay for them, or maybe all tasks do not require highly trained nurses, merely highly trained supervision. (Baly 1987, p. 56)

The gender order

National Health Service work is predominantly women's work, but it is controlled by men (Doyal 1985). Three quarters of the NHS workforce is female while 91% of general managers are men (Chiplin & Sloane 1982). In the most recent NHS changes to establish NHS Trusts we find that women are again grossly underrepresented. Fewer than 1-in-10 of chief executives is a woman, less than 7% occupy the chair and less than 25% of board members are women (Ashburner & Cairncross 1992).

While nursing is not solely a women's occupation, traditionally men made their significant contributions only in mental illness and mental handicap nursing (Carpenter 1977) while the professionalising thrust has resided in general hospital nursing. It is only with the rise of managerialism that men have made a significant contribution to nursing generally. Davies and Rosser (1986) found that up to 50% of senior nursing posts were occupied by men who constituted less than 10% of the workforce. As we described above, nursing has developed in the shadow of male medicine, to adopt the class structure of modern capitalism and the patriarchal structures and values in British society. The rise of male-nurse management now means that nursing is dominated by men from within nursing.

Davies and Rosser (1985) studied gender issues in both administrative and nursing personnel in a health authority. While women clustered in the lower grades, they did not feel discriminated against but were more dissatisfied than men about promotion and training prospects. This position can be understood by the social ideological models of economic rationality and patriarchal tradition. We can trace the low pay of nurses to their position as women who did not have to earn the family wage but only support themselves. Women's work is generally devalued and paid at low rates. Nurses have also always been regarded as a 'disposable' workforce (Mackay 1989) and so not worth investing in to maximise their potential. Women

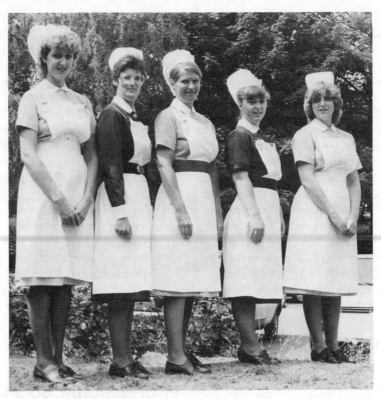

Fig. 11.1   Fed-up with their 'shop-assistant' type uniform, nurses designed their own style with different colours for wach grade. 'It will do wonders for the nurses' morale and professional image', said the Community Nursing Manager (courtesy of Nursing Times).

do not typically have careers, they are regarded as temporary although, with the extension of female employment during the 1960s and 1970s, expected to have jobs for an increasing period of their lives. Thus it was the demand for labour that permitted married nurses to obtain work.

Women typically have two kinds of labour, that in the domestic sphere which is unpaid and paid work (Yeandle 1984). The requirements of domestic life mean that women more often work part-time than men, with consequent downgrading. Yet they are resourceful in juggling two jobs, and positive about the possibility of promotion and making something of their jobs (Brannen & Moss 1991). What Davies and Rosser found was that in the NHS 'the whole way of thinking and way of organising work assumed it

was men who would fill the senior posts and that women were seen as women first and workers second' (Davies & Rosser 1985, p. 18). However, they found no evidence to support the notion that men were career minded and women were not. The difference lay in men being more prepared than women to put themselves forward for advancement, either because they felt more confident or were encouraged to do so. The prevailing gender order in society means that men and women occupy different assumptive worlds regarding career prospects. It remains to be seen whether the introduction of positive policies directed towards equal opportunities for women's advancement in NHS management (Department of Health 1992) change the balance of power since equal opportunities policies have not been implemented effectively (Equal Opportunities Commission 1991). The introduction of extended clinical career grades for nurses (DHSS 1988) may mean that women are more attracted to remaining 'at the bedside' where they continue to gain work satisfaction from caring for patients and, with current pay structures, to earn less than their managers.

In the meantime, the removal of the enrolled nurse grade, with its frustrations of nonadvancement and ambiguous status, and its replacement with the nurse support worker, with shorter preparation, will create cheaper options for the NHS. Those not able to enter Project 2000 courses will have to accept this lower status and less well paid employment, while greater attention will have to be given to retaining the services of the more costly graduates of the new nurse preparation in higher education.

The ethnic order

No less ubiquitous than gender and class-based differences is the influence of ethnicity. Ever since the colonialisation of the Developing World prior to and during the industrialisation of Europe and North America, slaves and then immigrant or migrant labour has been imported to undertake both 'productive' and 'unproductive' work. This enabled the indigenous male population to concentrate on higher status and higher paid 'productive' work. Thus in the postwar years of the 1950s large numbers of black workers were encouraged to emigrate from Developing World countries to the United Kingdom to fill vacancies in public-sector and service industries. Migrant workers became and have remained the backbone of the NHS ancillary workforce in many areas of the United Kingdom where there was a shortage of labour and relatively low levels of male unemployment (Doyal 1985, Doyal et al 1981). For black women the NHS continues to provide secure but poorly paid employment, and within the health sector black women are more likely to undertake the less skilled jobs (Doyal 1985, Doyal et al 1981). People from ethnic minorities are grossly underrepresented as nursing stu-

dents (Commission on Racial Equality 1987) and as nurses they are less likely to be successful in bids for promotion (Nursing Times 1987, Commission on Racial Equality 1988) and to achieve poorer gradings (Commission on Racial Equality 1992).

A Kings Fund Task Force concluded 'Racial inequality in the nursing profession is wide ranging and deep seated' (Kings Fund 1990, p. 38). Black nursing staff are more likely to be concentrated in 2nd-level grades and in elderly care and mental health care than in acute units, and to work night shift. A study of nurses' aides caring for old people in London and New York (Godlove et al 1980) found that in London 45% were noncaucasian and 73% had not been born in the United Kingdom. While London is atypical of the United Kingdom as a whole, these data point up the over-representation of ethnic minorities in the lowest level the least financially attractive and least prestigious nursing work.

PROFESSIONAL SOCIALISATION

The above discussion related to the place of nursing in the health division of labour. We now turn to how people become professionals.

As we would expect, different sociological perspectives give rise to very different views of what it means to become a professional. However, it is not only a matter of looking at the same things and explaining them differently. Different perspectives of professional socialisation have examined different phenomena. The functionalist position emphasised the socialisation of 'professional' trainees. From this point of view it is the process of socialisation which reconciles the opposition between the functioning of the social system and the actions of individual members of society. The core values are internalised through this process so that there is a correspondence between the norms and values of the system and the subjective meanings of the actors in it.

A functionalist view of medical education (Merton et al 1957) focused on the medical school and its faculty as a subsystem of the wider professional system. They regarded student doctors more as student-professionals than as students *per se*. They become professionals by a process within the professional system of the school, with didactic teaching as well as involvement with professionals as important features of the learning that develops them into 'full professionals'. According to this model, socialisation consists of transmitting professional culture to students who are eager to learn it through role relationships with the professional teachers, from whom they learn expectations of the professional role. For this to happen, teachers and other significant professionals who interact with students must uphold definitions of professional roles in their contact with students, and the training experience provided for students must enable them to see the connection between the skills they learn and the carrying out of the professional role. The emphasis therefore is on socialisation by professional education into a professional role. Simpson (1979) comments that this approach fails to consider whether what students learn formally persists into their work as professionals. Nor has it examined the students' motivation to pursue the professional role. A more fundamental criticism is that, rather than focus on a 'noble' profession, with respect of the 'establishment', greater sociological insights would be gained from considering professions as occupations, and identifying similarities among diverse occupations.

For interactionists the search for criteria of 'profession' is quite misconceived. Profession is regarded as a 'lay' term, which some occupations claim at some time under certain conditions. Despite the connotations of the term itself, there is nothing inherent in the work, training, values or whatever to distinguish occupations designated as professions. By the same token there is no assumption of consensus. Bucher and Strauss (1961) remark that 'the assumption of relative homogeneity within the profession is not entirely useful; there are many identities, many values and many interests.' Different segments press their own particular interests, for example, district nurses and health visitors, clinical level nurses and nurse managers. As always, the moral concern of interactionists is on what happens to the 'underdog' rather than the rhetoric of superordinates.

In line with their interests in day-to-day survival two interactionist studies of professional socialisation, Becker et al's (1961) *Boys in White* and Oleson and Whittaker's (1968) study of nursing students, focus on what happens to *students* and not on the professional role. By regarding students as students, they examine how they deal with the problems of getting through school and not as student-professionals. Oleson and Whittaker (1968) note that the important issues for analysis are the 'learner's self-awareness', situational management and integration of multiple roles and selves. They do not consider it useful to take the view that a professional is produced during professional education. It is not until individuals actually occupy that status that they can learn appropriate behaviour. Thus while students learn attitudes as well as skills and knowledge during professional education, these are not regarded as the major influences on the behaviour of practitioners. Rather they argue that the organisation of the environment *after* leaving professional education influences performance. The interactionists are more concerned with the here and now, how students cope with and negotiate demands of the curriculum and other experiences in professional school rather than what they might do once they are professionally qualified.

An essential feature of socialisation, however, is continuity and, in this case, the continuity of behaviour between the status of student and that of professional. The functionalists do not see this as problematic since the student acquires professional culture through the educational process and so membership is assured by provision of appropriate norms and attitudes as well as knowledge. The interactionists make no such assumption since behaviour in unknown future situations depends on transactions between individuals and the particulars of the situations they will meet. The student nurses, who move into the new status of being professionally qualified, will behave and respond to others behaviour according to the way they and others perceive roles at that time.

Simpson identifies three requirements for continuity of behaviour between the worlds of training and work:

1. Enough cognitive preparation for the person to perform their role.
2. Orientation that forms a person's perception of demands of the role and behaviour to meet the demands.
3. Motivation sufficient to make the transition from one situation to another. (Simpson 1979, p. 13)

These three requirements are regarded as dimensions of socialisation – education, orientation, and relatedness to the occupation. Conceiving socialisation as multidimensional involved Simpson in studying the processes of development of each distinct dimension and the conditions in which they develop. Important among the nursing students studied by Simpson was the timing of their experiences and how the students' orientations to the occupational role differed from ideology as well as their original expectations of nursing. However, Simpson (1979) suggests that the purpose of her study was not so much to understand the socialisation of students as such but was to test the efficiency of this multidimensional and dynamic model. So what do we understand of this socialisation process?

Davis (1975) advocates a model which relies on Hughes' earlier conceptualizations of how the status passage from layman to professional is achieved. It is like 'passing through the mirror … [to create] … the sense of seeing the world in reverse' (Hughes 1958, pp. 119–120). He deals with the subjective perceptions of those experiencing this process. This he calls *doctrinal conversion*, which describes the transition from the lay imagery of the novice entering nursing to the institutionally approved imagery of the qualifying student. Bearing in mind that this is an American study where the organisation of nurse education is somewhat different from that in the United Kingdom, Davis identifies six stages of transition.

Stage 1 – initial innocence

Student nurses arrive with a lay imagery of nursing comprising 'a strong instrumental emphasis on *doing* alongside a secularised Christian-humanitarian ethic of care, kindness and love for those who suffer' (Davis 1975, p. 242). This lay conception is at once at odds with what they are taught and what is expected of them. While they look forward to developing skills in practical procedures, they are asked to go to the wards to 'observe' patients and learn how to 'communicate' with them. Because they are taught few practical skills in the early weeks, time spent on the wards creates feelings of embarrassment, uselessness and personal inadequacy. They are unable to act as they imagine a 'real nurse' does. Comparisons with their lay ideals are of no help in understanding what is being asked of them by their teachers.

Stage 2 – labelled recognition of incongruity

At this stage students collectively share the problems with each other – in handling their feelings about not being taught what they expected and their inability to act as nurses rather than on a social level with patients. Large numbers openly question their choice of nursing and consider other occupations. This recognised misalignment of their own expectations and that of teaching staff causes some to leave while those who remain progress to other ways of dealing with the incongruity.

Stage 3 – psyching out

Next, students try to find out what their teachers want from them and how to provide it. This requires the setting aside of their initial imagery of nursing. The students then work to develop ways of identifying what is regarded as desirable behaviour by their teachers – either asking outright or noting what it is that makes a teacher 'light up' – and providing it. While this may be effective to satisfy teachers, it can leave students with a feeling of moral discomfort because they are discrediting their own initial and dearly held ideals. To relieve this feeling for themselves as well as to acknowledge to their peers that they are not *truly* as they appear before staff, students describe themselves as 'putting on a front'.

Stage 4 – role simulation

Role simulation is the performance of 'psyching out'. This entails highly self-conscious manipulative behaviour of students which aims at constructing teacher-approved performances of the nurse's role. It is not truly 'doing nursing' because it embodies self-consciousness, ego-alienation and play acting. The students were uncomfortable and insecure in their performances but, in order to win the approval of teachers, they simulated appropriate performances on the wards. In effect it was 'playing nurse' and not 'being nurse'. However, the more the success in playing constructive performances, the easier it is to gain the conviction that performances are authentic. The symbolic interactionists would say that this is due to the students' ability to adopt towards themselves the favourable responses which their performance in the new role elicits from others. If others regard this performance as trustworthy, competent and legitimate, the student becomes that status which the performances claim. So it develops that students fashion performances in front of others which are more in accord with the doctrinal emphasis of the school than with residual elements of their lay imagery of nursing. Rewards for such performances gradually dissipated feelings of hypocrisy or inauthenticity. They were on the way to 'becoming nurse'.

Stage 5 – provisional internalisation

Students had passed through the first four stages by the end of their first year. The next 2 years were taken up by moving from *provisional internalisation* of institutionally approved perspectives to their *stable internalisation*.

What characterises this stage as 'provisional' is that there exists an inability to be absolutely committed to the new cognitions, percepts and role orientations which guide institutionally approved behaviour. At this time doubts emerge about suitability of the nurse and the practical value of what is taught; with vacillation between accepting the school's doctrinal emphasis and rejecting it as excessive, misguided or inconsistent.

Progress to stable internalisation is assisted by professional rhetoric and the identification of unambiguous, positive and negative reference models. Professional rhetoric describes nursing as something very different to lay descriptions. Whilst students were disparaging of the rhetoric of their teachers, it served cognitively to structure nursing for them, and provided a scheme by which they could appraise their performance and communicate meanings to significant others. It assisted students to construct a coherent map from their fragmented experiences. At the same time the clinical instructors in the schools represented a positive reference model. These were the people whose rhetoric and professional outlooks the students assimilated in the process of doctrinal conversion. The negative models were the less well-educated nurses they met in the clinical settings to which they were assigned. They exemplified nursing ideals very different from the college teachers.

Stage 6 – stable internalisation

The students then reach the final stage of *stable internalisation*. The self image of the students is now very different to their initial lay imagery of themselves as nurses, and previous ideals and attitudes are suppressed. Once the students move into professional practice and away from the influences of the school then further revisions and transformations in identity will occur.

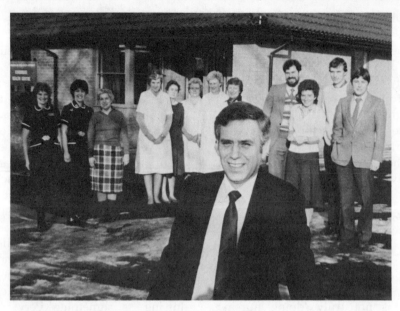

Fig. 11.2   Unequal status in the primary health care team (courtesy of Health Courant).

In the United States students receive a greater amount of their initial preparation in academic rather than clinical settings where they do not form part of the labour force. The transition into the staff-nurse role demands behaviour so different to that encountered as students that Kramer (1974) coined the term 'reality shock' to describe their experiences. Nursing students in the United Kingdom who also are no longer part of the workforce during initial preparation are similarly likely to need assistance to adjust to the staff-nurse role when, unlike their predecessors, they have not had clinical responsibilities as students.

British studies

Nursing students in the United Kingdom until recently have comprised an essential part of the nursing division of labour. Large parts of their preparation have taken place as pairs of hands in the clinical settings in which they worked and learned alongside other nursing students, nurses and nursing auxiliaries. This tradition leads to ambiguities of nurses' initial preparation as 'training', 'education' or 'work' (Macguire 1969).

During their courses students inhabit different organisational locales, and move back and forth between the clinical setting where nursing is done and the school where the scientific basis of nursing is transmitted. In one typical health authority and school, learning to be a nurse meant 'learning to negotiate quite contradictory conceptions of nursing held by different personnel in the nursing school and the hospital' (Chua & Clegg 1989, p. 111). Particularly in the school, there were strongly held beliefs about the scientific basis of nursing knowledge, while modern ideas about how to provide care based on managerial principles were promoted amidst an avowed need for academically able recruits. This ideology coexisted with older notions of nursing involving ritual obedience, hierarchical deference and authoritarian control, which also found expression in the school but were stronger in the wards. There was no neat split since even in the school being a 'good student' was closely linked with 'looking neat, tidy and respectable and showing appropriate respect for authority'. Other notions reminiscent of nursing's history lay in the stress on the 'good nurse' as self-motivated, sufficient to complete training, and able to stand the conditions imposed on students. Those who left were themselves regarded as responsible: that the system of training could be at fault was not considered. This is another example of victim blaming, akin to the labelling phenomenon we described in Chapter 8.

In the hospital, while senior managers were eager to promote the well-educated, detached scientific practitioner, the ward sisters and charge nurses downplayed these attributes. They stressed as key characteristics the desire to care and the possession of common sense. That is, getting the work done and being adaptable without the need for all the academic frills. This attitude put students in the position not of a colleague who was a student but a subordinate who needed to be controlled through authority, respect and discipline.

While Chua and Clegg (1989) examined the perspectives of those who controlled nursing education at the point of provision, these contradictory worlds of nursing, were found also by Melia (1987) who took the perspective of student nurses. Her focus was their descriptions of how they 'fitted in' during their training to cope with the expectations of the different segments encountered. The notion of segments relates to a subgroup within a profession:

It is composed of individuals who have in common some professional characteristics and beliefs which distinguish them from members of other segments. Members of a segment share specific professional identity; they also have similar ideas about the nature of their discipline, the relative order of activities it includes, and its relationship to other fields. (Bucher & Stelling 1977, p. 21)

The world of the nurse educator is different from that of the nurse or general manager which is again different from ward level staff. The different locales in which students become nurses are relatively distinct. Teachers do not perform nursing nor become involved in the multipeopled world of hospital wards. Sisters do not generally do classroom teaching, nor get involved in education committees. The two worlds are uncoupled and students moving from one to the other are socialised according to two different sets of criteria and expectations. The theory-practice distinction separates out the real basis of nursing work in looking after patients from what is taught in the classroom. However, Melia (1987) found that nursing is learned from unqualified staff rather than qualified nurses, and students with degree level education learn from those with less academic preparation and credentials. This creates difficulties for them in working out what constitutes the knowledge base of nursing work. One study found fewer students at the end of the first year of their course believed that research contributed to nursing's knowledge base. Perhaps more significantly none of their teachers subscribed to the belief (Wilson & Startup 1991). It is Melia's contention that, for students, what constitutes professionalised nursing are those tasks that nursing auxiliaries do not perform: those tasks of a more technical nature delegated from medical staff. This is in keeping with Freidson's (1975) view of those claiming 'professionalism' by virtue of working in close association with the medical profession.

Similarly, the wide range of settings in which nurses work creates more segmentation to which students have to adapt. Early evidence from students on new P2000 courses indicate that they 'do not feel like proper nurses' when they have community placements (Robinson 1991) and that too much time is spent in classroom teaching compared with time in the wards (Wilson & Startup 1991). Other writers have stressed students' concerns with authority and hierarchy relationships, and the tension created between this and initial expectations of nursing (Shaw et al 1984, Heyman et al 1984). While the quality of personal relationships with others is always important in how people feel about their jobs, students were concerned about the unjustifiable use of authority and unfair treatment by others. Both in Heyman's work and that by Melia, students had to learn the rules of the ward and find their place within it. In this, 'appearing to be busy' was stressed and, as found by Smith (1992), talking to patients did not constitute being busy.

As an essential part of the labour force students were there to get on with the work. A repeated finding is that a 'good' nurse is one who 'knows the ropes and pulls her weight' (Clarke 1978, p. 79). This applies to students and also has to be interpreted within the context of what constitutes nursing work. We touched on this topic in Chapter 10.

Secondary socialisation

There are comparatively few sociological studies of the socialisation of nurses beyond their formal initial education. The careers of graduates in nursing have been traced by their universities who want to find out what happens to this comparatively new and exclusive product in the nursing labour force (e.g. Sinclair 1984). However Johnson (1983) has shown that to plot careers through job lists is to miss important interactions between professional career and other aspects of the life career, often resulting in compromise decisions. This is especially so when women are faced with decisions about parenthood and career, but also when considerations other than work are important. To understand career behaviour, and within it socialisation into particular roles, it is important to go beyond situated microlevel analyses to include macrolevel notions. We have addressed issues of ethnicity, gender and class which bear on the structured nature of social life in general and working life in particular.

Socialisation as enculturation

It is evident that students graduate to nurse status with only a limited grasp of what the job entails. New graduates into the profession are called staff nurses, which is the same title as given to those with several years experience but who have not progressed up the nursing clinical hierarchy. While the clinical grading structure is intended to reward increased clinical responsibility and offers distinctions within the staff nurse grade, unlike the medical clinical career posts with their graded titles, there are no similar insignia to distinguish between the novice and more experienced staff nurse. For students becoming staff nurses, the meagre contact with the detail of the work of this grade means that they will experience 'reality shock' and have to cross that bridge after they have qualified.

This transition will be even more evident as new graduates of the P2000 courses will no longer assume the same kind of clinical responsibilities as those experienced by students who completed the older training. The process of learning new job responsibilities after transition is replicated when staff nurses become sisters. While continuity is an important feature of socialisation, discontinuities are repeatedly observed. Runciman noted that:

Some sisters remembered that, when they were staff nurses, they had been aware of the status or 'place' of the sister, but they had not understood the duties and responsibilities of the role or how to deal with them. The process of discovering about the range of responsibilities had been slow and sometimes painful ... 'hit and miss' learning had proved to be inefficient and costly and it seemed that each sister might meet the same difficulty and make the same mistakes as her predecessors. Supposedly reassuring remarks about 'taking a year to get into the job' has done little to lessen the feelings of insecurity or to help sisters cope with other people's altered expectations when status changed suddenly from staff nurse to sister. (Runciman 1982, p. 145)

Socialisation as acculturation

While the move from student to staff nurse to sister, or more recently ward manager, maintains a degree of situational stability in hospitals albeit with role changes, the transition from nursing to health visiting is characterised by marked discontinuity. All health visitors must be Registered Nurses but, like midwives, they claim a separate identity in official titles. Dingwall (1977) carried out an innovative study of the process of professional socialisation by constructing it from observing the actions of health visiting students and others towards them. This approach abandons the idea of socialisation as *enculturation* – the 'passive internalisation of an external normative order in abstraction from any broader social or historical context' (Dingwall 1977, p. 12). Rather, Dingwall adopts a perspective of socialisation as *acculturation* – 'a process by which newcomers to a group work to make sense of the surroundings and come to acquire the kinds of knowledge which would enable them to produce conduct which allowed established members of that group to recognise them as competent' (Dingwall 1977, pp. 12–13).

Dingwall's observations of health visitor students usage of 'profession' in order to establish their activity as profession rather than occupation gave rise to the following list:

A field health visitor is a professional because:

1. She is a certain sort of person, in that:
   a. She has certain ambitions and is committed to her occupation.
   b. She has certain personal qualities.
   c. She dresses in a certain fashion.
   d. She carries herself in a certain way.
   e. She uses a certain vocabulary of discourse.
   f. She uses certain kinds of transport.
2. She has autonomy in her work and knows what is best for her clients. It follows that:
   a. No other health visitor will interfere with her clients.
   b. No other health visitor will give her orders about her action towards her clients.
   c. No other health visitor will give her clients advice which might conflict with hers.
   d. She initiates her own contacts.
   e. She is self-critical.

   f. She enjoys her work and does not require to be stimulated to do it. But she does not work to excess at the expense of her own leisure.
3. She is a member of an occupation which:
   a. Selects its recruits.
   b. Has formal qualification.
   c. Is self-governing.
   d. Has its own body of knowledge.
   e. Has a history.
   f. Has research done on it.
4. She is responsible for supervising others' work:
   a. Clinic attendants.
   b. Health assistants.
5. She is equal to all other professionals but has a discrete area of work. Other professionals include:
   a. Social workers.
   b. Doctors.
   c. Teachers.
   d. University staff.
   e. Nurses.
   f. Various therapists.
6. She acts toward others on the assumption that they share this definition of her social location in an empirically identical, for all practical purposes, fashion. (Dingwall 1977, pp. 221–222)

Accomplishing profession

To accomplish health visiting requires demonstrating competent performance in the relevant elements of the list. Dingwall observed that competence did not follow a developmental model in the sense of later success being contingent on mastering earlier components. Rather it was a case of some aspects being more salient at particular times. While aiming for competence, the students adopted a perspective of 'getting through' – a concern with 'passing' rather than some drive for 'excellence'. This was associated with the fact that some students saw health visiting as filling in time until they married and had a family. Those who already had a family placed health visiting as a secondary concern to family life. Here was no orientation toward health visiting as a rung in a career ladder, except perhaps among male students. In any case, the mere possession of a certificate without any extra distinction was sufficient to guarantee a job at the end of the course. Competence in health visiting, however, is judged on the basis of *total personal evaluation* (Psathas 1968). For health visitors this means being assessed throughout their course – by the end-of-term examinations but also by fieldwork teachers, through case studies, and in individual tutorials with tutors. Competence is a matter not only of knowledge but also of conduct. The latter element is especially precarious for adult students since, because of the completeness of assessment, a judgement of incompetence reflects on the whole person. Dingwall describes how the student learned what was desirable to be judged as competent in the various elements in the list given on page 217. For example, a number of discussions focused on what health visitors would wear to be professional. 'Health visitors were only allowed to dress in the "professional" manner' (Dingwall 1977, p. 127). The same kind of learning about what is appropriate for professionals applies to the use of dialect and body position, for example, the inappropriateness of elbows on the table. Through their encounters with tutors, other professionals and fieldwork teachers, student health visitors learned 'doing health visitor' and in this way accomplished becoming a professional.

Dingwall's (1977) study is important because it raises issues about continuing education and socialisation for roles which follow after initial professional education.

SUMMARY

This chapter has covered some of the ground related to the concepts of career, occupation and profession and the place of nursing in the health division of labour. We have considered profession both as an occupation and as a status to which nursing aspires and which medicine has achieved. We discussed some different ways of thinking about the nature of professional control and its relation to clients who obtain services from professionals.

We then turned our attention to professionalism and used a historical analysis to describe how ideas about professionalism in nursing have changed from the time of Nightingale to the present day. Making comparisons of this kind is an important sociological technique, showing that society is dynamic and that changes in nursing are related to wider social changes. We stressed this particularly in relation to other occupational groups which may seek to maintain control over or aspire to the status of nursing and influence the division of labour within nursing. We considered changes in the culture of the health service in Britain with increased emphasis on managerialism and how this influenced the development of nursing. We also drew upon changes in ideas about the nature of nursing itself.

The relationship between profession and gender was associated with both the development of nursing professionalism and with career issues for women in our society. Ethnic differences which permeate society were related also to nursing careers, demonstrating inequality of opportunity.

The last section was devoted to professional socialisation, both of students in their initial transition to professional and from new professional to different roles within nursing. We compared different ways of conceptualising and studying socialisation. Findings were presented showing the discontinuities experienced by students and those changing their roles within nursing, and drew on studies carried out both in Britain and the United States.

In this chapter we have highlighted some of the social consequences of seeking and striving towards professional status and some of the conflicts which are an inevitable part of this process. What happens within occupations is a manifestation of social processes more generally and they in their turn influence changes in society at large.

FURTHER READING

Beardshaw V, Robinson R 1990 New for old? Prospects for nursing in the 1990s. Kings Fund, London

Dingwall R, Rafferty A M, Webster C 1988 An introduction to the social history of nursing. Routledge & Kegan Paul, London

Melia K 1987 Learning and working. The occupational socialisation of nurses. Tavistock, London

12

Doing sociological research

INTRODUCTION

In the preceding chapters of this book you have learned something of a number of broad sociological theories and we have applied their different perspectives to phenomena encountered in the social world. In so doing we have presented what counts as knowledge, generated by research applied to these phenomena. Some topics have been of a pervasive nature, like how societies may be considered as stratified collectivities and comprised of institutions like language and the family. In other ways we have introduced ideas and topics in which health professionals take a particular interest – concepts like health and illness, death and relationships with patients. We have also at times included a historical perspective, dealing with changes in the health service and the occupation of nursing.

Often these topics have been presented in a tentative way, representing the current state of knowledge. We have alluded to many empirical studies, carried out to generate what count as facts and knowledge in sociology. Knowledge is always in a state of evolution and what counts as knowledge changes over time. Like the other social elements referred to in the text, knowledge, in all disciplines, is socially constructed. In order to generate the knowledge of their particular discipline sociologists employ a variety of methods, ranging from those which are very similar to the methods of the natural sciences in terms of the logic employed through to

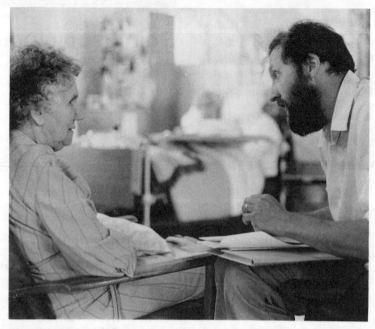

Fig. 12.1 Survey method using standardised interviews yielding comparable data (courtesy of Rik Walton).

what some might regard as common-sense interpretations of how society's members produce the social world in which they live. At one level then there is nothing distinctive about some of the methods used by sociologists, either in terms of the underlying logic or the techniques that they employ to generate data like interviews or analysis of records. However there are also distinctive methods which have been developed by social scientists, particularly related to qualitative research. These methods tend to shade across the social sciences and include social psychology and anthropology as well as sociology. It is the theory which is distinctly sociological rather than the method or its underlying logic.

There are many texts which give advice about doing sociological research and some are listed at the end of this chapter as further reading. Some are devoted to particular methods of doing research. For survey research we refer to the standard text of social survey methods prepared by Moser and Kalton (1971). and Hammersley and Atkinson (1983) and Strauss

and Corbin (1990) deal with qualitative methods. Roberts (1981) offers a feminist perspective on doing research, reflecting an explicit political as well as theoretical bias in methodology. In addition we suggest recent texts which describe the experience of doing research: Burgess (1990) and Shaffir and Stebbins (1991). These accounts assist in showing that the process of getting the bright idea and actually doing research often bears little resemblance to some glossy textbook stepwise prescriptions. These are all texts in the field of general sociology rather than applied to a particular context. There are, of course, specific texts applied to fields like education as well as health.

In practice, a range of methods is likely to be useful. In the introduction to *Doing Sociological Research*, Bell and Newby write 'No longer can there be one style of sociology with *one* method that is to be *the* method. Rather there are many' (Bell & Newby 1977, p. 10). They, like ourselves (Bond et al 1989) and others (e.g. Cook 1985) advocate methodological pluralism, i.e. the use of a variety of methods in sociological research.

This chapter describes these methodological divisions and links them with different sociological perspectives.

This methodological diversity should not come as any surprise given the range of different perspectives and theoretical positions in sociology. Just as sociologists view society from different perspectives, accept different theoretical assumptions and ask different questions, they also use different methods. There is a close relationship between a sociological perspective and the method used. As we shall demonstrate, particular perspectives are often committed to using particular research strategies to define, generate, collect and interpret empirical data. Indeed, Smith goes as far as to say 'methods and theory are inescapably connected' (Smith 1975, p. 27). This is often not obvious when theory is left inexplicit. Method here means not merely whether to use interviews or observation to collect data but more fundamentally whether to study causes or functions, whether to describe phenomena or explain them, or whether to determine the meaning of a phenomenon or examine the relationship between relevant variables.

Inevitably, theory gives rise to a particular definition of the problems to be studied, which influences the selection of method and subsequently the choice of particular techniques of data collection. We shall explore some of these considerations later in the chapter using the example of research on suicide but, first, let us consider briefly a difficult and major issue which faces all researchers and to which sociology researchers are particularly sensitised: the problem of epistemology.

EPISTEMOLOGY

Epistemology is that branch of philosophy which is concerned with the theory of knowledge. The central concern of epistemology is the question of how we *know* something to be true. It distinguishes between two kinds of knowledge: what we might call *public knowledge* and what we might call *private beliefs*. Public knowledge is that which is generally held to be the case, in contrast to private beliefs which is knowledge held by the individual in the sense of *knowing* or having a belief, opinion or faith. Epistemology addresses questions about the means by which we can say or know something or that it is so. It attempts to discriminate between public knowledge and private beliefs, and the process by which we come to have knowledge of the external world. An example is the process of changing the 'fact' that disease was caused by wicked spirits to the 'fact' that at least some disease is caused by microorganisms. How do we know that something is true? It is certainly not sufficient just to be told that this is the case, and sociologists face problems in making explicit the procedures they use to acquire sociological knowledge.

By virtue of the subject matter of the discipline, sociologists bring to their studies an awareness that they, like those they study, are social beings. They cannot but impart their own past experience, beliefs and attitudes into the social settings they study. In so doing they interpret social events and create social reality in the context of their own biography and actions and this may be at odds with the social reality of those they have studied. Sociologists, like every other human being, including all other scientists in every discipline, cannot be 'value-free'. Science is not value-free. This has major implications for how to 'do sociology' and handle sociological evidence. These are epistemological issues and they surface in different ways.

One major development has been the emergence of ethnomethodology. In Chapter 2, we said that ethnomethodologists were principally concerned with studying language as the means whereby society's members, and the ethnomethodologists themselves, gain an understanding of the methods society's members use to accomplish or produce social order. Thus, ethnomethodologists gain an understanding of what people themselves understand and know through language, which is regulated through social processes. Epistemologists have similar concerns. They attempt to understand what sociological concepts like class, status and power mean to the sociologist doing the research as well as to the subjects of the research. Thus, an understanding of class held by the sociologist and that held by the subject may be different and gained by different processes. We cannot take for granted that any sociological concept is understood and credited with the same meaning by subjects and researchers. Sociologists, as we indicated in Chapter 5 when discussing the family, will always face problems of this kind since most of the social phenomena they are concerned with will be familiar to them in their own private lives, and their private beliefs will influence their discovery of public knowledge.

A second epistemological concern is the close relationship between some political stances and sociology. Some critics regard sociology and sociologists as being politically biased. Marxist sociology is most often criticised. More recently feminist sociology has had the same treatment although other perspectives are often tarred with a similar brush. Is all sociology politically contaminated? Can it be otherwise since we all hold political beliefs, which may remain implicit, and sociologists, like other scientists, bring their political stance into their work? In this sense all science is influenced by political doctrines. This surfaces in such issues as linking heredity and intelligence and debates about the effectiveness of independent, comprehensive and grammar schools, or the effectiveness of market forces in creating health. Certainly, some people would regard all sociology as subversive and politically motivated.

There is no alternative to political influence in knowledge creation – be it through feminist research or any other way of generating knowledge. Since knowing itself is a political process, so knowledge is intrinsically political. The problem for sociologists of any persuasion is how to validate the knowledge that they produce (Cain & Finch 1981). Integral to all knowledge is political bias. There is generalised weakness in validity irrespective of the various constituent schools in sociology. What feminism has done is to make such problems explicit by recasting them

in the context of power relationships between men and women as well as between researcher and 'subjects' (Ramazanoglu 1992).

As well as political bias, much of the continued methodological debate in sociology centres on the distinctions between what might be termed broadly the qualitative-quantitative perspectives. These two broad perspectives are sometimes used to represent two fundamentally different approaches to studying the social world, encapsulating fundamentally different philosophical and political commitments and giving rise to different methodological approaches. In part, they arise from questions about the extent to which sociology should adhere to the positivist traditions of natural science.

Positivism

Over-simplifying, the method of *positivism* is what the natural sciences are supposed to do and is the foundation of statistical theory, exemplified by Popper's defence of quantitative methods in *The Poverty of Historicism* (Popper 1961). Positivism generally involves the setting up a hypothesis, for example, that working-class women are less likely to attend for antenatal care than middle-class women, which can be tested by statistical procedures to analyse relationships between variables. Put another way, positivism argues that there is no knowledge without experience of the external world as described by empirical data, for example, the proportion of working-class and middle-class women attending for antenatal care. Positivists argue that knowing is based on systematically collected data and not 'unreliable' individual descriptions based on beliefs or opinion about the use of antenatal care by working-class and middle-class women. This basic conception was elaborated by the early sociologists, particularly Comte, who stressed the appropriateness of the positive method for *all* sciences. All scientific knowledge should be acquired in the same manner. Those who subscribe to this position fail to recognise that experimental method is usually impracticable in sociology and that the phenomena studied by sociologists are not uniform, as are those studied by natural scientists. Making a variable like social class measurable is more complex than quantifying natural science variables, such as air pressure or atomic weight. Making variables measurable is called *operationalisation*.

Natural science

Like that of natural science, the aim of positivism is to reduce explanations of all phenomena to the smallest number of principles or laws. Positivists argue that given enough time and effort, sociologists should be able to uncover the laws which govern and explain social facts. In practice this means providing a sociological theory, at different conceptual levels (leading eventually to social laws). At the highest conceptual level are abstract postulates which cannot be given precise empirical definition – for example, 'social disadvantage causes ill health'. These postulates give rise to lower-level propositions in the form of hypotheses or predictions which can be tested in the real world – for example, 'there is a higher rate of maternal deaths among lower-class women'. Positivism therefore entails a uniform method of data collection which forces a definite mode of description and classification on the 'reality' being studied.

The principal components of the idealised scientific process advocated by positivism is shown in Figure 12.2. Data are collected about operational variables and hypotheses would then be upheld or rejected, depending on the findings. Through this process there is a quest for the smallest number of laws which will *explain* how things have worked in the past and *predict* how things will work in the future. At its simplest, if one kind of event has always been observed to have been followed by another event, then all future occurrences of the first event will produce the second. For example, in physics it has been shown that if you keep the pressure of a given gas constant, an increase in temperature will cause a corresponding increase in the volume of the gas. In sociology Janowitz

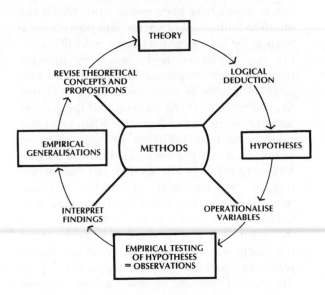

Fig. 12.2 Principal components of an idealised 'scientific' process (modified from Wallace, 1971. In: Bynner & Stribley 1979).

(1956) has listed a number of consequences of social mobility such as 'the greater the social mobility of a family, the greater the instability of the family'.

Deduction

Positivism therefore depends principally on being able to challenge predictions set up as hypotheses and attempting to falsify them because, if a prediction fails, then the theoretical proposition giving rise to it must be changed to take account of the findings. Any revision of theoretical concepts and propositions leads to revision of the sociological theory and the whole circular process begins once again. In a perfect and rational world this process is logically defensible.

Unfortunately, the world is neither rational nor perfect and a strict adherence to the positivists' position can be challenged on a number of grounds. Different views exist about what are proper tests and grounds for an adequate rejection of hypotheses. We each hold auxiliary beliefs about how phenomena work which can interfere with positive science and provide justification for *not* rejecting a theory. Scientific practice can be shown to be not very different from the logic employed in magical and religious practices in nonindustrialised societies. Evans-Pritchard (1950) showed that the Azande sorcerers were able to deal with what, to an outsider, would be falsifying or nonconfirming instances. If one person seeks, through magical means, to injure or kill another and that person remains in the best of health, explanations as to how this could be so are readily to hand. Something unknown 'went wrong' with the magic on this particular occasion when the oracle was consulted; the ritual incantation was not performed perfectly correctly; or the second person enjoyed access to even stronger magic than the first and was able to render his efforts ineffective. Giddens asks 'In what sense, if any, is Western science able to lay any claim to an understanding of the world that is more grounded in "truth" than that of the Azande?' (Giddens 1976, p. 138). Perhaps the Azande simply operate with a different overall meaning frame to that which we call science?

There are also criticisms of the logic underpinning positivism. Just because one event has been found to be consequent on another in the past, is that any justification for assuming that this will always be the case? Furthermore, just because one event comes after another it does not necessarily mean that the first *causes* the second or that they are bound together by some other, as yet undiscovered, law. The positivist scientist, however, can only assume that indeed this is the case and in so doing, is on the way to discovering a chain of events which will ultimately provide causes.

While positivists themselves produce such criticisms as a means of self-reform, sociologists have not been slow to find these arguments grounds for rejecting a positivist or scientistic approach to sociology. Atkinson (1978), whose work on suicide we shall deal with presently, provides a list of assumptions made by positivists together with the kinds of criticisms of positivism made by sociologists (Table 12.1).

These epistemological difficulties have caused a large number of sociologists to reject positivism. This has led Bell and Newby to question the standards by which sociologists now make decisions about what 'facts' to look at, how to examine them and how to evaluate other people's work. Positivism 'provided the normative standards by which sociological research was both judged and practised ... it no longer does so, hence sociology's troubles' (Bell & Newby 1977, p. 21). But, we may ask, is it necessarily a bad thing to have different logical and epistemological bases within sociology giving rise to methodological pluralism? Or is it a case of sociology, still a relatively young discipline, feeling pressured to present a sociology adhering to one generally accepted set of canons in order to gain acceptance by the 'academic' community? The basis for such questions lies in the character and stage of development of sociology as a discipline and the extent to which sociological methods are sufficiently cohesive to be shared by members of a 'scientific' community.

Kuhn and normal science

Kuhn's important treatise on physical sciences, *The Structure of Scientific Revolutions* (1962) gave rise to the idea that communities of scientists hold taken-for-granted and unexamined assumptions about what they should study and how it should be studied. They confine their attention to small scale puzzle-solving within the bounds of their assumptions. Kuhn referred to this shared agreement as a *paradigm* and those sharing it as a *community of scientists*. A shared paradigm produces criteria for judging and testing theories, with limits of acceptable margins of error and with exemplars of how to go about conducting similar research. When scientists operate within a paradigm they gain the support of their colleagues and are approved as doing *normal science*, for example, carrying out everyday routine scientific activity attempt-

Table 12.1 Summary statement of central assumptions and criticisms of positivism (From Atkinson, 1978)

Positivist assumptions	Criticisms
Social phenomena have an existence external to the individuals who make up a society or social group and can thus be viewed as objective facts in much the same way as natural facts...	Social phenomena are of an essentially different order to natural ones, owing to their symbolic nature and the subjective interpretations of social meanings by individuals in a society...
hence An observer can identify social facts relatively easily and objectively...	*hence* Identifying social phenomena is a very problematic exercise which involves the assumption that an action has a single unchanging meaning for all people, times and situations...
hence Numerical and other 'scientific' techniques can be adapted to 'measure' social facts...	*hence* Attempts to 'measure' will gloss over the above problems and lead to the imposition of observers' definitions on to a situation where the extent to which these are shared by actors under study is unknown...
hence Hypotheses which relate observer-defined variables can be tested...	*hence* To construct hypotheses is to assume that the problems listed above are either trivial or have been overcome...
hence Social theories can be constructed on the basis of discovered 'relationships' or tested by deducing testable hypotheses from some general theoretical statement...	*hence* The bid to explain social phenomena which are seldom adequately described in terms of actor orientations is at best premature and at worst a total misrepresentation of the problem of social reality...
hence Sociology can proceed with methodologies based on natural science models.	*hence* Sociology must develop alternative methodologies appropriate for studying subject matter which poses problems not faced by the subject matter of the natural sciences.

ing to solve the problems generated by the paradigm within which they are working, 'a strenuous and devoted attempt to force nature into the conceptual boxes supplied by professional education' (Kuhn 1962, p. 5). Kuhn contends that occasionally the orderly progress of science is disrupted by events which shatter the prevailing norm and, from a number of competing revisionary positions, a new conception of science is produced and a new paradigm emerges to reestablish a new normal science.

This explanation of the development of physical sciences is attractive to many sociologists – partly because its explanation is largely sociological, that is, one learns normal science through an educational process which socialises and indoctrinates, and through a professional training which further eliminates other possible approaches to science, while deviants are excluded and denied a career. It also suggests that, after its positivist critique, sociology has thrown up a number of competing paradigms (or perspectives as we have called them) and it is only a matter of time before sociology settles down to adhere to one of these as its appropriate basis. In this sense sociology may be regarded as *preparadigmatic*. There are a number of criticisms both of Kuhn's original treatise and its appropriate extrapolation to social science (Worsley 1974, Hawthorn 1976, Benton 1977). Perhaps the most powerful is that there never has been a sociology resembling normal science which has broken down so we cannot be going through a scientific revolution awaiting the emergence of a new dominant paradigm. There are no signs that one school or perspective is ousting the others. Indeed, we could say that British sociology is characterised by a healthy pluralism.

If there is no one acceptable way or agreement that one type of data is 'better' than another then this opens the door for different sociological methods to be applied as appropriate to different aspects of sociological problems. In the next part of this chapter we will deal with three different approaches to the study of suicide as a sociological phenomenon. We have selected this topic partly to reinforce the idea that what may be taken for granted by health professionals is a source of inspiration for sociological study, and what may be seen as a straightforward problem in definitional terms for psychiatrists and coroners, is in fact open to different interpretations. We have also selected suicide because it was one of the topics given early sociological treatment, yet it remains of sociological interest.

DURKHEIM AND A STRUCTURALIST TREATMENT OF SUICIDE

Durkheim was a structuralist and a positivist. Like Comte, he treated social facts as things to be regarded independently of the individuals who contribute to them (see Ch. 2). Durkheim used suicide as a means of showing that such apparently individual acts were more a matter for sociological treatment than the outcome of individual psychology. He was concerned to find the laws which govern suicide,

and particularly rates of suicide, within societies. To do this he developed several propositions or hypotheses at different levels of abstraction. The lowest level he could then put to the test against empirical data. These hypotheses are schematically summarised by Maris (1969) and progress from hypotheses at lower levels of generalisation (level III) through to propositions which encompass them, at level II and to a general theoretical premise at level I.

Having disposed of the extra social factors to his satisfaction, Durkheim proceeds to compound lower-level generalisations of the 'greater than', or ordinal scale variety from his statistics. Some of the more important 1st-level generalisations are listed below, roughly in the order of the appearance in *Suicide* (for the sake of brevity the symbol > is employed to mean 'tend to have a higher suicide rate than').

h1.   City dwellers > rural dwellers
h2.   The sane > the insane
h3.   Adults > children
h4.   Older adults > younger adults
h5.   In March through August > in September through February
h6.   In daytime > in the night
h7.   Protestants > Catholics > Jews
h8.   Majority groups > minority groups
h9.   Upper social classes > lower social classes
h10. The learned > the unlearned
h11. Males > females
h12. The unmarried > the married
h13. The married without children > the married with children
h14. Those in smaller families > those in larger families
h15. Bachelors > widows
h16. Those living in time of peace > those living in time of war
h17. Soldiers > civilians
h18. Elite troops > nonelite troops
h19. Those whose society is experiencing an economic crisis > those whose society is not experiencing an economic crisis

h20.   Those living in a period of rapid social change > those living in a period of slow social change

h21.   The rich > the poor

h22.   The morally undisciplined > the morally disciplined

h23.   Divorcees > nondivorcees.

Maris goes on to quote direct from *Suicide* (Durkheim 1952, p. 208) what he refers to as Durkheim's 2nd-level hypotheses from which all those listed above can be deduced:

H1.   Suicide varies inversely with the degree of integration of religious society.

H2.   Suicide varies inversely with the degree of integration of domestic society.

H3.   Suicide varies inversely with the degree of integration of political society.

Finally, on the 3rd-level, Durkheim posits a grand hypothesis intended to subsume all previously mentioned hypotheses. This hypothesis (which is also a grand empirical generalisation if we can assume that the previous hypotheses were true and that the determination of the common denominator of them were accurate) states that:

H.   Suicide varies inversely with the degree of integration of social groups of which the individual forms a part (Maris 1969, pp. 32–33, quoted in Atkinson 1978, pp. 12–13).

To repeatedly test and fail to falsify these hypotheses would provide grounds for their acceptance as laws governing suicidal behaviour. More generally this would uphold the positivist view that it is possible to isolate theories and their propositions which will ultimately provide an explanation for human conduct and events. The fact that individuals subjectively experience such events and attribute different meaning to them could be ignored in the quest for such social laws. Durkheim was concerned with finding ways of operationalising the concepts he was working with so that he could measure them and carry out statistical tests of the relationship between them in order to challenge

and ultimately strengthen his theoretical exposition of suicide.

To be able to do this it is necessary to accept that suicide, as the dependent variable, like each of the independent variables – integration of religious society, integration of domestic society and integration of political society – is indeed 'thing-like' and sufficiently easy to operationalise and internally consistent to use as a concept. Thus all suicides and all official categorisations of suicide are treated as if they are the same. Durkheim therefore independently defines what suicide *really* is; 'suicide is applied to all cases of death resulting directly or indirectly from a positive or negative act of the victim himself, which he knows will produce this result' (Durkheim 1952, p. 44). He assumes all official statistics are derived from the uncomplicated application of this definition.

Durkheim, like most sociologists had to rely on descriptive research since it is not acceptable to set up experiments to change the way society functions and examine the consequent suicide rates. What he had to do was to rely on published official statistical data and carry out an analysis of the relationship between them, for example, variable analysis or multivariate analysis, relying on the assumption that if there is a consistent relationship between variables then one is causing the other to happen. This process entailed collecting the suicide rates for different European countries and quantifying measures for his other variables, for instance marriage rates, the amount of divorce, the extent to which a country is Protestant or Catholic or Jewish, whether there is an economic crisis. He posed questions like the extent to which suicide is linked to religious persuasion. To test this he had to identify countries in which a particular religious group predominated, for example, Italy, highly Catholic, or Germany, highly Protestant. Even if there were different suicide rates in these two countries it could be a matter of other aspects of nationality – Italian or German – rather than the predominant religious affiliation. To overcome this problem Durkheim had to seek areas within countries where different religions predominated. In Germany, Bavaria had the fewest suicides and most Catholics and within the provinces of Bavaria there was a direct relationship between suicide rates and the proportion of Protestants and an inverse relationship to the proportion of Catholics. This is diagrammatically expressed:

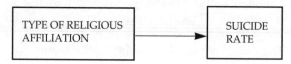

The more often Durkheim found this kind of relationship, the more certain were his claims that the empirical data indicate a casual link between the variables. Thus, rather than setting out to find examples or cases which would challenge and falsify his hypothesis (Popper's view of the process of scientific enquiry), Durkheim actually relies on accumulating more evidence to support his contentions.

His theory, going from lower to higher levels of abstraction as outlined above, was that it was not the fact of being Protestant or Catholic which influenced the individuals committing suicide but that these different religions influenced the degree of integration of communities – Protestantism encouraging individualism and Catholicism fostering close community ties. This variable he called social integration and is shown as:

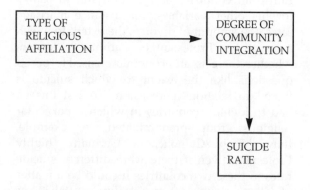

It is social integration which is a collective property, a social fact. This same process is worked through for domestic integration:

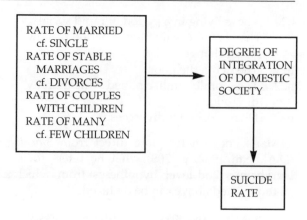

Thus, by testing more and more of such relationships Durkheim strengthened his proposition that one cause of one kind of suicide was insufficient societal organisation, specifically, integration. He produced a social explanation of suicide which also permitted prediction. He similarly characterised other types of suicide in the same way, but these do not need to concern us here. What is important, however, is the degree of clarity of these major variables or social facts. Acceptance of this theory rests not only on the logic of the relationships between the variables but more so on accepting that suicides and the integration of social groups are adequately conceptualised and measured. There is little point in having appropriate logic applied to inadequately operationalised concepts. Yet a British Medical Journal Editorial commenting on the increase in suicides among young men and a decrease among young women (see Fig. 12.3) refers to Durkheim's theory: 'We may have to turn to sociological theory. Changes in society may have resulted in young men becoming less integrated with and supported by those around them with the reverse pattern in women'. (Hawton 1992, p. 1000)

Some of those who followed the Durkheimian approach to suicide while adhering to the positivists' tradition have challenged his interpretation of social integration. For example, Gibbs and Martin (1964) clearly recognised the ambiguities in his treatment of social integration and consequently the lack of a rigourous test of his theory. What Gibbs and Martin did was to

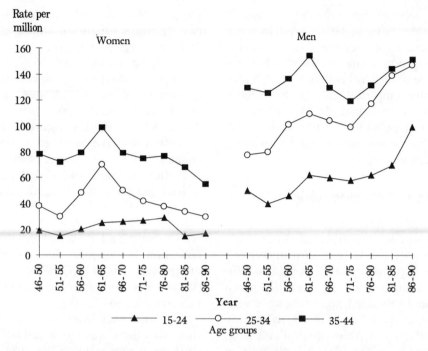

Fig. 12.3 Reported suicide rates: per million population by gender and age 1946–1990, England and Wales (Charlton et al 1992).

attempt a better operationalisation of social integration as the 'stability and durability of relationships' within a population. (As Douglas (1967) notes, they could equally well have chosen the volume or the extent of relationships, for example, frequency of contact, as part of such a definition and no explanation is given for choosing not to do so.) They also decided to focus on status rather than role conflict on the assumption that this is the fundamental determinant of the stability and durability of social relationships within a population. The picture presented by Gibbs and Martin is one of an individual experiencing a role configuration within which are so many role conflicts that the individual will wish to leave it. If they are unable to do so by other means then they make the ultimate departure by suicide – at least they commit suicide with more frequency than those with less role or status conflict. These reinterpreted variables then form the kind of hypothesis provided here:

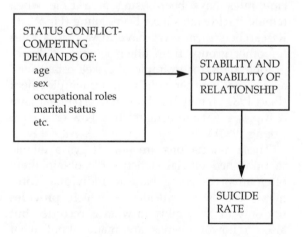

Douglas has pointed up a number of basic flaws in this reinterpretation of social integration which Gibbs and Martin devised because they considered it to be more measurable and hence provide a better test of Durkheim's theory. Gibbs and Martin provide no indication of what they believed to actually *cause* this hypothesised relationship, probably because it would ultimately have to be reduced to some kind of collective consciousness or individual personality to produce suicide. Thus, what sets out to improve upon Durkheim's work by providing a better empirical test of his theory through better operational definitions of the concepts, in fact provides no test of it at all. Durkheim's theory remains a theory awaiting sound empirical testing.

The meaning of suicide data

The other major and related criticism of Durkheim's work is his interpretation of suicide itself and the use of data from official sources. Atkinson (1978) points out that published official statistics about suicide are normally given as numbers and tabulated according to a very limited range of variables. Trends in suicide deaths for England and Wales are available from mortality statisitics since 1911 (Charlton et al 1992). Data on suicide are reported routinely according to age and gender. Recent analysis reveals that for the first time since 1911 male suicide rates have been rising at a time when female suicide rates have been falling (Fig. 12.3). Researchers themselves have to work out rates for other groups from other sources of demographic data, for example, the well-established association between suicide and unemployment (Platt 1984), family breakdown (Dorpatt, Jackson & Ripley 1965) and drug misuse (Fowler, Rich & Young 1986).

These associations are not always available in published official statistics. To obtain them often involves going back to individual coroners' records of suicides – which provides not only for variability in what is recorded but also in how decisions are made about what to record. Thus, suicide data have been derived from official sources which have compiled records in a variety of ways, and because of this they are not equivalent. Deaths officially recorded as having 'undetermined causes' are often suicides (Holding & Barraclough 1978) and suicides among children are considered to be seriously underrecorded. In 1990, for exam-

ple, of 3950 recorded suicides there were only two instances of suicide among children under 15 years of age (OPCS 1991).

We have to deal with this problem also in relation to interpreting official statistics about gestation age as an indicator of late booking of different social classes for antenatal care. Table 12.2 provides figures obtained from Scottish data. We were so impressed by the changes which had taken place in the overall reduction in 'late bookers' that we wrote to the official source, in this case, Information Services Division of the Scottish Health Service Common Services Agency, to check that the figures issued were correct and to ask about their method of collection. It transpires that the 1971 figures we quoted were based on data collected on about 44 000 women who offered a 'certain' date for last menstrual period (LMP).

Our letter back from the source stated 'I don't think that there was much validation of the data in those earlier days' (Cole 1984). That is, the LMP was that given by the women themselves and this was combined with date of delivery to produce the calculated gestation date for time of first booking for antenatal care. The 1981 data were based on *married* women only, and gestational age at booking was arrived at by calculating backwards from the clinical estimate of gestation at delivery, given in weeks, and subtracting the number of weeks between the date of booking and the date of delivery. This method has been adopted to help eliminate the 'nonsense' gestations which were the result of irregular menstrual cycles and postpill amenorrhoea. We must conclude, therefore, that it may be how the statistics are arrived at as much as, or rather than, changes in behaviour which explains a larger reduction in apparently 'late bookers'. The same holds for other social phenomena. Are there differences in how suicides are recorded in different countries or systematic variations in applying the categorisation to men and women?

To accept official data also avoids questioning the substance of what is to be studied, for example, what is meant by suicide and how it is to be studied. This central assumption of agreed defi-

Table 12.2 Percentage of married women making a late antenatal booking (after more than 21 weeks gestation)

	Scotland	
Social class	1971[1]	1981[2]
I Professional	28	11
II Managerial	35	12
III Skilled manual and nonmanual	36	12
IV Party skilled	39	15
V Unskilled	47	18

Sources:
1. Brotherston Sir J 1976 Inequality: is it inevitable? In: Carter CO, Peel J (eds) Equalities and inequalities in health. Academmic Press, London, p. 85

2. Information Services Division 1983 Unpublished Tables

nitions made by positivists leaves no room to question whether suicides as perceived in official data are a complete record, or whether official definitions of what constitutes suicide are universally shared. (We can say the same about late booking and many other apparently unproblematic concepts.) Legal definitions, official categorisations and researchers' theoretical conceptions of suicide do not necessarily coincide. Probable differences in the definitions underpinning suicide give rise to the important problem of the validity of suicide data as well as their reliability.

In terms of validity we are questioning whether one official definition of death as suicide is necessarily the same as any other, be it official, sociological, theoretical or lay definition, and whether any one is any more correct or relevant. Reliability poses questions about the consistency of such definitions between individuals and cultures and over time, and whether there is a 'true rate' to which official rates approximate. In suicide research it is not just a matter of finding the 'error rate' in the statistics. Douglas (1967) adds a further dimension to the problem of official statistics. Picking up

Durkheim's notion of social integration, Douglas proposed a possible connection between social integration, rates of concealment and attempted concealment of suicide, and the influence this may have on suicide rates. If official rates in part depend upon rates of concealment and if rates of concealment are highest among the more socially integrated, then Durkheimian theory may be more to do with the data entered as official suicide rates rather than any 'real' rate. This gets us back to the question of what constitutes a 'real' suicide and so the problems of validity and reliability are compounded. Douglas makes the point as follows: 'We shall never be very sure about the reliability of official statistics, and certainly not about their validity, until a great many good studies have been made of the methods used by officials to categorise deaths, their assumptions, their methods of collecting data and tabulating it, and of the "real" community rates of suicide' (Douglas 1967, p. 297). This of course raises the question of whether the 'real' rate *is* potentially knowable, but we are then faced with the issue of whose definition of reality should be the focus of such a concern.

Social definitions of suicide

For any research to be done on the subject of suicide a death must be categorised as suicide and this involves someone making this decision. One approach to suicide research arising from this problem is to attempt to gain an understanding of how officials, in this case coroners, actually go about the process of making decisions to categorise a death as suicide rather than as an accident, misadventure, homicide or returning an open verdict. An empirical issue is *how* the categorisations are done and not how well they are done, or how closely they match to any official definition of suicide or ideal conception of how they should be done. This approach involves no longer taking officially generated data at its face value, and treating it as 'hard, objective data' about incidents, but attempting to investigate the complexities of social processes and interactions which lead to official categorisations of deaths as suicide. At the same time, it involves attempting to 'understand' or 'appreciate' the meanings which those involved attribute to their own actions and to the actions of others – including in this case those of the deceased. In following this approach the definition of suicide becomes not the content of law or that which is written in the coroner's handbook or even that provided by the researcher. Rather, it is empirically grounded and evolves from examining the actions of those involved in deciding what constitutes suicide as they go about their everyday work. This interpretation of the issue removes some of the problems of validity and reliability inherent in the criticisms of the positive approach outlined above. It is not, however, without its own problems, as we shall see.

ATKINSON AND AN INTERACTIONIST APPROACH TO SUICIDE

Atkinson (1978) examined *how* some deaths are categorised as suicides. In using an interactionist perspective he was concerned with observing and recording at first hand the various social processes which were involved in the work of coroners who have legal responsibility for categorising deaths referred to them. However, categorising deaths involves medical as well as legal concerns and so interaction takes place between two sets of professionals – doctors, on the one hand and, on the other, coroners who are usually lawyers (and their clerks who are members of the police force). This interaction is of continuous importance, especially in the initial stage because, for a death to be referred to a coroner in the first place, others must make the decision about whether it is violent, unnatural or 'a sudden death, the cause of which is unknown'. However, a death may be sudden but not unexpected; to be referred to a coroner it must be both 'sudden' and 'unnatural'. These quotation marks are used because what constitutes a sudden or an unnatural death is not predefined but itself is socially constructed. Coroners' investigations leading to categorisation of deaths involve a number of different kinds of activities, many carried out by the coroner's officer. These include not only inquests but also examining the scene of death, identification of the deceased, interviews with relatives and other witnesses, arranging and attending post-mortems and collecting the evidence together to write reports.

In his initial overtures with coroners while he was setting up his study and before he began his formal data-collection, Atkinson found that officials could see nothing interesting or problematic in what for them was a straightforward activity. They saw categorisation of deaths as an orderly procedure rather than one in which there was any ambiguity or uncertainty. This interpretation of their work was one reason Atkinson did not pursue his research using a method well used by those who regard the definition of the problem as unproblematic. That is, he did not resort to questionnaires or interviews asking coroners standardised questions about how they went about their activities because this would have yielded only a generalised account of the 'ordinary' and perhaps some references to what is regarded as 'ordinary' by contrasting this to what coroners regard as 'extraordinary'. While interviews or questionnaire data would certainly have yielded some pointers, this method would not have been suitable as a means of finding out how decisions are made *in practice* compared with in theory. To achieve this understanding demanded a much wider set of data from diverse sources in order to find out the kind of social and interpretative processes involved in the categorisation of deaths. These data certainly included interview material, not of a standardised variety but interviews which sought to elaborate and clarify observed events. Other forms of data used by Atkinson included analysis of coroners' written reports, newspaper reports of suicides and, most important, first-hand observation of the work of the coroner's officer and inquests.

From the mass of data collected, Atkinson found that coroners must search for specific pieces of evidence to confirm the verdict of suicide and to reject other possible verdicts. The search for 'clues' involved a whole range of sources – the remains, including suicide notes and threats as well as the body, the mode of dying, location and circumstances of the death and the biography of the deceased person. These 'clues' however are interpreted against and in the light of a variety of taken-for-granted assumptions about what constitutes a 'typical' suicide or a 'typical suicidal biography'. Therefore suicide notes and other 'relics' are not interpreted independently but in conjunction with all other 'clues'. Nothing in itself would be sufficient – even what may be regarded as a 'suicide note' must be interpreted by the finders in the context of other 'clues'. Thus clues have to be 'read' (Garfinkel 1967b) and it is only when they have been 'read' that they can be used as evidence or 'facts'. Thus 'clues', once they are interpreted or considered as 'facts' about the case, are then given the status of facts about the case for the purposes of deciding whether it is indeed a suicide. No mode of death is entirely unequivocal, although hanging or inhaling exhaust fumes from a car are almost always taken as a definite indicator of suicide. Mode of death suggests what other types of evidence should be sought and directs other activi-

ties. An explanatory model of each death is built up and to be categorised as suicide, no part of it must be inconsistent with the coroner's ideas about what constitutes a typical suicide.

What Atkinson is saying is that coroners hold a view of what constitutes a typical suicide; this is their 'meaning' of suicide. Coroners construct their own common-sense theories of what is suicide and it is this which guides the kind of information sought and its interpretation.

Interactionists' methods

We can see that interactionists and structuralists conceive the problem of suicide very differently. Interactionists seek explanations of how specific groups of individuals interpret and define suicide, in other words, how the meaning of suicide is socially constructed. Rather than pursue the studies at a societal or macro-sociological level they carry out much finer-textured analysis at the point where the action takes place in an endeavour to interpret what is happening. Typically data are collected in one or a narrow range of settings to provide a case study, which involves researchers observing and inevitably taking part in what is happening even though they may retain 'observer' status.

This kind of research owes a great deal to anthropologists who studied cultures other than their own. Malinowski (1922) provides three main principles for this type of research: any researcher must espouse scientific values, must live among the people being studied and must apply a number of techniques for collecting and ordering data and presenting evidence. A distinction is drawn between the data collected, for example the particular question the coroner asks relatives of the deceased at an inquest, and the researchers' *interpretation* of that data, for example, that the question reflects the coroner's attempts to reconstruct the deceased person's biography in terms of propensity to commit suicide. Thus, interactionist sociology can also be called *interpretative* sociology. It relies on *inference*; for example, the inference that a person kneeling in a place of worship is *at prayer* involves assumptions about the social significance of posture, the locale in which the act is taking place and the relationship between locale and religious belief. Problems arise in qualitative social research in connecting observation and interpretation. The purpose of the research is 'to grasp the native's point of view, his relation to life, to realise *his* vision of *his* world' (Malinowski 1922, p. 25, original italics). The problem, therefore, is one of knowing that the interpretation provided by the researcher is faithful to the point of view of the subjects of the study, that it *is* their version of their world.

This approach in sociology, while studying our own society, has come to be known as ethnography. The researcher is involved in collecting data at first hand, using participant observation or, more generally, field methods. It relies on making observations as they happen, following these up by informally interviewing informants, collecting written records which are relevant and then turning these into usable data.

In the example quoted of Atkinson's work on suicide this involved him in observing a range of settings, interviewing some of the participants as well as using coroners' records and newspaper cuttings. One of the difficulties, however, is what to observe and what to make of the data. As Atkinson himself said elsewhere about the research strategies adopted by interactionists: 'a funny story here, an apt quote from a "subject" there, a few extracts from a newspaper or television. Indeed it sometimes seemed that anything one happened to stumble across would do, so long as it seemed relevant in some way to the arguments being presented' (Atkinson 1977, p. 42). Collecting data need not be as sloppy as this, but it does raise the problems mentioned earlier of the epistemological status of ethnographic research and how it addresses problems of reliability and validity. Hammersley's (1992) account of problems of ethnographic research provides a useful summary.

Interactionists criticise positivist structuralists because of the way they operationalise and measure theoretically relevant concepts. Positivists at least indicate before they begin empirical studies what they regard as relevant concepts, how they are operationalised and how they relate theoretically. Interactionists, on the other hand, are likely to set out without an explicit theoretical model to guide their data-collection, and have to generate theory as they go along, interpreting the data they have and creating hypotheses which will provide pointers for new data to be collected. These new data are thus used to test the hypotheses generated. This process of going from data to theory is called *analytical induction*. The term was used by Znaniecki (1934) to *describe* what *actually* happens in doing the research which *begins* with collecting data. More recently it has been used to attempt to specify how it is legitimate to arrive at general propositions by abstracting 'essential features' of observed cases of phenomena. This is not the same as 'data dredging'(Fig. 12.4) or 'data snooping', otherwise called innumerative induction from survey research data, which relies on collecting a large number of cases and developing categories and empirical generalisations strictly on the basis of the data to hand. Rather analytic induction involves abstracting out of empirical data and generating categorisations which are then tested against subsequently collected data. It abstracts from a given concrete case the features which are essential to its definition and generalises them to new cases. The stages in this abstract procedure of theory construction are described by Robinson (1951) as:

1. A rough definition of the phenomenon to be explained is formulated.
2. A hypothetical explanation of the phenomenon is formulated.
3. One case is studied in the light of the hypothesis.
4. If the hypothesis does not fit the facts, either the hypothesis is reformulated, or the phenomenon to be explained is redefined so that the case is excluded.
5. Practical certainty may be attained after a small number of cases have been examined, but the discovery by the investigator or any

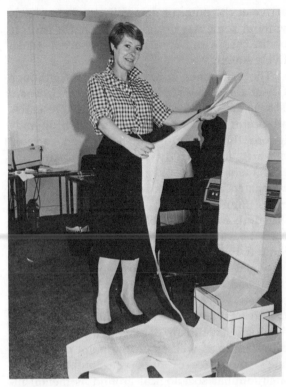

Fig. 12.4 Research yielding large quantities of numerical data may become nothing more than 'data dredging' exercises (courtesy of Nursing Standard).

other investigator of a single negative case disproves the explanation and requires a reformulation.

6. This procedure of examining cases, redefining the phenomenon and reformulating the hypothesis is continued until a universal relationship is established, each negative case calling for a redefinition or a reformulation. (Robinson 1951, p. 813)

The procedure calls for successive reformulation of hypotheses. The essential feature of analytical induction is to establish which conditions must be in existence before a phenomenon occurs, leading to the identification of characteristics *all* of which are present when the phenomenon occurs and, when the characteristics are *not* present, the phenomenon does not occur. Through this method *practical* certainty, rather

than claims for universality, is achievable. The researcher searches for exceptions, cases in which, within the established conditions, the phenomenon does not occur or cases when, in their absence, it does. These cases would form the focal point for a new examination of the prevailing explanation, with an extension of knowledge. In this way induction always progresses from the basis of observations to generate or test theory. While grounded theory (Glaser & Strauss 1967, Strauss 1987) and analytic induction are advocated for theory development and testing, there are few examples of this actually being carried out.

Lindesmith's (1968) research on opiate addiction provides a clear illustration of the method to produce explanatory propositions. He conducted 70 in-depth interviews with heroin addicts to produce case studies. Lindesmith concluded that the power of the opiate habit is derived basically from the effects which follow the withdrawal of the drug rather than upon any positive effects which its presence in the body produces. Addiction only occurs when opiates are used to alleviate withdrawal distress. After this distress has been properly understood or interpreted by the individual experiencing it, addiction is quickly and permanently established through further use of the drug. If individuals fail to conceive of their distress as withdrawal distress brought about by the absence of opiates, they do not become addicted.

The analytic method followed is best described as setting up a series of critical case studies, leading to successive revision of the guiding theory. Each hypothesis set up based on findings in earlier cases studied, could then be tested against subsequent cases and repeated when any negative case was found. An initial hypothesis was that individuals who do not know what drug they are receiving do not become addicted and that they become addicted when they know what they are getting and have taken it long enough to experience withdrawal distress. This initial hypothesis was destroyed by a negative case. A doctor, who had received morphine for several weeks and was fully aware of the fact, did not become addicted.

Lindesmith had to reformulate and set up a second provisional hypothesis that persons become addicts when they recognise or perceive the significance of withdrawal distress which they are experiencing, and that if they do not recognise withdrawal distress they do not become addicts regardless of other considerations. This hypothesis had to be revised when cases were found in which individuals who had experienced and understood withdrawal distress did not use the drug to alleviate the distress and never became addicts. The revision of this hypothesis involved shifting the emphasis from the individuals' recognition of withdrawal distress to their use of the drug to alleviate the distress after this insight had occurred. No negative cases were subsequently found.

He concluded that 'this theory furnishes a simple but effective explanation, not only of the manner in which addiction becomes established, but also in the essential features of addiction behaviour, those features which are found in all parts of the world, and which are common sense to all cases' (Lindesmith 1947, p. 165). Lindesmith's aim was to produce *universal* generalisations which would apply to all cases which could be studied. Finding a single negative case caused either reformulating the hypothesis or redefining the phenomenon of addiction. This is possible because the process is one of building types or classifications out of the data as one goes along rather than being established *a priori*.

Some would argue that concepts and observations are not so independent, that concepts are not just developed out of observations but neither are they imposed as *a priori* categories. Lachenmeyer writes 'theories are not developed deductively or inductively, but *both* deductively and inductively. There is constant interplay between the observation of realities and the formation of concepts, between research and theorising, between perception and explanation. The genesis of any theory is best described as a reciprocal development of observational sophistication and theoretical precision' (Lachenmeyer 1971, p. 61). In reality there may be a synthesis of approaches since the researcher is unlikely to arrive at the point of data collection completely without some *a priori* notion or what is *likely* to be the case with hypotheses and concepts tentatively stated.

The researcher is not a *tabula rasa* although Glaser and Strauss in their *Discovery of Grounded Theory*, an important text on inductive research, advocate that investigators 'at first, literally ignore the literature of theory and fact on the area under study, in order to assure that the emergence of categories will not be contaminated by concepts more suited to different areas. Similarities and convergencies with the literature may be established after the analytic core of categories has emerged' (Glaser & Strauss 1967, p. 37). The question is the extent to which researchers impose concepts on their data and seek data which fit preselected concepts.

Those favouring deductive rather than inductive logic have made damaging attacks on logical grounds as well as on the point of keeping one's mind free of prior conceptualisation in such familiar sociological ground as mental illness and social stratification. Today it would be extremely difficult to conduct a sociological study of the management of dying patients without being influenced by Glaser and Strauss' work already described in Chapter 10.

We come therefore to the same kind of issue that confronted us with positivist research – namely the precision of the concepts used and their relationships with theory. Bulmer contends that, 'Interpretative procedures tend to be weak in providing justifications for particular conceptualizations. There is often a shared assumption that the concepts used are fruitful and make sense in the particular analysis being done' (Bulmer 1979, pp. 673–674). This assumption leaves aside the whole question of the meaning and intersubjective validity of concepts, as well as the point at which it can be assumed that concept formation is sufficiently complete to stop seeking new data. We are also left with the problem of the extent to which the interpretative studies carried out by interactionists can be generalised beyond the locales in which they take place. This has implications for how health care professionals read studies using these methods and consider their relevance to their own place of work.

More seriously still, interactionist studies may be said to be as deterministic as those of positivists because the researcher, albeit using different logic and methods, attempts to define and make causal statements about how it *really* is in the world. Just as the positivists provide a theoretical account of objective reality which is devoid of reference to the meaning of phenomena to the individuals involved, so interactionists attempt to understand these meanings but they are filtered and *interpreted* by the researcher. Are interactionists therefore simply providing a different version of reality and is it any better a version than that provided by positivists? Cicourel (1964) contends that the reasoning, interpretations and interactional skills used to produce such explanations are largely unexamined and themselves should be the basis for sociological investigation. Furthermore, since they are likely to resemble those of the subjects they study, the appropriate field for study should be the taken-for-granted and unexamined methods which members – including sociologists – use to produce the shared meanings and collective behaviour which characterise and constitute social life. This is clearly an ethnomethodological viewpoint.

GARFINKEL AND AN ETHNOMETHODOLOGICAL TREATMENT OF SUICIDE

Atkinson's study indicated that coroners had their own common-sense theories about suicide which guided their subsequent actions in categorising deaths. Atkinson wrote:

There appeared to be a convergence between common sense and expert theorising about suicide, and that there were good reasons why the latter was in line with the former. For if coroners regarded evidence, for example, depression or social isolation as strong indicators that a suicide had taken place, it was hardly surprising that statistical analyses based on their decisions would 'discover' such connections. It was still a puzzle as to what the import of this was for their practice of claiming that such correlations

supported general explanatory theories. ... In short, the positivist legacy was still evident in this continued concern to make causal statements about how it *really* is in the world; to replace one kind of determinism with another. ... At the heart of the final paradigmatic crisis in the research was the problem of what to make of the apparent convergence between common sense and expert theorising about suicide, and in particular whether the implication of this was that the layman's charge against sociology to the effect that it was no more than common sense was, after all, perfectly justified. (Atkinson 1977, p. 44)

Ethnomethodologists would of course agree with this to the extent that sociologists must use the same process as anyone else to make sense of a potentially senseless world. Garfinkel called this *practical sociological reasoning* and it is the way that such reasoning takes place that is the heart of their concerns. Related to this are problems of categorisation and description. This applies not only to the status and adequacy of categorisations by researchers as referred to above but also to the analysis of how people go about constructing categories in their everyday lives in order to proceed. Ethnomethodologists' concern with suicide therefore stems not from an interest in the subject *per se* (and as such this bears resemblance to Durkheim's use of suicide merely as a topic by which he pursued methodological interests) but in *describing* the methods used in a practical situation which demands choice and decision-making. Similar kinds of situations include jury deliberations of negligence cases and clinic staff selection of patients for outpatient psychiatric treatment (Garfinkel 1967a). In each of these the central analytic issues are the nature of practical sociological reasoning and reflexivity, concepts which we described in Chapter 2.

Garfinkel (1967b) studied coroners and suicide investigators working for the Los Angeles Suicide Prevention Centre (SPC). The staff of SPC carried out what were referred to as 'psychological autopsies' in which they had to cope with unclassified deaths which were referred to them as equivocal – the same problem as studied by Atkinson. The nature and manner of this practical sociological reasoning is best summed up by Garfinkel in the following way:

SPC inquiries begin with a death that the coroner finds equivocal as to *mode* of death. They use the death as a precedent by means of which various ways of living in society that could have terminated with the death are searched for and read 'in the remains' – in the scraps of this and that, such as the body and its trappings, medicine bottles, notes, bits and pieces of clothing, memorabilia: anything that can be photographed, collected and packaged.

Other 'remains' are collected too: rumours, passing remarks, and stories – material in the 'repertoire' of whomever might be consulted through the common work of conversations. These 'whatsoever' bits and pieces that a story or a rule or a proverb might make intelligible are used to formulate a recognizably coherent, standard, typical, cogent, uniform, planful, i.e. a professionally defensible, and thereby for members *recognizably* rational, account of how the society worked to produce these remains. This point will be clearer if the reader consults a standard textbook in forensic pathology. In it he will find the inevitable photograph of the victim with a slashed throat. Were the coroner to use that 'sight' to suggest the equivocality of the mode of death he might say something such as this: 'In the case where a body looks like the one in that picture, you are looking at a suicidal death because the wound shows the "hesitation cuts" that accompany the great wound. One can imagine these cuts are the remains of a procedure whereby the victim first made several preliminary trials of a hesitating sort and then performed the lethal slash. Other courses of action are imaginable, too, and so cuts that look like hesitation cuts can be produced by other mechanisms. One needs to start with the actual display and imagine how different courses of action could have been organized such that *that* picture would be compatible with it. One might think of the photographed display as a phase-of-the-action. In any actual display is there a course of action with which that phase is uniquely compatible?' *That* is the coroner's question. (Garfinkel 1967b, p. 176)

It is by using the concept of reflexivity that Garfinkel provides an understanding of how it was the officials were producing decisions which had to be 'justifiable' and 'reasonable' in the 'circumstances'. He uses the main features of the work of SPC to do so – the organised character of the work that they do and the particular problem of investigating equivocal deaths.

In carrying out their work, Garfinkel showed that the organisational arrangements were taken for granted and not commented upon, yet at the same time they were continually being made visible so that others could agree the grounds for actions. The grounds for such activities are not distinct from them but are situationally embedded in the activities to which they relate. This reflexivity is also clearly manifested in the production of clear rational accounts for what were initially referred because they were 'equivocal deaths'. Garfinkel makes the important point that the accounts of a particular death as this or that type of death are constitutive features of the death. The 'remains' and 'relics' which are 'read' in arriving at an account of death which is 'rational for all practical purposes' are not just already there but are all that is there to provide grounds for classifying a death as suicide. In other words, the 'relics' which are selected and defined as 'relics' suggest a proposed categorisation, and the proposed categorisation is then checked by reference to the relics. With reference to such procedures:

Coroners and SPC staff have to start with *this* much; *this* sight; *this* note; *this* collection of whatever is at hand. And *whatever* is there is good enough in the sense that whatever is there not only *will* do but *does*. One makes whatever is there do. By this is not meant that an SPC investigator is too easily content or that he does not look for more when he should. What is meant rather is that the 'whatever' it is that he has to deal with is what will be used to find out, to make decidable the way that society operated to produce *that* picture, to have come to *that* scene as its end result. In this way the remains on the slab serve not only as a precedent but as a goal of SPC inquiries. *Whatsoever* SPC members are faced with must serve as the precedent by means of which they read the remains in order to see how the society could have operated to have produced what it is that they have 'in the end', 'in the final analysis', and 'in *any* case'. What the inquiry can come to is what the death came to. (Garfinkel 1967b, p. 177)

Members of the SPC, as in all other imaginable settings, are engaged in 'monitoring' descriptions derived from the features of the setting by reference to the features of the same setting. In this way the methods used by members to test hypotheses, rule out alternatives, develop

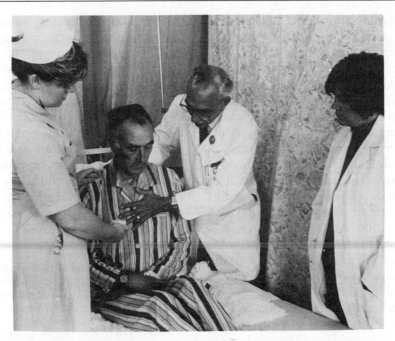

Fig. 12.5   Researchers resort to the ubiquitous while coat beloved of hospital workers while collecting data. They may be in the group but not of the group (courtesy of Rik Walton).

theories and construct categories are the same as those used by sociologists – in other words, reflexivity is central to practical sociological reasoning.

Ethnomethodologists' methods

The heading for this section may provide a clue as to why Garfinkel and his colleagues, as far as we can ascertain, provide no clear instructions or programme for how to do ethnomethodological studies or what they might look like. Rather they urge us to examine the studies themselves. Because ethnomethodology sets out with questions about *how* rather than *why* social order is accomplished, and seeks to provide generalised descriptions which go beyond the context in which empirical data were generated, they avoid the position that there could be any recipe for doing ethnomethodology. Researchers have to develop methods of analysis which are the same as those used by the subjects of their study, to produce or accom-

plish the situations being studied through their joint everyday reasoning. They are not seeking to provide an account of reality 'out there', independent to or different from those involved in it.

In order to achieve this kind of analysis Payne et al (1981) point to two basic rules which ethnomethodologists follow. One is to regard the subject matter as 'anthropologically strange' – that is, as an anthropologist would study some alien culture. How ethnomethodologists 'see' the order in the settings they are studying poses questions about their own social competence and the whole issue of reflexivity with their data.

Second, social actors in a setting are not regarded as 'rule-governed dopes' following a set of imposed rules. Rather ethnomethodologists present actors as interpreters of rules. Rules may apply but they will require extension, adaptation and modification to suit each unique situation. In this sense members produce culture rather than are produced by it.

These basic considerations have given rise to two strands of empirical work. One takes conversational analysis as its subject matter. This approach rejects the inevitably incomplete nature of the data presented in ethnographic studies as well as their dependence on the competence of the ethnographer for their solutions and analytic organisation. They reflect the researchers' descriptions and interpretations.

Conversational analysis depends on making its data, in its raw state, publicly available. This depended on the development of tape recorders to provide a faithful, albeit decontextualised, reproduction. Both the data and the procedures by which ethnomethodologists arrive at some interpretation of it are made available for scrutiny and evaluation. In order to carry out the analysis, ethnomethodologists make use of knowledge shared with other members of their culture and display this in their efforts to account for particular collections of talk. They make public both the analysis and the uncontaminated, unprocessed data from which it was produced. Conversational analysts do not seek out the exceptional or extreme. Rather they choose the most 'obvious' social phenomena as a topic. That is, that we can usually talk to each other effectively and amicably. Conversational analysis seeks to describe the processes which make possible an apparently uninteresting sociological phenomenon, for example, everyday conversation. This depends on an analysis of how order is achieved in verbal interaction and those features which enable an appearance of intelligibility of what is going on among competent participants.

Recorded talk is potentially the soundest and least contaminated of all data. Moreover, it is data which can be reproduced at the depression of a tape recorder's switch. What conversational analysts ultimately seek to do is to describe the context-free structure of talk. They have therefore studied turn-taking, opening and closing exchanges, topic change and maintenance, and the design of question and answer sequences. As Atkinson and Drew (1979) say, they are concerned with the '95%' which is common to all settings rather than the '5%' which is context-specific.

The second major ethnomethodological stance is that of ethnomethodological ethnography. Unlike the conversational analysts, they are concerned with the content and substance of conversation, not only its structural features. Payne et al write 'the ethnomethodological ethnographer starts from the question of how the participants in some event find its character and sustain it, or fail to, as a joint activity. He proceeds by a systematic process of inductive reasoning to specify the actors' models of their everyday social world which can be consulted to generate the observable conduct' (1981, p. 134). This approach is very close to the ethnographic tradition in anthropology:

A society's culture consists of whatever it is one has to know or believe in order to operate in a manner acceptable to its members, and to do so in any role that they accept for any one of themselves ... culture is not a material phenomenon; it does not consist of things, people, behaviour or emotions. It is rather an organization of these things. It is the forms of things that people have in mind, their models for perceiving, relating and otherwise interpreting them. ... Given such a definition it is impossible to describe a culture properly simply by describing behaviour or social, economic and ceremonial events and arrangements as observed material phenomena. What is required is to construct a theory of the conceptual models which they represent and of which they are artifacts. We test the adequacy of such a theory by our ability to interpret and predict what goes on in a community as measured by how its members, our informants, do so. A further test is our ability ourselves to behave in ways which lead to the kind of responses from the community members which our theory would lead us to expect. Thus tested, the theory is a valid statement of what you have to know in order to operate as a member of the society and is, as such, a valid description of its culture. ... The relation of language to culture is that of part to whole. Theory and method applicable to one must have implications for the other. (Goodenough 1964, pp. 36–37, quoted in Payne et al 1981, p. 135).

It is the stress on actors' models as opposed to a researcher's selective interpretation of these models which distinguishes ethnomethodological ethnography from its predecessors.

The explication of actors' models depends on the standing of the ethnomethodologist on the margins of the social group being studied. That is, the group being studied is regarded as anthropologically strange. Collecting and interpreting data involves a continuous interchange of cultural frames – now taking the perspective of the member and now that of the stranger. The reflexivity engendered itself becomes a source of data by enhancing knowledge of the phenomenon being studied through the same intimacy of knowledge of it as the members themselves have. The data presented are more analytic than descriptive, and less a product of the filtering and interpretation by the researcher than in typical ethnographic reports. They also claim to be closer to that used by conversational analysts by presenting *key* conversations or the context in which conversations take place in as complete a form as possible. An example of this kind of research is Strong's (1979a) *The Ceremonial Order of the Clinic* which contains a methodological appendix. This includes an account of the identified basis of the social rules adhered to by participants in over 1000 paediatric consultations. The logic is clearly inductive, going from the data to generate propositions which explain them and which are subsequently tested out with other data. However, the initial cases were selected according to survey sampling methods and the study is comparative, both in terms of cases within the same clinic as well as internationally using clinics in the United Kingdom and the United States. Furthermore, Strong (1988) argues that by drawing on other studies of medical consultation that the bureaucratic format predominates in all medical consultations in the United Kingdom public health service. While the data treatment and analytic logic are essentially ethnomethodological, the study overall included elements of different methodological research practices.

In general terms, it can be argued that the ethnomethodologists, by their commitment to explicating as far as possible the relationship between data and its analysis, are being more 'scientific' in their approach than are sociologists using other perspectives and their associated methods of hypothesis testing.

A FEMINIST PERSPECTIVE

Readers may have noticed a male bias in our descriptions of perspectives, theories and methods. The major theorists are all male. Only in feminist sociology is there a predominance of female writers. One way of taking a feminist standpoint is to produce knowledge which makes explicit the gendered meanings and relationships of which we may not be aware and which sociology has generally ignored. While taking a feminist standpoint exposes male-centredness and hence power differentials in social life, it also raises the problems of how to make both sociological knowledge and feminist knowledge convincing (Ramazanoglu 1989).

Feminist sociologists have expressed methodological preferences which are concerned with the role of *experience in method* (Du Bois 1983). They have a greater orientation to studies which are qualitative and adopt nonhierarchical approaches which avoid treating the researched as 'objects' and which avoid subordinating them as subjects (Ramazanoglu 1992). This does not mean that feminists do not carry out quantitative studies, but that they raise issues of the often insensitive nature of quantitative research and that some of these insensitivities can be remedied (Webb 1984, Hunt 1986, Eichler 1988). A feminist approach to studying suicide could involve a consideration of the differential ways of treating the suicides of men and women or the differential consequences of bereavement by suicide compared with loss by deaths due to natural causes. These studies would be likely to involve close working with the individuals concerned, drawing on their experiences, and with the researcher acknowledging that sharing experiences can be counted as data.

METHODOLOGICAL PLURALISM

In this chapter we have tried to demonstrate the interdependence of methods and sociological perspectives. Indeed, method *is* a perspectival component. However, often methods are taught in a prescriptive, cookery-book fashion, with recipes requiring certain ingredients processed in a variety of ways to produce the final product.

Feminist writers have made evident that much sociological knowledge, as well as knowledge more generally, has depended on male-centred sociological categories of thought and reason. However, even amongst feminists 'Different methodologies will produce different sorts of knowledge. When feminists disagree methodologically, they also disagree politically' (Ramazanoglu 1989). An extreme position was taken by Feyerabend (1975) who argues that scientists should follow no methodological rules, either inductive or deductive, and that, in reality, scientists frequently change their rules, what they are doing and how they are doing it. For him, there is no point in subscribing to any of the positions we have outlined and he argues *against* method.

This radical position finds little favour with traditional philosophies of science, with prescriptive approaches to how science should be done or with pragmatists attempting to carry out studies. However, debates about the status of sociological knowledge and the methods used to provide it are not confined to the philosophical and sociological communities. In 1982 Sir Keith Joseph, Secretary of State for Education, decreed that no longer did we have a Social *Science* Research Council but an Economic and Social Research Council. The work funded or undertaken by the then SSRC did not match to *his* normative expectations of science. This raises questions, therefore, for society about the status of knowledge generated by sociology and other forms of social research.

We retain our stance that methodological pluralism is warranted in sociology and advocated for other disciplines studying the social world. Different methods have their place provided one knows what questions to ask and emphasis is placed on the relevance and the validity of the ensuing research. Indeed, we try to practise what we preach in carrying out health services research. In carrying out an extensive evaluation of long-stay accommodation for elderly people, we have used both the most rigorous of traditional clinical experiments, the randomised-controlled trial as well as sample surveys and ethnographic case studies to provide data relevant to different kinds of questions concerning health service policy (Bond et al 1989).

We are left in the position of saying that sociology is about studying a social world that is external to sociologists but of which they are part, and which is experienced by them in systematic ways. These ways differ, providing *different* conclusions. However, without exception, they involve systematic observation, recorded data collection, generating propositions, and testing them to provide confirmation or falsification. They also involve attempting to make these processes public.

FURTHER READING

Barrat D, Cole T 1991 Sociology projects: a student's guide. Routledge & Kegan Paul, London

Brewer J, Hunter A 1989 Multimethod research: a synthesis of styles. Sage, Beverly Hills

Hammersley M, Atkinson P 1983 Ethnography: principles in practice. Tavistock, London

Shaffir W B, Stebbins R A (eds) 1991 Experiencing fieldwork: an insider view of qualitative research. Sage, Beverly Hills

13

Appreciating sociology

INTRODUCTION

We have found this a difficult book to write – not just because it has been a time-consuming enterprise which has permeated our private and professional lives, but because we wanted sociology and its application to health to be understood by any health professional who happens to read it. At the same time, we have tried to avoid trivialising its subject matter into a series of 'social facts' or empirical findings divorced of their theoretical context. In other words, we realised from the outset that we would need to satisfy the often conflicting perspectives of the professional sociologist and the nonsociologist health professional. Sociology is renowned for its jargon and often incomprehensible language. Many of the critics of this feature of sociology suggest that this is a method of making the subject more mysterious in order to give it an inflated sense of importance. We suspect that there is a lot of truth in this view but also recognise that every discipline, whether in the social or natural sciences, has a specialised terminology and language. Specialised language is a necessary characteristic of advanced study whether it is about society, the human body, quantum physics or computing. In writing this book we have tried to demystify sociology and at the same time show why its language has to be more specific than that used in everyday speech and writing in order that the meaning of its concepts can be more precisely defined and shared. Because sociology deals with topics familiar to all of us the need for this precision is not always recognised, particularly when dealing with topics like social class or profession. In the same way sociological investigation is sometimes accused of telling us things we already knew.

A WAY OF LOOKING

Sociology is just one way of looking at the world in which we live and act out our daily lives. We saw in Chapter 1 how other social sciences can observe the same phenomenon from different perspectives, providing a variety of insights into the world in which we live. The views of the natural sciences should also not be excluded since, as we hope we have shown, they often take for granted a particular view of society upon which their own particular areas of knowledge and scientific enterprise focus. Thus, for example, geologists in their quest for oil-bearing rocks take for granted society's need for oil in particular and for energy in general. It is their own and others' definitions of what society needs which is directing their scientific endeavours.

Sociology, we have argued, is not the monopoly of sociologists. Indeed, we have suggested that sociology is for all those who are interested in society or deal with people in their everyday lives. The first people to attempt a sociological view of health and illness in Britain predated professional sociologists just as barbers predated surgeons. In the section devoted to the study of health at the first annual conference of the British Sociological Association in the early 1950s only one of six speakers was a professional sociologist. Of the other five, four were medical doctors and one was a medical administrator (Illsley 1980). Many of the early patrons of a sociology of health and illness were clinicians and epidemiologists, while the founder of medial sociology in Britain, Raymond Illsley, was an ex-economist and town planner interested in social class and poverty. Nowadays, some sociologists might argue that the activities of these early pioneers were not sociology at all but social epidemiology. But, as we saw in Chapter 1, sociology has many perspectives and social epidemiology is one of them. Researchers involved with the rapidly expanding applied discipline of health services researcher apply many of the ideas and concepts generated by sociology in their studies, offering sociology *in* health care.

Different ways of looking

In an introductory text about sociology we see it as important to try not to take sides with a particular perspective but, at the same time, it is also extremely difficult not to do so. With such a variety of sociological perspectives to choose from any omission will be viewed by our critics as favouring a particular perspective or perspectives. Throughout this book we have tried to adopt an eclectic approach to our subject matter. Wherever possible we have provided different views of the social world, often juxtaposing the more conservative views of the functionalists with those of the Marxists or ethnomethodologists or feminists. As with all theory there is no single correct approach. Theories are judged in terms of their usefulness in generating ideas and their explanations, not their correctness.

A major consequence of choosing any particular perspective is that it asks different questions, uses different methods and very often gets different answers to the other approaches. We illustrated this characteristic of sociology particularly with the example of mental illness in Chapter 2, when introducing different sociology perspectives, and again in the last chapter in relation to suicide. In our treatment of different aspects of health care we have drawn attention to contrasting sociological perspectives, identified the kinds of questions asked, described the kinds of research methods used and reported a variety of answers. We hope that this has been enriching even though, inevitably, it has made the sociology more complex. These are the kinds of problems sociologists deal with all the time.

These different ways of looking and conceptualising involve a critical examination of the world in which we live. Like all academics, it is the purpose of sociologists to examine things critically. However, whereas geologists and meteorologists focus on such topics as the long-term effects of volcanic activity on weather patterns and historians criticise theories about why Napoleon eventually lost his empire, sociologists normally describe and explain the structures and functions of current everyday life – your life and our lives. In this sense, sociologists have to conceive everyday events as problems warranting investigation. Few people will feel threatened by the activities of geologists, meteorologists or even historians, since they are discussing events and knowledge which do not impinge directly and obviously on us. The work of sociologists has a more direct bearing. This applies at different levels in society. At the macro-level there may be a critical examination of the relationships between the activities of large-scale social institutions like the food and tobacco industries, or social structures like occupation or class on health and ill health. At the meso-level are studies about the working of institutions like hospitals or health centres, or the construction of social data like suicide rates or waiting lists. At the micro-level sociologists have studied interpersonal relationships between professionals and their clients. Being involved in sociological research and reading about its findings can threaten people; it can make them feel uncomfortable at a personal level and give rise to the comment that there is nothing sociologists can add to personal knowledge of a situation. If general managers *know* how their units function or nurses *know* how they provide care to families what can sociologists possibly tell them?

So what?

A second normal response to the reporting of much sociology is not one of feeling threatened but one of 'So what?'. A number of sociological studies have met with this reaction. However, further research had often identified the initial findings as facts of greater practical and theoretical significance than was obvious at first. In the '50s and '60s, when the rate of unemployment was relatively low, sociological research on the relationship between unemployment and health was treated as insignificant and irrelevant. There were also attempts to squash this research, just as more recently there were attempts at the highest level not to fund research on sexual behaviour as it related to sexually transmitted disease and HIV infection because the work was not considered likely to provide any useful information to deal with the problem. Admittedly the findings of the early studies of unemployment and health were equivocal. There was little evidence that unemployment caused ill health, since there were so few unemployed people and ill health itself was likely to be the cause of some of the unemployment. The dramatic increase in unemployment rates in the late '70s, throughout the '80s and in the early '90s makes the earlier research no less equivocal, but the findings have proved to be highly relevant both theoretically and practically.

Similarly, in the late '70s there was immense activity by sociologists with ethnomethodological and phenomenological leanings in the study of the language used in interactions between clients and professionals. In their infancy, these studies produced numerous 'obvious' and 'trivial' findings, which were regarded as irrelevant to the practitioners concerned. Yet these same findings are becoming more acceptable to many practitioners who have attempted to change educational practices in such fields as interviewing techniques, health promotion activities and counselling, in order to influence the way in which professionals interact with and talk with clients. Indeed, in the past 10 years issues in communication have become an increasingly important feature of the curriculum of almost every health professional's initial professional education. One of the problems of much sociological data is that, because it is about everyday life, it seems obvious and even trivial when spelt out in a research report. But, like hindsight in all aspects of our lives, we may ask, 'Why did we, as members of society, not see it before?'.

Table 13.1   Reported research projects ranked by level of funding in 1990 by substantive category listed in *Medical Sociology in Britain* in 1982 and 1990

Research topic	Rank	1990[1] Amount £000	N	1982[2] Rank	N
HIV/AIDS	1	2763	32	–	–
Mental health	2	1620	8	13	10
Health services	3	729	27	11	11
GP/primary care	4	706	19	4	23
Pregnancy/reproduction	5	638	13	3	27
Chronic illness/disability	6	419	20	1	28
Women and health	7	405	9	9	13
Addiction	8	378	10	–	–
Health beliefs	9	344	16	15	8
Hospitals	10	294	11	16	7
The elderly	11	252	10	5	23
Nursing	12	249	9	2	27
Children and health	13	140	6	7	14
Ethnicity and health	14	91	6	–	5
Inequalities and health	15	61	5	–	–
Terminal care	16	–	6	–	6

Sources:
1. Field D, Woodman D (eds) 1990 Medical sociology in Britain: a register of research and teaching, 6th edn. British Sociological Association, Medical Sociology Group, Table 1, p. 115
2. Field D, Clarke B A, Goldie N 1982 Medical sociology in Britain: a register of research and teaching, 4th edn. British Sociological Association, Medical Sociology Group, pp. 79–131

As we observed in Chapter 5, when discussing the problems in carrying out studies about the family we *take for granted* much of what happens in our everyday worlds. In the same way as we may often refuse to accept what may be happening to ourselves, we are often able to see the same thing happening to others. We notice when other people are bad-tempered or tired but will not readily recognise the symptoms in ourselves. We may recognise immediately the characteristics of marital stress in our friends or colleagues but not in ourselves. Sociology then is one means of sensitizing us to facts and issues in our public and private lives, which we would otherwise take for granted.

Although we use and have developed sociology as an academic subject in order critically to examine the world around us, and to sensitize ourselves to things which we take for granted, we also recognise that it is a product of the society in which we live. To survive in the jungle of the educational marketplace sociology must present a saleable product. Funding for socio-logical research will therefore tend to reflect the needs of society in general and of government in particular. These needs are reflected in the cur-rent research being undertaken by sociologists concerned with health and illness. The latest Register of research of the Medical Sociology Group (Field & Woodman 1990) shows not only the extent to which sociology is taught in the various educational establishments for different health professionals, but also the extent to which research activities reflect the interests of society. Table 13.1 shows the reported amount of funds received by 'sociologists' by substantive category with the number of entries within the category. There are 16 main categories and there is, of course, also an 'other' category. To some extent such categorisation will be fairly arbi-trary. For example, a study, in which we are both involved, evaluating continuing-care acco-mmodation for frail elderly people (Bond et al 1989), is classified under 'the elderly' but it could equally well have been put in at least three other categories: nursing, hospitals and health services. Nevertheless, the categories shown provide a useful indication of the inter-ests that sociologists have in health care.

It is not only the interests of sociologists which influences what they study. In our increasingly market-driven academic world, it is the availability of funding and 'customers' which determine the nature of sociological work. This can be clearly illustrated by the sub-stantial amount of research funding awarded for social and behavioural aspects of the study of HIV infection. Since the 1982 edition of the Register (Field et al 1982), reported in our first edition, the league table of substantive cate-gories has changed markedly, reflecting political priorities and the marketplace for health ser-vices research. For example, it is worth noting that the second largest category with 27 entries reported in 1982 consisted of research projects about 'nursing and related occupations'. In

1990, only seven entries were in this category compared with 32 within the 'AIDS/HIV' cate-gory. Similarly, in 1982, 'the elderly' category recorded 23 entries and ranked joint fourth with 'general-practitioner based studies'. In 1990, 'GP/primary care' remained a high priority to funding agencies with 27 entries but 'the elderly' was no longer in favour with only 10 entries. Of course, as the editors of the Registers point out these data depend on people making the effort to provide information and their interpretation of what their own research is about! Never-theless, we suspect that these changes in fashion for sociological research mirror reality quite well.

ACHIEVEMENTS OF SOCIOLOGY IN HEALTH CARE

It is difficult to extol the achievements of socio-logy. Many of the achievements of natural scien-tists end up as new technology, such as the combustion engine or the cardiac monitor, and we can recognise their scientific origins. It is more difficult to attribute changes in social life in general, or the provision of health services in particular, to sociological achievements. Many of the contributions of sociology are not tangible and, when they are, the time lag between the ini-tial theoretical idea and social change is so great that the change will be embodied in society's rules and expectations. Yet work like that car-ried out by Stacey and her colleagues (Stacey et al 1970, Hall & Stacey 1979) on the welfare of children in hospital has left its mark on service provision in this sector.

The same may be said at the other end of the age spectrum. It is now over 30 years since Townsend (1962) published his influential book *The Last Refuge*, which described and was highly critical of the institutional environment of resi-dential homes for elderly people which pro-duced damaging effects on their lives (see Ch. 7). In the intervening years there have been a range of arguments and ideas about insti-tutions, some subversive to institutional care, then a resurgence of the notion that while insti-

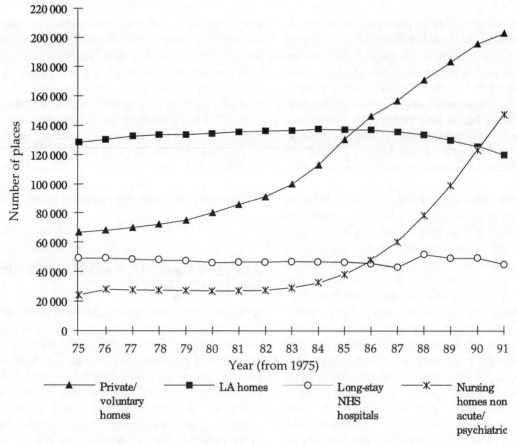

Fig. 13.1 Increase in residential care/continuing care places (Laing & Buisson 1991).

tutional living may have harmful effects on residents this is because of poor resourcing and staffing, bad management practices and administration, inadequate education and poor equipment. There have been some improvements in some aspects of the quality of institutional life (Willcocks et al 1987), and the policy of creating nursing homes and community care while reducing the number of hospital beds for the long-term care of people with learning disabilities, who are mentally ill and frail elderly people, probably owes something to findings about the inadequacies of long-term care in hospitals (Bond & Bond 1993). Yet Booth (1985) has found that the main effects on residents in residential homes are not related to how homes are run: it is being in an institution *per se* which has overwhelmingly negative consequences. Yet the residential and nursing home industry flourishes, as shown in Figure 13.1.

The findings from sociological studies are interpreted in political and policy contexts which are constructed by the societies in which we live. Sociological knowledge is only one of many potential influences on society and the welfare policies which influence our lives. Health professionals themselves, some with more influence than others, also make contributions from their particular perspectives.

It would be extremely difficult to catalogue individual sociological studies which have been major influences in shaping society. Unlike the 'breakthroughs' we hear of in biomedical or physics research, which can be transferred into technological advances, sociological contributions operate more as enlightenment, adding in a gradual way to understanding social processes. We should like to identify just some of the themes in this book, which may have sensitized health professionals to look at taken-for-granted phenomena in a different and perhaps more enlightened way. In doing so we will attempt to address those themes which are part and parcel of the work of health professionals.

Medical and social models

In Chapter 1 we described two different and extreme models of health – the medical model and the social model. We saw in Chapter 4 how a social model helped us to understand the social causes of illness and some of the difficulties in applying a medical model to preventing illness and promoting health. We also described, in Chapter 8, a social model which helps us to understand an individual's reactions to health or ill health.

We have argued that the practice of health care is dominated by the medical model, which encapsulates the perspective of the medical profession and other professions related to medicine. The emphasis of the medical model is on illness, disease or ill health and the need for medical treatment, rather than on health or normality. In some ways these differences are encapsulated in the distinction between disease prevention and health promotion. As well as focusing on health rather than disease, we have argued that health professionals might find it helpful to consider illness, the causes of illness and patients' responses to their illness from viewpoints other than medical ones. It is difficult to establish the extent to which the concept of the social model in health has sensitized health professionals to think in different ways. In general conversation with health professionals we have noticed a change in the attitudes of some health professionals over the last 20 years of our professional lives. One general physician,

in describing to one of us the emergence of AIDS and HIV infection in his professional life, admitted that the social model of illness was essential in understanding and providing health care to sufferers of AIDS. Another discussion with orthopaedic surgeons highlighted the recognition that the medical model had many weaknesses. They suggested that if they adopted the medical model too rigidly they would be operating on thousands of knees which were not impairing, handicapping or disabling to their owners!

There is also increasing attention now being given to considerations of quality of life as well as saving life at the cost of quality, and to the social and functional outcomes of treatments rather than only physiological effectiveness (McDowell & Newell 1987, Bowling 1992, Wilkin et al 1992). Examination of the curricula of newly developing courses and redrafting of established curricula for health professionals may provide some indication of the extent to which a variety of perspectives on health are being advocated by teachers as well as demonstrated in practice. Certainly, the influence the social model has had on the work of the World Health Organization is not insignificant, as a glance at some of their publications will quickly establish.

Inequalities in health

Both epidemiology and sociology have made major contributions to the analysis of inequalities in health, as is evident from the report *Inequalities in Health* (DHSS 1980, Townsend & Davidson 1982, Townsend et al 1988). An understanding of inequalities in health requires an understanding of social class. We tend to take the concept of social class, like that of the family, for granted and to use it in a variety of ways. In Chapter 3, we emphasised the importance of social class in particular and social stratification in general. Social class has often been used as a panacea to *explain* a variety of human behaviour and this has been the case in understanding health and illness. Many writers have suggested that social class is a *cause* of illness. We disagree. Lower social class is a characteristic of people who are more likely to be *ill*, not a cause of their ill health.

Understanding social class and the real causes of inequality in health is a central concern of sociology which should be of interest and value to all of those concerned with the health of the nation. At an interpersonal level, studies of social class have helped health professionals to understand the difficulties they have in communicating and interacting with patients from different social backgrounds who, as well as showing linguistic differences, will probably also have a different perspective on health, ill health and health care. We have described the scepticism and fatalism of some patients about the benefits of measures to prevent ill health. Blaxter (1983) also found that people simply do not believe that there are differences in health between the rich and the poor. The rich and famous succumb to cancer, stroke, dementia and Parkinson's disease and statistical proof about health inequalities have little salience for the person in the street or even politicians. At one level, health education and health promotion efforts need to recognise the differences between social groups and target their efforts in socially appropriate ways to the groups concerned. However, there needs to be a questioning of the assumption that poor people can choose healthy lifestyles in the face of poverty and its consequences.

The problems of health inequalities require political action, however. Yet in the *Health of the Nation* (Secretary of State for Health 1992) which provides a strategic approach to health in the United Kingdom, social inequalities receive scant attention at the expense of individual health behaviour. A sociological understanding can assist health professionals at all levels to contribute to the reduction of health inequalities by adopting a positive approach to the problems faced by disadvantaged clients and patients. This can range from structural inputs, like the number of district nurses and health visitors provided in areas according to established need, to the siting of help centres and tailoring parenting education specifically to the needs of prospective parents. However, the basic prob-

lem is one of poverty and that demands political action, which in turn depends on political action stemming from a national desire to reduce inequality. In the United Kingdom there is simply no such desire.

Social epidemiology

We have suggested that the social model is helpful in the understanding of the aetiology of illness. In Chapter 4 we focused on two kinds of sociological analysis, both of which informed health professionals about the relationship between a variety of social factors and health. First, we described the relationships between illness and social structure using the tools and methods of social epidemiology. Second, we discussed a model of the origins of health which relates health outcomes to the characteristics and life experiences of the individual.

The importance of both of these analyses can be illustrated in our understanding of prevention. In Chapter 4, we suggest that primary prevention is principally a social activity over which health professionals have little direct control but which social policies influence through the distribution of resources between and within groups. However, within this overarching constraint health professionals have a role to play in health education in aspects like preventing accidents and encouraging sensible eating habits. An understanding of social processes should equip health professionals to more readily comprehend the difficulties that many of us have in conforming to a rational lifestyle which maximises our health status and potential. Sociology, however, will not directly assist in changing the layout of roads or introducing speed restrictions to prevent accidents.

The family

In Chapter 5, we used the family as an example of how sociology sensitizes us to three aspects of society which we take for granted. Within the context of the notion that the family is the basic unit in health and medical care we discussed three important issues. First, that the way we generally describe the family as a husband and wife with 2.2 children is not particularly useful. The increasing trend toward 'serial' marriage, single-parent families and different forms of group living, suggests that the family is a more complex social structure than conventional wisdom generally accepts. Second, we observed that the theoretical basis to the study of the family is still in its infancy and does not reflect the real world as documented by epidemiologists and demographers, as well as sociologists. Third, we argued that conventional wisdom about the family is not always a good indicator of the relationship between health and illness, both in the way we promote and maintain health, and in the way the family reacts and copes with illness, particularly chronic illness, in one of its members.

We suggest that the study of the family as the basic unit in health and medical care has assisted health professionals in caring for patients and their families. This interest in the effects of illness on family life, and in the effects of the family on illness and health behaviour, is likely to become an even more central concern of health professionals as the emphasis on community care for those with mental illness, learning disability and physical and mental frailty in later life increases. Sociology will continue to add to our understanding of the various social mechanisms involved.

Social construction

General to sociological understanding is the idea that all human actions are socially constructed. In Chapter 3, we showed that old age is a social category defined by society. The importance of the ideal of social construction is illustrated by the way such a social category can impinge on the quality of life of elderly people. Thus, for example, different categories of elderly people receive different benefit entitlements.

At the individual level, we saw in Chapter 9 how these social constructions reflect what sociologists call typifications. Throughout our lives we typify in order to know how to react to and with individuals in different social categories. We described how staff typify patients according to their social and work-related characteristics as well as their medical characteristics, and how patients are treated on the basis of these typifications. Thus, sociology helps us to understand how, as individuals, we continually reconstruct the social world around us and how these typifications reflect society's construction of social categories.

The fact that we react to people in social categories challenges the idea that it 'all boils down to personalities' and that we treat people as individuals. To say that we treat people as individuals in our professional or private lives is to ignore the fact that we first make assumptions about people from their obvious social characteristics and often get no further using these as the basis for relationships. Associated with individuals within social categories are, among other things, that different definitions of the situation will exist; that different roles with specific obligations are being enacted; that different expectations are involved; and that different sets of values are adopted. Because of this we can appreciate that conflicts are a normative and even useful feature of social life, present in our interactions with our children, with patients and clients and with other professionals. Seen in this way conflict is inevitable.

Similarly, we tend to apportion blame to others for the work they apparently create for us or which they carry out ineptly, for the unreasonable demands they apparently make on us and for the trouble they apparently cause. Taking the perspective of the other is likely to yield a very different picture, which is why many educational programmes ask students to role play patients, to experience life from a wheelchair or with muffled ears or darkened eyes. It is much more difficult to try to adopt the role of someone in poverty, with learning disabilities, with different ethnic or religious backgrounds or of a different gender. Behind the interpretations of events that all of us make in our social and working lives, lie sociological explanations of why particular states of affairs exist and why they are interpreted in different ways by different people. These explanations transcend personal psychology.

Grasping this point will not provide immediate solutions to work problems. Indeed, it can complicate and raise new problems by suggesting that we should take more account of what are others' views of a particular situation. The recent rise of consumerism in the health service, if taken seriously, will have major and often uncomfortable consequences for health policy makers and providers. However, understanding that competing perspectives do exist and that individuals will interpret events from their own social, political and economic stance, may help to make more bearable those forms of social interaction which are stressful and have negative connotations. They may also give rise to more helpful, workable and widely acceptable solutions to problems.

USING SOCIOLOGY

We exemplified some problems of interaction in Chapter 9, specifically in relation to sociological features of the management of pain, and in Chapter 10 in relation to dying, death and bereavement. Carrying out sociological research, and using its findings to gain an understanding of the interpersonal aspects of the work of health professionals, may go some way towards providing relevant services to assist those patients or staff who experience such problems to overcome them. As well as heightening awareness that difficulties may exist locally, with deleterious consequences for patients and staff alike, sociologically derived knowledge can be used at the level of policy decisions about, for example, whose responsibility it is to identify bereaved people at risk of social or psychiatric breakdown and to organise services so that supportive interventions are available to those judged as requiring care. Sociological approaches are also relevant at the micro-level in assessing forms of interaction between, for example, midwives and women at antenatal clinics, midwives and women during labour, or midwives and women after the delivery of a stillborn baby.

Sociological knowledge may make a number of contributions in circumstances like these. First, in pointing out that problems of inter-

action with patients are especially difficult when competing perspectives exist, when the organisation is not 'geared up' to deal with them and when the contexts in which they occur involve highly salient social values. These have been identified in a number of different settings and are more than a reflection of idiosyncratic strengths or deficits among individuals involved. They demonstrate that particular features of work may require greater attention than that given to them in the past and that their analysis requires an appreciation of their social context.

Second, the findings of sociological research may be used in policy development at a range of levels as a means of developing appropriate and workable solutions from the variety of possibilities that might exist. Appropriateness in this sense will be as much a matter of available skills, talents and resources as what empirical studies have shown to be desirable.

Third, sociology may be used in education to encourage staff to explore their own and others' feelings about the subject, and to point to processes and facts which may assist in promoting action learning. Group rather than individual learning should increase the likelihood that possible solutions are acted upon. Sociological knowledge about particular concerns facing health professionals may have relevance at any level in the structure of health care organisations – at regional and unit levels to devise appropriate policies about how resources may be allocated and services organised; within primary health care and ward teams to decide the appropriate professional to take responsibility for particular features of care; in hospital wards to agree means by which interactional difficulties may be identified and resolved; by individual professionals to ascertain the nature and extent of family support for patients with different kinds of problems. At an individual level, too, a reading of the sociological literature on specific topics may help to extend awareness and understanding of the concerns currently faced.

In this book we have concentrated largely, but by no means exclusively, on sociology directly generated by and linked to health problems and the professions which are directly involved. Health care is a complex institution and is able to benefit from studies in other areas of society. In Chapter 5, we discussed some theoretical issues in the sociology of the family and then, in Chapter 6, demonstrated their relevance to health issues; in Chapter 11, the sociology of occupations was helpful in understanding nursing and the other health professions. The structure of nursing has been influenced by models drawn from industrial organisation and management. An understanding of nursing and some other paramedical work as women's work, and the strong influence of paternalism and capitalism discussed in Chapter 11, has emerged from feminist writers. This topic has recently also become an increasing concern among women doctors.

To gain an understanding of the ways in which individuals, professional groups and organisations are involved in health care work necessitates taking into account other features of our society, as well as the views of *all* those who contribute to it. Throughout this book we have attempted to enrich this understanding by showing the relevance of sociology. We entitled this chapter 'Appreciating sociology'. We trust that you do appreciate it!

Glossary
and
References

GLOSSARY

In the text of the glossary, words appearing in italics are themselves defined.

Acculturation: the process of contact between *cultures* by which an individual or group is assimilated into the existing culture and which, in turn, modifies the existing culture. The term is used on pages 216–217 to refer to the socialisation process of newcomers to a professional group who conduct themselves in a manner by which established group members recognise them as competent.

Action: action is distinct from *behaviour* in that it involves meaning or intention.

Ageing: as well as being a genetically programmed process of living organisms, social gerontologists are concerned with ageing as a process linked with the social and demographic structure of human groups; as an aspect of personal status in the life cycle; as a component of stratification in terms of generational membership and as a contemporary social problem raising questions about exploitation, victimisation and stigmatisation. Important are the criteria by which an individual is *labelled* 'elderly'.

Alienation: the estrangement of individuals from themselves and from others. It was originally used by Marx to denote human estrangement rooted in existing *social structures* which denied people their essential human nature. It is now more widely used to denote discontent with society, feelings of moral breakdown in society, feelings of powerlessness and the dehumanisation of large scale organisations.

Assumptive world: used to describe our image or our perception of the environment in which we live.

Attitude: a relatively stable set of beliefs concerning an object and resulting in an evaluation of that object. Attitudes are not necessarily related to behaviour.

Authority: a type of *power* in which people willingly obey commands because they regard the exercise of power as legitimate.

Awareness context: in interactionist theory, interaction between individuals takes place in awareness contexts – what each knows about the identity of the other and his own identity in the eyes of the other, including what each knows about particular events and situations. This term is referred to on pages 183–186 in relation to dying.

Behaviour: used by psychologists to describe observable conduct in response to stimuli. It disregards the subjective aspects of conduct. Sociologists use the term *action* to distinguish meaningful activity from behaviour.

Bourgeoisie: in Marxist theory, a description of the middle or ruling classes in capitalist society who are assumed to be interested in preserving capitalism in a struggle with the working class.

Bureaucracy: a concept first defined by Weber to describe a form of administration. His *ideal type* includes a high degree of specialisation and a clearly defined division of labour with tasks distributed as official duties; a hierarchical structure of authority with clearly circumscribed areas of command and responsibility; the establishment of a formal body of rules to govern the operation of the organisation; administration based on written documents; impersonal relationships between organisational members and with clients; recruitment of personnel on the basis of ability; promotion on the basis of seniority or merit; a fixed salary; and the separation of private and official income.

Career: a concept denoting a progression of events which relate to each other. It is often used to describe a sequence of jobs, which may be either structured or unstructured. It may also apply to other sequences of events in the *life career*, such as the patient career.

Career contingencies: Goffman introduced this term to describe points in a *career* at which mechanisms are triggered affecting the course of the career.

Caste: a caste system is a form of *social stratification* in which castes are hierarchically organised and separated from each other by rules of ritual purity.

Class: in Marxist theory, class is used to describe two opposing social groups: the *bourgeoisie* and the *proletariat*. In Weberian theory, a person's class position is the location which he shares with those who are similarly placed in the processes of production, distribution and exchange.

Class, ascribed: the position of an individual in terms of the social standing into which he is born and over which he has no control, rather than the position he attains by his own achievements.

Clinical uncertainty: exists when there is a real uncertainty about clinical matters and when information of this kind may be withheld to avoid revealing that uncertainty exists among health professionals.

Community: this term is one of the most elusive and vague used by sociologists. It is now used largely without specific meaning. It may refer to a set of people resident in a geographical area. It may also include elements of a sense of belonging as in 'community spirit'; a self-contained unit in which all of the daily work and nonwork activities of a community take place; collections within a particular social structure which are often rural or 'preindustrial'. Thus, notions of 'therapeutic community' or 'care in the community' contain slightly different elements.

Community care: this term refers to the trend of replacing large and often geographically remote institutional facilities with smaller units of residential provision. More recently, it has been used to refer to the fact that carers reside in the community.

Concept: in general usage the term mainly means notion or idea. It may be defined as the name for the members of a given class of objects of any sort, or as the name of the class itself. More simply, concept refers to a descriptive property or relation.

Conflict: social conflict assumes various forms. Competition describes conflict over the control of resources or advantage desired by others where physical violence is not employed. Regulated competition is resolved within a framework of agreed rules. Other conflicts may be more violent and not bound by rules, in which case they are settled by the opposing parties mobilising their *power* resources.

Correlation: it is normal to record a variety of data simultaneously in sociological research. When one datum provides information about the other they are said to be associated or correlated. All measures of correlation indicate the strength of the association between two or more variables. The fact that two variables are correlated does not establish that one is antecedent to or causes the other.

Cultural group: the collection of people who share the same *culture*.

Culture: a collective noun which describes the symbolic and learned aspects of human society, including language, custom and convention, and by which human *action* can be distinguished from the *behaviour* of other primates.

Culture of poverty: used by Oscar Lewis to describe an impoverished way of life which is remarkably stable and persistent and which is passed down from generation to generation along family lines.

Deduction: a process by which valid conclusions can be logically deduced from valid premises. Rarely are sociological arguments strictly deductive in form, even if they claim to be.

Definition of the situation: the importance of the subjective perspectives of social actors for the objective consequences of social interaction is often summarised in sociology by the notion of defining the situation. One implication of the *concept* is that the 'truth' or 'falsity' of beliefs (definitions of the situation) are not important issues and what matters is the outcome of social interaction.

Design, prospective: a study design in which data are collected as events occur.

Design, retrospective: a study design in which data are collected after the events have occurred.

Deviance, primary: in *labelling theory*, primary deviance refers to the act of labelling by another actor who is accepted by the social group as having the *authority* to do so.

Deviance, secondary: in *labelling theory*, secondary deviance refers to the effect the label has on both the people being labelled and other people around them.

Enculturation: the process of *socialisation* as the passive *internalisation* of an existing normative order, in abstraction from any broader social or historical context.

Ethnic group: conceptual confusion surrounds the distinctiveness of the terms 'ethnic group', *'cultural group'*, 'racial group' and *'caste'*. Sociologists have generally rejected the notion that human groups can be unambiguously defined in terms of their genetic constitution. Social groups are more commonly defined by reference to a shared culture such as language, customs and institutions. A group which claims ethnic distinctiveness is different from one which has had distinctiveness imposed on it by a politically superior group in the context of a political struggle. Ethnicity may, therefore, become the basis for racial separation or for political subordination.

Ethnomethodology: the term literally means 'peoples' methods', invented by Garfinkel to describe a branch of sociology which criticises other perspectives that impose sociological categories on the ordinary person. For ethnomethodologists other perspectives in sociology redescribe what ordinary people do, treating these accounts as deficient. Ethnomethodology aims to study how people ('members') construct their social world and how the orderly nature of that world is achieved. It examines how 'members' work continuously to make sense of others. Yet, despite this, the way in which the world is constructed is entirely taken for granted. Ethnomethodology as a sociological perspective is discussed on pages 31–33.

Expressed emotion: the concept of expressed emotion was developed by Brown et al (1972) to describe the emotional atmosphere of the family of people with schizophrenia. More recently Gilhooly and Whittick (1989) have used the term to describe the number of critical comments made by family caregivers about their caring relationship with relatives with dementia.

Fact: an observed phenomenon – a thing, an event, a measurement.

Fact, social: not all facts about human behaviour are necessarily social facts; a *fact* is only social in so far as it exists externally to the individual and exercises constraint over him.

Family: perhaps the most loosely defined term in the sociologist's vocabulary. *Marriage*, parenthood and residence comprise the three central elements of the family. The important characteristic of these elements is that they are neither necessary nor sufficient parts of a definition but do, in various combinations, delineate a definition of the family.

Family, conjugal: used to define a social group consisting of a man and woman and their dependent offspring. The central element of the conjugal family is parenthood.

Family of marriage: a kinship term which refers to the kin grouping of ego, his or her spouse and their children.

Family of origin: a kinship term which refers to the kin grouping of ego, his or her parent(s) and sibling(s).

Frame: a term coined by Goffman to provide for the analysis of ongoing social actions proceeding within a socially constructed frame. This social framework permits actors to structure interactions, to negotiate, and to attribute meaning to their experience. When actors operate within mutually defined frames this is conducive to a high level of intersubjective communication. Goffman's use of frame is described on pages 149–151.

Function: in *functionalist theory*, the consequences of the existence or operation of a unit for other units in a social system are referred to as 'its function'.

Function, latent: in *functionalist theory*, a functional relation which is neither intended or recognised.

Function, manifest: in *functionalist theory*, a functional relation having a recognised value.

Functional alternatives: in *functionalist theory*, Merton identified the need to get away from the conservative tendency to argue that something is indispensable for the well-being of society. There are different and equally successful ways of providing for functions.

Functional autonomy: in *functionalist theory*, the degree to which the parts of a social system are self-sustaining and may survive independently of the system of which originally they were a part.

Functional uncertainty: when uncertainty is imputed into circumstances in which there is no real doubt, for social purposes, this is functional uncertainty.

Health field concept: draws on the *medical* and *social models* of health and illness. Health is attributable to four main elements: human biology, including those aspects of mental and physical health which are a direct consequence of the basic biology of the individual; environment, including all matters related to health which are external to the human body and over which the individual has little or no personal control; lifestyle, including those decisions made by individuals themselves, which have implications for their health; and health care organisation, which consists of the quantity, quality, arrangement, nature and relationships of people and resources in the provision of health care.

Ideal type: used by Weber to make explicit the procedure by which social scientists formulate general abstract concepts such as *bureaucracy* or *career*. Ideal types are thus hypothetical constructs formed by emphasising aspects of behaviour and institutions which are observable. 'Ideal' signifies 'pure' or 'abstract' rather than normative. The precise relationship between ideal types and their empirical referents remains obscure.

Ideology: a system of interdependent ideas (beliefs, traditions, principles and myths) held by a social group or society which reflects, rationalises and defends its particular social, moral, religious, political, or economic institutional interests or commitments.

Illness behaviour: coined by Mechanic to describe the social facts which influence the ways individuals view signs and symptoms, and the kinds of action engaged in to deal with them.

Impression management: a method of achieving *social mobility* through the manipulation of status symbols and personal attraction.

Indexicality: ethnomethodologists argue that all actions and utterances are indexical, that is, they depend for their meaning on the context in which they occur. This feature means that actors will normally make sense of action and utterances of others by referring to their context.

Induction: a process by which truth of a proposition is made more probable by accumulations of confirming evidence. It cannot ever be ultimately valid because there is always the possibility of unconfirming evidence.

Institution: widely used to describe social practices that are regularly and continuously repeated; are sanctioned and maintained by social *norms*; and which have a major significance in the social structure. The concept has been defined by Berger and Berger as 'a regulatory pattern which is programmed by society and imposed on the conduct of individuals.'

Institution, total: a place of confinement or partial confinement in which all aspects of life are conducted under the control of a single *bureaucratic authority*. Examples of total institutions are: prisons, hospitals, army camps and boarding schools.

Institutionalisation: the process whereby social practices become sufficiently regular and continuous to be described as *institutions*. This process also permits social practice to modify existing institutions. The term is sometimes used to describe the effects of an institution on social behaviour, so that individuals act out a narrow and repetitive range of behaviour.

Internalisation: this concept refers to the process by which an individual learns and accepts the social *values* and *norms* of conduct relevant to his or her social group or wider society.

Kinship: an anthropological term which describes the social relationships deriving from blood ties (real and supposed) and *marriage*. Kinship is a universal feature of societies and usually plays a significant role in the *socialisation* of individuals and in the maintenance of group solidarity. In complex societies, kinship normally forms a fairly small part of the totality of social relations which make up the social system.

Legitimacy: Weber uses the term in his analysis of power. Legitimacy means that people accept *authority* as just and that those endowed with authority are given it rightfully. Weber identified three ideological bases of legitimacy: traditional, charismatic and legal-rational, which may confer authority on power holders.

Life career: this concept may be referred to as the life cycle to describe the development of a person through childhood, adolescence, midlife, old age and death. However, this does not relate to biological maturation but to transitions through socially constructed categories of age, and to variations in social experience of ageing. The length and importance of these stages varies between cultures, and between men and women who have different social experiences during biological ageing.

Marriage: the relation of one or more men with one or more women which is recognised by custom or law and which involves certain rights and duties, both in the case of the parties entering the union and in the case of the children born of it.

Maternal deprivation: refers to the absence of a stable, continuous and affectionate relationship between a mother and child. In functional theory, it is suggested that the absence of such a relationship may lead to an increase in social pathology, such as mental illness or delinquency. This theory has important implications for women in society. It implies that women should remain at home to look after young children, a position which has been described as an ideology for keeping women out of the labour force.

Model, medical: the medical model of health assumes that improvements in the health of the population and the quality of health care are attributable to the art and science of medicine.

Model, social: the social model of health emphasises the social rather than the biological contexts in the aetiology of disease and illness and their treatment and care.

Negotiated order: in interactionist theory, a concept which regards social phenomena, particularly organisational arrangements, as emerging from ongoing processes of interaction between people. The interaction process involves constant negotiation and renegotiation of the terms of social action, stressing the fluidity and uncertainty of social arrangements.

Neonatal mortality rate: the proportion of deaths in the first 4 weeks of life.

Norm: norms are prescriptions serving as common guidelines for *social action*. Human behaviour exhibits certain regularities which are the product of adhering to common expectations or norms. In this sense, human action is 'rule governed'. A social norm is not necessarily actual behaviour and normative behaviour is not simply the most frequently occurring pattern. Since the term refers to social expectations about 'correct' or 'proper' behaviour, norms imply the presence of *legitimacy*, consent and prescription. Deviation from norms is punished by sanctions. Norms are acquired by *internalisation* and *socialisation*. The concept is central to theories of social order.

Normative: explanations or theories which assume that the *norms* and *values* of the sociologist hold true.

Organisation: a relatively stable pattern of social relationships of individuals and subgroups within a social system or social group, based upon systems of social roles, norms and shared meanings that provide regularity and predictability in social interaction. The term often refers to specific social groups, such as a factory, school or hospital.

Organisation, formal: a highly organised group having explicit objectives, formally stated rules and regulations, and a system of specifically defined roles, each with clearly designated rights and duties.

Organisation, informal: the system of personal relationships that develops spontaneously as individuals interact within a *formal organisation*.

Paradigm: a scientific *paradigm* refers to the shared agreement or shared assumptions of a community of scientists.

Perinatal mortality rate: the proportion of stillbirths and deaths in the first 4 weeks of life.

Power: the ability of an individual or group to carry out its wishes or policies, and to control, manipulate, or influence the behaviour of others, whether they wish to cooperate or not. The agent who possesses power has resources to force his will on others. These resources often stem from social relationships and the individual's position in a group or society. The terms power, authority and influence are sometimes defined as authority terms implying the ability of one person to change the behaviour of another. In this sense, power is widely diffused through society rather than being concentrated in a ruling elite.

Power, coercive: a type of *power* in which the holder of power can compel the actions of subordinate individuals or groups by the use or the threat of physical force. This can be acceptable to people if they believe it is administered by appropriate office-holders.

Power, expert: a type of *power* based on the subject's belief that the holder of power possesses superior knowledge and ability.

Power, legitimate: a type of *power* which is the result of an individual's position within a social system or social group. It stems from the *moral authority* of a particular position in the group.

Power, referent: a type of *power* which relates to the prestige of individuals and which, to some extent, relates to the *status* of a person in the social system or social group.

Power, reward: a type of *power* which derives from the exertion of influence by controlling rewards or resources valued by the subject.

Prevention: three types have been delineated – primary prevention involves taking measures in order to prevent disease or injury from occurring; secondary prevention refers to health care measures which are concerned with identifying and treating ill health; and tertiary prevention is concerned with mitigating the effects of illness and disease which have already occurred.

Profession: in *functionalist theory*, an occupation which may be identified by the following attributes – the use of skills based on theoretical knowledge; education and training in these skills; the competence of professionals ensured by examinations; a code of conduct to ensure professional integrity; performance of a service that is for the public good; and a professional association that organises members. These criteria can also be used to measure the degree to which occupations are professionalised.

Proletariat: in Marxist theory, the equivalent to the working class who, in capitalist society, are in conflict with the *bourgeoisie*.

Reflexivity: in *ethnomethodology*, this concept refers to the essential interdependence of the circumstances members attribute to social events and their descriptions or accounts of what the events themselves entail. When members take part in a social occasion they use the features of the occasion to make visible to others what is happening and also to make the features themselves come about.

Rites de passage: a term denoting public ceremonies celebrating the transition of an individual or group to a new *status*. Such rites are typically associated with transitions in the *life career*, marked by ceremonies like marriage or retirement parties.

Role: people occupying particular social positions behave in ways expected of that position rather than their own individual characteristics. Roles are the socially defined attributes and expectations associated with social positions.

Role conflict: exists when incompatible expectations are held. It can occur at two levels. (1) When an individual perceives a difference between how he thinks he should act out a particular *role* and how he perceives he actually acts out the role. Conflict also occurs when he perceives an incompatibility between performing certain prescriptions of one of his roles and carrying out those of another of his role. (2) At a group level conflict occurs when different actors perceive the same role in different ways.

Role making: in interactionist theory, role making is the process of creating and modifying expected behaviour in interaction. Rather than roles being fluid and indeterminate, role making produces consistent patterns of behaviour.

Role taking: in interactionist theory, roles are depicted as the outcome of a process of social interaction that is tentative and creative. Individuals imaginatively engage in role taking new roles and, in so doing, work out their own roles.

Role set: in functionalist theory, the term describes the array of roles and expectations that any individual will confront while taking a particular role.

Roles, multiple: describes the fact that most people are engaged in acting out various roles.

Self-fulfilling prophecy: a false *definition of the situation* or belief regarding a social situation which, because one believes it and one acts upon it, actually manifests itself as a truth, further strengthening the belief.

Sentimental order: in interactionist theory, interactions between individuals in social groups produce collective sentiments, which are not internal subjective feelings but overt observable signs of solidarity between individuals. The *sentimental order* is the level at which these signs are expressed at any one time in response to social circumstances influencing the group. Sentiments are an essential feature of social exchange.

Sick role: a concept originally formulated by Parsons in which illness is regarded as a form of social *deviance* and the ill individual adopts a specific *role*. The sick role is described on pages 145–146.

Social change: social change is so ubiquitous and varied in form that it has lost importance as a general concept. Its importance as a distinct area for sociological study has its roots in functionalism, where the object was to explain the causes and course of changes like the French political and English industrial revolutions, to reveal the 'laws of motion' of society. The theories of Marx and Weber attempted different explanations of large scale social evolution. Attention was subsequently turned to more detailed studies of smaller social units. There is general agreement that change is the normal condition of society everywhere though theoretical disputes as to the nature of change remain.

Social control: broadly indicates an aspect of sociology concerned with the maintenance of order and stability. There is broad agreement that this is achieved through a combination of compliance, coercion and commitment to social *values*. In contemporary sociology, the concept is primarily encountered in the analysis of *deviant behaviour* where it is an aspect of *labelling* theory. It is agreed that, paradoxically, attempts to increase coercive social control tends to amplify *deviance* rather than reduce it. The implication is that social control depends more on the stability of social groups, community relations and shared values than it does on mere coercion.

Social mobility: refers to the movement of individuals between different social strata, usually defined occupationally in Western societies. Unlike the situation in *caste* or estate, movement from one *status* to another can be achieved by means which are in the control of the person.

Social stratification: this key concept reflects sociologists' interest in the basic principles of social organisation. The concept refers to social differentiation which produced hierarchical ranks or strata. All members of society will belong to a strata. Within each strata all are equal, but strata are superior and inferior relative to each other and these differences are recognised and sanctioned. Different approaches to social stratification are described on pages 37–63.

Social structure: refers to the enduring, orderly and patterned relationships between elements of a society. Within sociology there is considerable debate about what these elements should be – people, *roles* or social institutions. Social structure is an abstract theoretical concept and therefore cannot be used as an explanation for any social phenomena.

Socialisation: used to describe the process by which people learn to conform to social *norms*, thus making possible an enduring society and the transmission of culture between generations. The process has been conceptualised in two ways. (1) Socialisation as the *internalisation* of social norms by a process which is self-imposed rather than imposed by means of external regulation. The norms are thus part of the individual's personality and he therefore feels a need to conform. (2) Socialisation may be conceived as an essential element of social interaction on the assumption that people want to enhance their self-image by gaining acceptance and status in the eyes of others. Individuals therefore become socialised as they guide their own actions to accord with the expectations of others.

Socialisation, anticipatory: the internalisation of the rights, obligations and expectations of a social *role* preparatory to assuming it.

Sociology, naturalistic: an approach to sociology which questions the assumption that our social surroundings can be subjected to 'scientific' laws, as are our physical surroundings. The approach emphasises the distinction between *action* and *behaviour* and the importance of seeing and understanding from the actor's point of view. The approach is theoretical rather than empirical, and has a different approach to method than that employed in studying the natural sciences.

Sociology, scientistic: an approach to sociology which is grounded in the belief that the logic and methods used in studying natural sciences should be employed also in sociological studies. The approach is empirical rather than theoretical.

Standard mortality ratio: the number of deaths, either total or cause specific, in a given occupational group expressed as a percentage of the number of deaths that would have been expected in that occupational group, if the age-and-sex-specific rates in the general population had obtained.

Status: used in two ways in sociology. (1) Status describes the position in a social system as in 'child' or 'grandparent'. Status refers to what the person is whereas the related concept *role* refers to the behaviour expected of people occupying a status. (2) Status is used as a synonym for prestige, when social status denotes a position in a publicly recognised hierarchy of social worth. Weber's use of the term status group is described on page 40.

Status passage: in *symbolic interactionism*, used to describe the process of changing from one status to another. Glaser and Strauss, in attempting to create a formal theory, suggested that properties which would have to be considered in such a change include whether or not the transition is regularised, scheduled, prescribed – desirable, reversible, collective, voluntary, legitimate or disguised.

Stigma: in *labelling theory*, refers to a relationship of devaluation in which one individual is disqualified from full social acceptance. Stigma is a social attribute which is discrediting for an individual or group. It can be physical (a blemish), documentary (a prison sentence) or contextual (bad company), as well as ascribed or achieved. Its sociological significance lies in the analyses of information management, *deviance* and mechanisms of *social control*.

Subculture: describes the system of *values*, *attitudes*, modes of behaviour and lifestyles of a social group which is distinct from, but related, to the dominant *culture* of a society. While there is a great diversity of subcultures in modern society, the concept has been most used in the study of *ethnic groups*, youth and *deviance*.

Symbolic interactionism: a major sociological perspective deriving from the study of the self-society relationship as a process of symbolic communications between social actors. This perspective is described on pages 28–32.

Theory: used loosely in social science and may mean no more than a set of assumptions, *concepts* or relatively abstract inquiry distinguished from empirical research or practical recommendations. More fully developed, a theory is a set of interrelated principles and definitions that serves conceptually to organise selected aspects of the empirical world in a systematic way. The foundation of a theory consists of a set of basic assumptions and axioms from which are derived logically interrelated and empirically verifiable propositions. Although usage varies, the propositions that comprise a theory may be regarded as scientific laws if they have been sufficiently verified to be widely accepted, or as hypotheses if they have still to achieve verification. In either case, the propositions which comprise a theory are constantly subject to further empirical testing and revision. Through the process of *deduction*, a theory provides specific hypotheses for research and, through *induction*, research data provide generalisations to be incorporated into and modify theory. The essence of theory is that it attempts to explain a wide variety of empirical phenomena in a parsimonious way.

Theory, action: an analysis of *action* which begins with the individual actor. It proceeds in terms of individual actors in typical situations by identifying actors' goals, expectations and *values*; the means of achieving these goals; actors' interpretation of the situation and other elements. Action theory as applied to the analysis of organisations is described on pages 122–123

Theory, functionalist: a major sociological perspective which emphasises the interdependence of various elements of societies. Functionalism accounts for a social activity by referring to its consequences for the operation of some other social activity, institution, or society as a whole. Functionalism is described on pages 18–22.

Theory, labelling: this theoretical perspective considers sociological explanations of deviance which treats deviance, not as a product of individual psychology or genetic constitutions but of *social control*. Two important aspects of labelling theory are *primary deviance* and *secondary deviance*. Labelling theory is discussed on pages 135–137.

Theory, middle-range: coined by Merton, who regarded useful sociological theory as lying between minor working hypotheses and major conceptual schemas.

Theory, systems: in organisational theory, a *functionalist* perspective which emphasises explanations of behaviour in terms of the interaction of systems attempting to satisfy their organisational goals.

Trajectory: refers to the curve described for an object moving under the action of given forces. In sociology, it is used to describe the course and timescale of events associated with phenomena like dying and pain.

Typification: a major concept in phenomenological sociology, used to denote that the great bulk of all knowledge in our life world is typified, that is, it refers not to the individual or unique qualities of things or persons but to their typical features. Typification is the process by which people typify the world about them.

Values: ideas that people hold to be right or wrong. In *functionalist theory*, values are accepted as statements to which each group member assents and is committed, and which provide a standard for judging specific acts and goals.

REFERENCES

Abel-Smith B 1960 A history of the nursing profession. Heinemann, London

Abrams P 1978 Community care: some research problems and priorities. Social Care Research, London, p 78–99

Abrams P S, Abrams R, Humphrey R, Snaith R 1989 Neighbourhood care and social policy. HMSO, London

Alaszewski A 1977 Doctors and paramedical workers: the changing pattern of interprofessional relations. Centre 8 Paper. Health and Social Services Journal B1–B4

Alexander J C 1985 Neofunctionalism. Sage, London

Allan J L, Townley R R W, Phelan P D 1974 Family response to cystic fibrosis. Australian Paediatric Journal 10: 136–146

Altschul A 1972 Patient nurse interaction: a study of interaction patterns in acute psychiatric wards. Churchill Livingstone, Edinburgh

Anderson R 1988 The quality of life of stroke patients and their carers. In: Anderson R, Bury M (eds) Living with chronic illness: the experience of patients and their families. Unwin Hyman, London, p 14–42

Anderson R 1992 The aftermath of stroke: the experience of patients and their families. Cambridge University Press, Cambridge

Anderson R, Bury M 1988 Living with chronic illness: the experience of patients and their families. Unwin Hyman, London

Antonovsky A 1979 Health, stress, and coping. Jossey-Bass, San Francisco

Antonovsky A 1987 Unraveling the mystery of health: how people manage stress and stay well. Jossey-Bass, San Francisco

Armitage P 1983 Joint working in primary health care. Nursing Times, Occasional Paper 79: 75–78

Armitage S K 1981 Negotiating the discharge of medical patients. Journal of Advanced Nursing 6: 385–389

Armstrong D 1976 The decline of the medical hegemony: a review of government reports during the NHS. Social Science and Medicine 10: 157–163

Armstrong D 1982 The doctor-patient relationship 1930–80. In: Wright P, Treacher A (eds) The problem of medical knowledge: examining the social construction of medicine. Edinburgh University Press, Edinburgh, p 109–122

Armstrong D 1983 The fabrication of nurse-patient relationships. Social Science and Medicine 17: 457–460

Ashburner L, Cairncross L 1992 Just trust us. Health Service Journal 14 May: 20–22

Ashworth P 1980 Care to communicate: an investigation into problems of communication between patients and nurses in intensive therapy units. Royal College of Nursing, London

Atkinson J M 1977 Coroners and the categorisation of deaths as suicides: changes in perspective as features of the research process. In: Bell C, Newby H (eds) Doing Sociological Research. Allen & Unwin, London, p 31–46

Atkinson J M 1978 Discovering suicide: studies in the social organisation of sudden death. Macmillan, London

Atkinson J M, Drew P 1979 Order in court: the organisation of verbal interaction in judicial settings. Macmillan, London

Averill JR 1968 Grief: its nature and significance. Psychological Bulletin 70: 721–748

Backer B A, Hannon M, Russell N A 1982 Death and dying: individuals and institutes. John Wiley & Sons, New York

Backett K C 1990 Studying health in families: A qualitative approach. In: Cunningham-Burley S, McKeganey N P (eds) Readings in medical sociology. Routledge & Kegan Paul, London, p 57–84

Baer H A 1981 The organisational rejuvenation of osteopathy: a reflection of the decline of professional dominance in medicine. Social Science and Medicine 15A, 5: 701–711

Baker D 1983 'Care' in the geriatric ward: an account of two styles of nursing. In: Wilson-Barnett J (ed) Nursing research: ten studies in patient care. John Wiley & Sons, Chichester, p 101–117

Balint M 1956 The doctor, his patient and the illness. Pitman, London

Baly M 1987 Florence Nightingale and the nursing legacy. Croom Helm, London

Baxter J 1988 Gender and class analysis: the position of women in the class structure. Australian and New Zealand Journal of Sociology 24: 106–123

Bayley M 1973 Mental handicap and community care: a study of mentally handicapped people in Sheffield. Routledge & Kegan Paul, London

Beardshaw V, Robinson R 1990 New for old? Prospects for nursing in the 1990s. King's Fund Institute, London

Becker H 1952 Social class variations in the teacher-pupil relationship. Journal of Educational Sociology 25: 451–465

Becker H S 1967 History, culture and subjective experience: an exploration of the social basis of drug induced experiences. Journal of Health and Social Behaviour 8: 163–176

Becker H S 1971 The nature of a profession. In: Becker H S (ed) Sociological work. Aldine, Chicago

Becker H S, Geer B, Hughes E C, Strauss A L 1961 Boys in white: student culture in medical school. University of Chicago Press, Chicago

Beech B A, Claxton R 1980 Health rights handbook for maternity care. Association for Improvements in the Maternity Services and The Birth Centre, London

Bell C, Newby H 1971 Community studies: an introduction to the sociology of the local community. George Allen & Unwin, London

Bell C, Newby H 1977 Doing sociological research. Allen & Unwin, London

Benner P, Wrubel J 1988 The primacy of caring. Addison-Wesley, Menlo Park

Benoliel J Q 1978 The changing social context for life and death decisions. Essence 2: 5–14

Benton T 1977 Philosophical foundations of the three sociologies. Routledge & Kegan Paul, London

Berger B, Berger P L 1983 The war over the family: capturing the middle ground. Hutchinson, London

Berger P L 1966 Invitation to sociology: a humanistic perspective. Penguin, Harmondsworth

Berger P L, Berger B 1976 Sociology: a biographical approach. Penguin, Harmondsworth

Birch J 1975 To nurse or not to nurse: an investigation into the causes of withdrawal during nurse training. Royal College of Nursing, London

Blackburn A M 1989 Problems of terminal care in elderly patients. Palliative Medicine 3: 203–206

Blaxter M 1983 The causes of disease: women talking. Social Science and Medicine 17: 59–69

Blaxter M 1984 Equity and consultation rates in general practice. British Medical Journal 288: 1963–1967

Blaxter M 1990 Health and lifestyles. Routledge & Kegan Paul, London

Blaxter M, Paterson E 1982 Mothers and daughters: a three generational study of health attitudes and behaviour. Heinemann, London

Bloch M, Parry J 1982 Death and the regeneration of life. Cambridge University Press, Cambridge

Bloor M 1976 Professional autonomy and client exclusion: a study in ENT clinics. In: Wadsworth M, Robinson D (eds) Studies in everyday medical life. Martin Robertson, London, p 52–68

Bloor M, Samphier M, Prior L 1987 Artefact explanations of inequalities in health: an assessment of the evidence. Sociology of Health & Illness 9: 231–264

Blumer H 1969 Symbolic interactionism perspective and method. Prentice-Hall, Cliffs, New Jersey

Bond J 1992 The politics of caregiving: the professionalisation of informal support. Ageing and Society 12: 5–21

Bond J, Bond S, Donaldson C, Gregson B, Atkinson A 1989a Evaluation of an innovation in the continuing care of very frail elderly people. Ageing and Society 9: 347–381

Bond J, Cartlidge A M, Gregson B A, Barton A G, Philips P R, Armitage P, Brown AM , Reedy B L E C 1987 Interprofessional collaboration in primary health care. Journal of the Royal College of General Practitioners 37: 158–161

Bond J, Gregson B A, Atkinson A 1989b Measurement of outcomes within a multicentred randomised controlled trial in the evaluation of the experimental NHS nursing homes. Age and Ageing 18: 292–302

Bond S 1978 Processes of communication about cancer in a radiotherapy department. Unpublished PhD thesis, University of Edinburgh

Bond S 1983 Nurses' communication with cancer patients. In: Wilson-Barnett J (ed) Nursing research: ten studies in patient care. John Wiley & Sons, Chichester

Bond S, Bond J 1993 Evaluation of continuing care accommodation: an overview of the nursing staff survey. Report 60. Centre for Health Services Research, University of Newcastle

Bond S, Bond J, Fowler P, Fall M 1991 Evaluating primary nursing, Part II. Nursing Standard 5: 37–39

Bond S, Bond J, Fowler P, Fall M 1991 Evaluating primary nursing, Part III. Nursing Standard 5: 36–39

Bond S, Bond J, Fowler P, Fall M 1991 Evaluating primary nursing, Part I. Nursing Standard 5: 35–39

Booth C 1892 Pauperism: a picture and the endowment of old age, an argument. Macmillan, London

Booth C 1894 The aged poor in England and Wales: condition. Macmillan, London

Booth T 1985 Home truths: old people's homes and the outcome of care. Gower, Aldershot

Booth T, Simons K, Booth W 1990 Outward bound: relocation and community care for people with learning difficulties. Open University Press, Milton Keynes

Bott E 1971 Family and social network, 2nd edn. Tavistock, London

Bottomore T B, Rubel M 1965 Karl Marx: selected writings in sociology and social philosophy. Penguin, Harmondsworth

Bowlby J 1971 Attachment and loss, Vol. 1. Attachment. Penguin, Harmondsworth

Bowling A 1992 Measuring health: a review of quality of life measurement scales. Open University Press, Milton Keynes

Bowling A, Cartwright A 1982 Life after a death: a study of the elderly widowed. Tavistock, London

Boyce W T 1985 Social support, family relations and children. In: Cohen S, Syme S,L. (eds) Social support and health. Academic Press, Orlando, Florida

Brannen J, Moss P 1991 Managing mothers. Unwin Hyman, London

Braverman H 1974 Labour and monopoly capital: the degredation of work in the twentieth Century. Monthly Review Press, New York

Brechling B G, Kuhn D 1989 A specialised hospice for dementia patients and their families. Journal of Hospice Care May/June: 27–30

British Medical Association 1977 Royal Commission on the National Health Service. Report of Counsel to the Special Representative Meeting, London, 9th March 1977. Submission of evidence. British Medical Journal 1: 299–334

Brocklehurst J C, Morris P, Andrews K, Richards B, Laycock P 1981 Social effects of stroke. Social Science and Medicine 15A: 35–39

Brooking J 1986 Patient and family participation in nursing care: the development of a nursing process measuring scale. King's College (PhD thesis), London

Brotherston Sir J 1976 The Galton Lecture: 1975. Inequality: is it inevitable? In: Carter C O, Peel J (eds) Equalities and inequalities in health. Academic Press, London

Brown A, Kiernan K 1981 Cohabitation in Great Britain: evidence from the General Household Survey. Population Trends 25: 4–10

Brown G W, Andrews B, Harris T, Adler Z, Bridge L 1986 Social support, self-esteem and depression. Psychologica Medicine 16: 813–831

Brown G W, Birley J L T, Wing J K 1972 Influence of family life on the course of schizophrenic disorders: a replication. British Journal of Psychiatry 121: 241–258

Brown G W, Harris T 1978 Social origins of depression: a study of psychiatric disorder in women. Tavistock, London

Brown G W, Harris T O 1989 Life Events and illness. The Guildford Press, London

Brown G W, Prudo R 1981 Psychiatric disorder in a rural and an urban population: aetiology of depression. Psychological Medicine 11: 581–599

Buchan I C, Richardson I M 1973 Time study of consultations in general practice. Scottish Health Service Study No. 27. Scottish Home and Health Department, Edinburgh

Bucher R, Stelling J 1969 Characteristics of professional organisations. Journal of Health and Social Behaviour 10: 3–15

Bucher R, Stelling J G 1977 Becoming professional. Sage, Beverly Hills

Bucher R, Strauss A 1961 Professions in process. American Journal of Sociology 66: 325–334

Buck M 1963 The language disorders. Journal of Rehabilitation xxix: 37–38

Buckenham J, McGrath G 1983. In: The social reality of nursing. ADIS Health Science Press, Balgowlah, Australia

Bulmer M 1979 Concepts in the analysis of qualitative data. Sociological Review 27: 651–677

Burgess R G 1990 Reflections on field experience. JAI Press, London

Burkitt D P, Trowell H C 1975 Refined carbohydrate foods and disease: some implications of dietary fibre. Academic Press, London

Bynner J M 1969 The young smoker: a study of smoking among schoolboys carried out for the Ministry of Health. Government Social Survey No. SS 383. HMSO, London

Bynner J, Stribley K M 1979 Social research: principles and procedures. Longman & Open University Press, London

Cain M, Finch J 1981 The rehabilitation of data. In: Abrams P, Deem R, Finch J, Rock P (eds) Practice and progess: British sociology 1950–1980. Allen & Unwin, London

Calnan M 1982 Non-governmental approaches to the control of cancer. In: Alderson M (ed) The prevention of cancer. Edward Arnold, London, p 210–226

Calnan M 1987 Health and illness: the lay perspective. Tavistock, London

Calnan M 1990 Food and health: a comparison of beliefs and practices in middle-class and working-class households. In: Cunningham-Burley S, McKeganey N,P. (eds) Readings in medical sociology. Routledge & Kegan Paul, London, p 9–36

Campbell E A, Cope S J, Teasdale J D 1983 Social factors and affective disorder: an investigation of Brown and Harris's model. British Journal of Psychiatry 143: 548–553

Carpenter M 1977 The new managerialism and professionalism in nursing. In: Stacey M, Reid M, Heath C, Dingwall R (eds) Health and the division of labour. Croom Helm, London, p 165–193

Carpenter M 1978 Managerialism and the division of labour in nursing. In: Dingwall R, McIntosh J (eds) Readings in the sociology of nursing. Churchill Livingstone, Edinburgh, p 87–103

Carpenter M 1980 Asylum nursing before 1914: a chapter on the history of labour. In: Davies C (ed) Rewriting nursing history. Croom Helm, London

Carson R 1963 Silent spring. Hamish Hamilton, London

Carstairs V, Patterson P E 1966 Distribution of hospital patients by social class. Health Bulletin XXIV: 59–65

Cartwright A 1967 Patients and their doctors: a study of general practice. Routledge & Kegan Paul, London

Cartwright A 1970 Parents and family planning services. Routledge & Kegan Paul, London

Cartwright A 1991a Changes in life and care in the year before death 1969–1987. Journal of Public Health Medicine 13: 81–87

Cartwright A 1991b The role of hospitals in caring for people in the last year of their lives. Age and Ageing 20: 271–274

Cartwright A 1991c The role of residential and nursing homes in the last year of people's lives. British Journal of Social Work 21: 627–645

Cartwright A, Anderson R 1979 Patients and their doctors 1977. Journal of the Royal College of General Practitioners, Occasional Paper 8. Journal of the Royal College of General Practitioners, London

Cartwright A, Hockey L, Anderson J 1973 Life before death. Routledge & Kegan Paul, London

Cartwright A, O'Brien M 1976 Social class variations in health care and in the nature of general practitioner consultations. In: Stacey M (ed) The sociology of the National Health Service. Sociological Review Monograph No. 22. University of Keele, p 77–98

Cartwright A, Seale C 1990 The natural history of a survey: an account of the methodological issues encountered in a study of life before death. King Edward's Hospital Fund for London, London

Caudhill W A 1958 The psychiatric hospital as a small society. Harvard University Press, Cambridge, Mass

Central Health Services Council 1959 The welfare of children in hospital. Report of the Committee. HMSO, London

Central Statistical Office 1992 Social Trends 22. HMSO, London

Challis D J 1981 The measurement of outcome in social care of the elderly. Journal of Social Policy 10: 179–208

Challis D, Davies B 1986 Case management in community care. Gower, Aldershot

Chamberlain G 1980 The pre-pregnancy clinic. British Medical Journal 281: 29–30

Charles N, Kerr M 1985 Attitudes towards the feeding and nutrition of young children. Health Eduction Council, London

Charlesworth A, Wilkin D, Durie A 1984 Carers and services: a comparison of men and women caring for dependent elderly people. Equal Opportunities, Manchester

Charlton J, Kelly S, Dunnell K, Evans B, Jenkins R, Wallis R 1992 Trends in suicide deaths in England and Wales. Population Trends 69: 10–16

Charlton J, Kelly S, Dunnell K, Evans B, Jenkins R 1993 Suicide deaths in England and Wales: trends in factors associated with suicide deaths. Population Trends 71: 34–42

Chen E, Cobb S 1960 Family structure in relation to health and disease: a review of the literature. Journal of Chronic Diseases 12: 544–567

Chiang B N, Perlman L V, Epstein F H 1969 Over-weight and hypertension: a review. Circulation 39: 403–421

Chiplin B, Sloane P.J. 1982 Tackling discrimination in the workplace: an analysis of sex discrimination in Britain. Cambridge University Press, Cambridge

Chua W F, Clegg S 1989 Contradictory couplings: professional ideology in the organisational locales of nurse training. Journal of Management Studies 26: 103–127

Chua W F, Clegg S 1990 Professional closure: the case of British nursing. Theory and Society 19: 135–172

Cicourel A V 1964 Method and measurement in sociology. Free Press, New York

Clark J M 1983 Nurse-patient communication – an analysis of conversations from surgical wards. In: Wilson-Barnett J (ed) Nursing research: ten studies in patient care. Wiley, Chichester, p 25–56

Clarke M 1978 Getting through work. In: Dingwall R, McIntosh J (eds) Readings in the sociology of nursing. Churchill Livingstone, Edinburgh, p 67–86

Clay T 1987 Nurses: Power and politics. Heinemann, London

Cole S K 1984 Personal communication

Colledge M 1982 Economic cycles and health: towards a sociological understanding of the impact of the recession on health and illness. Social Science and Medicine 16: 1919–1927

Comaroff J, Maguire P 1981 Ambiguity and the search for meaning: childhood leukaemia in the modern clinical context. Social Science and Medicine 15B: 115–123

Commission on Racial Equality 1987 Ethnic origins of nurses applying for training: a survey. CRE, London

Commission on Racial Equality 1988 South Manchester District Health Authority: a report of a formal investigation. CRE, London

Commission on Racial Equality 1992 Clinical nurse grading: the costs of a 'colour blind' approach. CRE, London

Cook T D 1985 Postpositivist critical multiplism. In: Shotland L, Mark M.M. (eds) Social science and social policy. Sage, Beverly Hills, CA, p 21–62

Copp LA 1974 The spectrum of suffering. American Journal of Nursing 74: 491–495

Cornwell J 1984 Hard-earned lives: accounts of health and illness from East London. Tavistock, London

Cowie B 1976 The cardiac patient's perception of his heart attack. Social Science and Medicine 10: 87–96

Crawford M P 1973 Retirement – a rite-de-passage. Sociological Review 21: 447–461

Crombie D L 1984 Social class and health status: inequality or difference. Journal of the Royal College of General Practitioners, Occasional Paper 25. Journal of the Royal College of General Practitioners, London

Cuff E C, Payne C G F 1979 Perspectives in sociology. Allen & Unwin, London

Cuff E C, Sharrock W W, Francis D W 1990 Perspectives in sociology, 3rd edn. Unwin Hyman, London

Cumming E, Henry W E 1961 Growing old: the process of disengagement. Basic Books, New York

Davey Smith G, Bartley M, Blane D 1990 The Black Report on socioeconomic inequalities in health ten years on. British Medical Journal 301: 373–377

Davies C 1976 Experience of dependency and control of work: the case of nurses. Journal of Advanced Nursing 1: 273–282

Davies C 1977 Continuities in the development of hospital nursing in Britain. Journal of Advanced Nursing 1,2,: 479–493

Davies C 1980 Rewriting nursing history. Croom Helm, London

Davies C 1983 Professionals in bureaucracies: the conflict thesis revisited. In: Dingwall R, Lewis P (eds) The sociology of the professions: lawyers, doctors and others. Macmillan, London, p 177–194

Davies C, Rosser J 1985 Equal opportunities for women in the NHS. Report on an ESRC/DHSS project grant no. RDB/1/19/2. University of Warwick, Coventry

Davies C, Rosser J 1986 Processes of discrimination: a study of women working in the NHS. HMSO, London

Davis A, Strong P 1976 The management of a therapeutic encounter. In: Wadsworth M, Robinson D (eds) Studies in everyday medical life. Martin Robertson, London, p 123–137

Davis F 1963 Passage through crisis: polio victims and their families. Bobs-Merrill, New York

Davis F 1975 Professional socialisation as subjective experience: the process of doctrinal conversion among student nurses. In: Cox C, Mead A (eds) A sociology of medical practice. Collier-Macmillan, London, p 116–131

Davis K, Moore W E 1945 Some principles of stratification. American Sociological Review X: 242–249

Davitz L J, Davitz J R 1981 Nurses' response to patient's suffering. Springer, New York

Day P, Klein R 1983 Two views of the Griffiths Report. British Medical Journal 287: 1813–1816

Day R, Day J V 1977 A review of the current state of negotiated order theory: an appreciation and a critique. In: Benson J,K (ed) Organisational analysis: critique and innovation. Sage Publications, London, p 128–144

De Swann A 1990 Affect management in a cancer ward. In: The management of normality. Routledge & Kegan Paul, London, p 31–56

De Vries R G 1981 Birth and death: social construction at the poles of existence. Social Forces 59: 1074–1093

Department of Health 1991 The patient's charter. HMSO, London

Department of Health 1992 Women in the NHS: an implementation guide to opportunity 2000. (EL92) 14. HMSO, London

Department of Health and Social Security 1972 Management arrangements for the reorganised National Health Service. HMSO, London

Department of Health and Social Security 1980 Working group on inequalities in health. DHSS, London

Department of Health and Social Security 1982 Ageing in the United Kingdom. DHSS, London

Department of Health and Social Security 1983 Report of the NHS management inquiry. (The Griffith's Report, DA (83) 38). HMSO, London

Department of Health and Social Security 1986 Community nursing review. Neighbourhood nursing—a focus for care. HMSO, London

Department of Health and Social Security 1987 The role and preparation of support workers to nurses, midwives and health Visitors and the implications for manpower and service planning. HMSO, London

Department of Health and Social Security 1988 Review Body for nursing staff, midwives, health visitors and the professions allied to medicine. Fifth report on nursing staff, midwives and health visitors. (Chairman, Sir James Cleminson), Cmnd 360. HMSO, London

Dex S 1985 The sexual division of work: conceptual revolutions in the social sciences. St. Martin's Press, New York

Dick-Read G 1958 Childbirth without fear: the principles and practices of natural childbirth. Heinemann, London

Dingwall R 1976 Aspects of illness. Martin Robertson, London

Dingwall R 1977 The social organisation of health visitor training. Croom Helm, London

Dingwall R 1980 Problems of teamwork in primary care. In: Lonsdale S, Webb A, Briggs T L (eds) Teamwork in the personal social services and health care. Croom Helm, London, p 111–137

Dingwall R, Murray T 1983 Categorisation in accident departments: 'good' patients, 'bad' patients and children. Sociology of Health and Illness 5: 127–148

Dingwall R, Rafferty A M, Webster C 1988 An introduction to the social history of nursing. Routledge & Kegan Paul, London

Dopson L 1990 Nursing without nurses. Nursing Times 86, 14: 46–48

Dorpatt T L, Jackson J L, Ripley S H 1965 Broken homes and attempted suicide. Archives of General Psychiatry 12: 213–216

Douglas J D 1967 The social meaning of suicide. Princeton University Press, Princeton

Douglas J D 1976 Understanding everyday life. In: Douglas JD (ed) Understanding everyday life: toward the reconstruction of sociological knowledge. Routledge & Kegan Paul, London, p 3–44

Douglas M, Nicod M 1974 Taking the biscuit: the structure of British meals. New Society 30: 744–747

Doyal L 1985 Women and the National Health Service: the carers and the careless. In: Lewin E, Olesen V (eds) Women, health and healing: toward a new perspective. Tavistock, London, p 236–269

Doyal L, Hunt G, Mellor J 1981 Your life in their hands: migrant workers in the National Health Service. Critical Social Policy 2: 54–71

Doyal L, Pennell I 1979 The political economy of health. Pluto Press, London

Doyle D 1980 Domiciliary terminal care. The Practitioner 224: 575–582

Du Bois B 1983 Passionate scholarship: notes on values, knowing and method in feminist social science. In: Bowles G, Duelli Klein R (eds) Theories of women's studies. Routledge & Kegan Paul, London

Duff R S, Hollingshead A B 1968 Sickness and society. Harper & Row, New York

Dunham H W, Faris R E C 1965 Mental disorders in urban areas. University of Chicago Press, Chicago

Dunnell K, Cartwright A 1972 Medicine takers, prescribers and hoarders. Routledge & Kegan Paul, London

Durkheim E 1915 The elementary forms of the religious life. George Allen & Unwin Ltd, London

Durkheim E 1952 Suicide. Routledge & Kegan Paul, London

Durkheim E 1964a The division of labour in society. Free Press, New York

Durkheim E 1964b Rules of sociological method. Free Press, New York

Eddie S, Davies J A 1985 The effect of social class on attendance frequency and dental treatment received in the General Dental Service in Scotland. British Dental Journal 159: 370–372

Edwards R B 1984 Pain and the ethics of pain management. Social Science and Medicine 18: 515–523

Eichler M 1988 Non-sexist research methods: a practical guide. Allen & Unwin, Boston

Elias N 1985 The loneliness of the dying. Blackwell, Oxford

Elkin F 1960 The child and society: the process of socialisation. Random House, New York

Ellis R 1980 Social skills training for the interpersonal professions. In: Singleton W, Spurgeon P, Stammers R (eds) The analysis of social skill. Plenum Press, New York

Ellis R 1988 Competence in the caring professions. In: Ellis R (ed) Professional competence and quality assurance in the caring professions. Chapman & Hall, London, p 43–57

Engel G 1961 Is grief a disease? Psychosomatic Medicine 23: 18–22

Equal Opportunities Commission 1991 Equality management: women's employment in the NHS. Equal Opportunities Commission, London

Ettinger R C W 1965 The prospect of immortality. Scientific Book Club, London

Etzioni A 1969 The semi-professions and their organisation. The Free Press, New York

Evans-Pritchard E 1950 Witchcraft, oracles and magic among the Azande. Oxford University Press, Oxford

Evers H K 1981 Tender loving care? Patients and nurses in geriatric wards. In: Copp L A (ed) Care of the ageing. Churchill Livingstone, Edinburgh, p 46–74

Fagerhaugh SY, Strauss A 1977 Politics of pain management: staff-patient interaction. Addison-Wesley, California

Fairhurst E 1981 What do you do? Multiple realities in occupational therapy and rehabilitation. In: Atkinson P, Heath C (eds) Medical work: realities and routines. Gower, Farnborough, p 171–187

Faulkner A 1980 Communication and the nurse. Nursing Times Occasional Papers 21 (76): 93–95

Feyerabend P 1975 Against method: outline of an anarchistic theory of knowledge. New Left Editions, London

Field D 1989 Nursing the dying. Tavistock/Routledge & Kegan Paul, London

Field D, Clarke B A, Goldie N 1982 Medical sociology in Britain: register of research and teaching, 4th edn. British Sociological Association Medical Sociology Group, London

Field D, Woodman D 1990 Medical sociology in Britain: a register of research and teaching, 6th edn. British Sociological Association, Medical Sociology Group, London

Finch J 1989 Family obligations and social change. Polity Press, Cambridge

Finch J, Groves D 1980 Community care and the family: a case for equal opportunities. Journal of Social Policy 9: 487–511

Finch J, Mason J 1990 Filial obligations and kin support for elderly people. Ageing and Society 10: 151–175

Fisher M J Y, Calvert E J, Mychalkin W 1983 Patterns of attendance at developmental assessment clinics. Journal of the Royal College of General Practitioners 33: 213–218

Fitton F, Acheson H W K 1979 The doctor-patient relationship in general practice. HMSO, London

Ford P, Walsh M 1990 Nursing: rituals, research and rational actions. Scutari, London

Forster D P 1976 Social class differences in sickness and general practitioner consultations. Health Trends 8: 29–32

Forster M 1989 Have the men had enough? Penguin, Harmondsworth

Foster K, Wilmot A, Dobbs J 1990 General household survey 1988. HMSO, London

Foucault M 1973 The birth of the clinic. Tavistock, London

Foucault M 1979 The history of sexuality, Vol. 1. Translated by R. Hurley. Allen Lane, London

Foucault M 1980 Power and knowledge. In: Gordon C (ed) Selected interviews and other writings 1972–1977. The Harvester Press, London

Fowler R C, Rich C L, Young D 1986 San Diego suicide study. II: Substance abuse in young cases. Archives of General Psychiatry 43: 962–965

Fox A J, Goldblatt P O, Jones D R 1985 Social class mortality differentials: artefact, selection or life circumstances? Journal of Epidemiology and Community Health 39: 1–8

Fox J 1989 Health inequalities in European countries. Gower, Aldershot

Fox J, Goldblatt P 1982 Longitudinal study: socio-demographic mortality differentials. HMSO, London

Freidson E 1970 Professional dominance. Atherton, New York

Freidson E 1975 Profession of medicine: study of the sociology of applied knowledge. Dodd, Mead & Co, New York

Freidson E 1983 The theory of professions: state of the art. In: Dingwall R, Lewis P (eds) The sociology of the professions. Lawyers, doctors and others. Macmillan, London, p 19–37

French J R P, Raven B 1968 The bases of social power. In: Cartwright D, Zander A (eds) Group dynamics: research and theory. Harper & Row, New York, 3rd edn., p 259–269

Froggatt P 1989 Determinants of policy on smoking and health. International Journal of Epidemiology 18: 1–9

Gamarnikow E 1978 Sexual division of labour: the case of nursing. In: Kuhn A, Wolpe A,M. (eds) Feminism and materialism: women and modes of production. Routledge & Kegan Paul, London, p 96–123

Garcia J 1982 Women's views on antenatal care. In: Enkin M, Chalmers I (eds) Effectiveness and satisfaction in antenatal care. Heinemann, London

Garfinkel H 1967a Studies in ethnomethodology. Prentice Hall, Englewood Cliffs, NJ

Garfinkel H 1967b Practical sociological reasoning: some features in the work of the Los Angeles Suicide Prevention Centre. In: Shneidman E S (ed) Essays in self-destruction. Science Home, New York, p 171–187

Gaze H 1987 Man appeal: men in nursing. Nursing Times 83, 20: 24–29

Gelsthorpe L 1992 Response to Martyn Hammersley's paper 'On feminist methodology'. Sociology 26: 213–218

Gerth H H, Mills C W 1948 From Max Weber: essays in sociology. Routledge & Kegan Paul, London

Gibbs J P, Martin W T 1964 Status integration and suicide. Oregon University Press, Evgene, Oregon

Giddens A 1973 The class structure of the advanced societies. Hutchinson, London

Giddens A 1976 New rules of sociological method: a positive critique of interpretative sociologies. Hutchinson, London

Giddens A 1989 Sociology. Polity Press, Cambridge

Gilhooley M L M, Berkeley J, McCann K, Gibling F, Murray K 1988 Truth telling with dying cancer patients. Palliative Medicine 2: 64–71

Gilhooly M L M, Whittick J E 1989 Expressed emotion in caregivers of the dementing elderly. British Journal of Medical Psychology 62: 265–272

Gilroy P 1987 There ain't no blacks in the Union Jack: the cultural policies of race and nation. Hutchinson, London

Glaser B G, Strauss A L 1965 Awareness of dying. Aldine, Chicago

Glaser B G, Strauss A L 1967 The discovery of grounded theory: strategies for qualitative research. Aldine, New York

Glaser B G, Strauss A L 1968 Time for dying. Aldine, Chicago

Glass D V 1954 Social mobility in Britain. Routledge & Kegan Paul, London

Godlove C, Dunn G, Wright H 1980 Caring for old people in New York and London: the 'nurses' aide' interviews. Journal of the Royal Society of Medicine 73: 713–723

Goffman E 1961 Asylum: essays on the social situation of mental patients and other inmates. Anchor Books, New York

Goffman E 1968 Stigma: notes on the management of spoiled identity. Penguin, Harmondsworth

Goffman E 1971 The presentation of self in everyday life. Penguin, Harmondsworth

Goffman E 1974 Frame analysis: an essay on the organisation of experience. Penguin, Harmondsworth

Goldblatt P 1988 Changes in social class between 1971 and 1981: could these affect mortality differentials among men of working age? Population Trends 51: 9–17

Goldblatt P 1989 Mortality by social class, 1971–85. Population Trends 56: 6–15

Goldthorpe J 1980 Social mobility and class structure in modern Britain. Clarendon Press, Oxford

Goldthorpe J H 1983 Women and class analysis: in defence of the conventional view. Sociology 17: 465–488

Goldthorpe J H, Hope K 1974 The social grading of occupations: a new approach and scale. Clarendon Press, Oxford

Goldthorpe J H, Payne C 1986 Trends in intergenerational class mobility in England and Wales 1972–1983. Sociology 20: 1–24

Goodenough W H 1964 Cultural anthropology and linguistics. In: Hymes D (ed) Language in culture and society: a reader in linguistics and anthropology. Harper & Row, New York, p 36–39

Gordon I 1951 Social status and active prevention of disease. Monthly Bulletin of the Ministry of Health 10: 59–61

Gorer G 1965 Death, grief and mourning. Gresset, London

Graham H 1991 The concept of caring in feminist research: the case of domestic service. Sociology 25: 61–78

Graham J M 1983 Experimental nursing homes for elderly people in the National Health Service. Age and Ageing 12: 273–274

Gray P G, Todd J E, Slack G L, Bulman J S 1970 Adult dental health in England and Wales in 1968, SS 411. HMSO, London

Green H 1988 Informal carers. HMSO, London

Green J M, Coupland V A, Kitzinger J V 1990 Expectations, experiences and psychological outcomes of childbirth: a prospective study of 825 women. Birth 17, 1: 15–24

Gregson B A, Cartlidge A M, Bond J 1991 Interprofessional collaboration in primary health care organisations. Occasional Paper No. 52. Journal of the Royal College of General Practitioners, London

Griffin T 1991 Dying with dignity. Office of Health Economics, London

Gubrium J F, Holstein J A 1990 What is family? Mayfield Publishing Company, Mountain View, California

Haavio-Mannila E 1986 Inequalities in health and gender. Social Science and Medicine 22: 141–149

Habermas J 1972 Knowledge and human interests. Heinemann, London

Hall D J 1977 Social relations and innovations: changing the state of play in hospitals. Routledge & Kegan Paul, London

Hall D, Stacey M 1979 Beyond separation: further studies of children in hospital. Routledge & Kegan, London

Ham C 1985 Health policy in Britain. Macmillan, London

Hammersley M 1992 On feminist methodology. Sociology 26: 187–206

Hammersley M, Atkinson P 1983 Ethnography: Principles in practice. Tavistock, London

Hamnett C, McDowell L, Sarre P 1989 Restructuring Britain: the changing social structure. Sage Publications, London

Handy C 1989 The age of unreason. Business Books, London

Hannay D R 1979 Factors associated with formal symptom referral. Social Science and Medicine 13A: 101–104

Hardey M, Crow G 1991 Lone parenthood: coping with constraints and making opportunities. Harvester Wheatsheaf, London

Hargreaves D H 1977 The process of typification in classroom interaction. British Journal of Educational Psychology 47: 274–284

Harris C C, Stacey M 1969 A note on the term 'extended family'. In: Stacey M (ed) Comparability in social research. Heinemann, London, p 56–64

Harrisson S 1977 Families in stress: a study of the long-term medical treatment of children and parental stress. Royal College of Nursing, London

Hart E 1991 Ghost in the machine. Health Service Journal 101: 20–22

Haskey J 1988 Trends in marriage and divorce, cohort analyses of the proportion of marriages ending in divorce. Population Trends 54: 21–28

Haskey J 1990a Children in families broken by divorce. Population Trends 61: 35–42

Haskey J 1990b Identical address at marriage and pre-marital cohabitation: results from linking marriage registration and census records. Population Trends 59: 20–29

Haskey J 1991 Estimated numbers and demographic characteristics of one-parent families in Great Britain. Population Trends 65: 35–47

Haskey J, Kelly S 1991 Population estimates by cohabitation and legal marital status: a trial set of new estimates. Population Trends 66: 30–44

Haskey J, Kiernan K 1989 Cohabitation in Great Britain: characteristics and estimated numbers of cohabiting partners. Population Trends 58: 23–32

Hawthorn G 1976 Enlightenment and despair: a history of sociology. Cambridge University Press, Cambridge

Hawton K 1992 By their own hand. British Medical Journal 304: 1000

Hayward J 1986 Report of the nursing process evaluating working group. King's College, Nursing Education Research Unit, London

Heady J A, Heasman M A 1959 Social and biological factors in infant mortality: studies on medical and population subjects, No. 15. HMSO, Table 5A, London

Hearn J 1982 Notes on patriarchy, professionalisation and the semi-professions. Sociology 16: 184–202

Heath A, Evans G 1988 Working class conservatism and middle-class socialists. In: Javell R, Witherspoon S, Brook L (eds) British Social Attitudes: The 5th Report. Gower, Aldershot, p 53–69

Henderson V 1966 The nature of nursing. Collier Macmillan, London

Hertz R 1905 La representation collective de la mort. Sociologique

Hertz R 1960 Death and the right hand: a contribution to the collective representation of death. Translated by R & C Needham. Cohen & West, London

Herzlich C 1973 Health and illness. Academic Press, London

Herzlich C, Pierret J 1987 Illness and self in society. Johns Hopkins, Baltimore

Heyman R, Shaw M P, Harding J 1984 A longitudinal study of changing attitudes to work among nurse trainees in two British general hospitals. Journal of Advanced Nursing 9: 297–305

Himsworth H 1984 Epidemiology, genetics and sociology. Journal of Bio-Social Science 15: 159–176

Hinton J 1972 Dying. Penguin, Harmondsworth

Hockey J 1990 Experiences of death: an anthropological account. Edinburgh University Press, Edinburgh

Holding T A, Barraclough B M 1978 Undetermined deaths – suicide or accident? British Journal of Psychiatry 133: 542–549

Hollingshead A B, Redlich F C 1958 Social class and mental illness: a community study. John Wiley & Sons, New York

House A 1987 Mood disorders after stroke: a review of the evidence. International Journal of Geriatric Psychiatry 2: 211–221

Hughes E C. 1958 Men and their work. Free Press, Glencoe, Illinois

Hunt A 1986 Use of quantitative methods in researching issues which affect women. Methodological Issues in Gender Research 10: 12–19

Hunt M 1990 Caring for the terminally ill at home. Nursing Standard 4, 39: 23–26

Illich I 1975 Medical nemises: the expropriation of health. Calder and Boyars, London

Illsley R 1955 Social class selection and class differences in relation to stillbirths and infant deaths. British Medical Journal II: 1520–1524

Illsley R 1980 Professional or public health? Sociology in health and medicine. The Nuffield Provincial Hospitals Trust, London

James N 1989 Emotional labour: skill and work in the social regulation of feelings. Sociological Review 37: 15–42

James P M C 1965 The problem of dental caries. British Dental Journal 119: 295–299

James V 1986 Care and work in nursing the dying: a participant study of a continuing care unit. Unpublished PhD thesis. University of Aberdeen, Aberdeen

Janowitz M 1956 Some consequences of social mobility in the United States. Transactions of the Third World Congress of Sociology 3 191–201

Jeffrey R 1979 Normal rubbish: deviant patients in casualty departments. Sociology of Health and Illness 1: 90–107

Jellife D B, Jellife E F P 1978 Human milk in the modern world. Oxford University Press, Oxford

Jenkins P M, Feldman B S, Stirrups D R 1984 The effect of social factors on referrals for orthodontic advice and treatment. British Journal of Orthodontics 11: 24–26

Jenkins-Clarke S 1992 Measuring nursing workload: a cautionary tale. Discussion Paper 96. Centre for Health Economics, University of York, York

Jervis J 1957 On the office and duties of coroners. 9th edn. Sweet & Maxwell, London

John A L 1961 A study of the psychiatric nurse. Churchill Livingstone, Edinburgh

Johnson M 1983 Professional careers and biographies. In: Dingwall R, Lewis P (eds) The sociology of the professions: lawyers, doctors and others. Macmillan, London, p 242–262

Johnson T 1977 The professions in the class structure. Allen & Unwin, London

Johnson T J 1972 Professions and power. Macmillan, London

Kane R L, Klein S J, Bernstein L, Rothenburg R 1986 The role of the hospice in reducing the impact of bereavement. Journal of Chronic Diseases 39: 735–742

Kane R L, Wales J, Bernstein L, Leibowitz A, Kaplan S 1984 A randomised controlled trial of hospice care. The Lancet i: 890–894

Kaplan D M, Smith A, Grobstein R, Fischman S E 1973 Family mediation of stress. Social Work July: 60–69

Kasl S V, Cobb S 1966 Health behaviour, illness behaviour and sick-role behaviour. I. Health and illness behaviour. Archives of Environmental Health 12: 246–266

Kasl S V, Cobb S 1966 Health behaviour, illness behaviour and sick-role behaviour. II. Sick-role behaviour. Archives of Environmental Health 12: 531–542

Katz F E 1969 Nurses. In: Etzioni A (ed) The semi-professions and their organisation. The Free Press, New York, p 54–81

Kavanaugh R 1972 Facing death. Penguin, Baltimore

Kelly MP, May D 1982 Good and bad patients: a review of the literature and a theoretical critique. Journal of Advanced Nursing 7: 147–156

Kesey K 1973 One flew over the cuckoo's nest. Picador, London

King's Fund 1990 Racial equality: the nursing profession. Equal Opportunities Task Force, Occasional Paper No. 6. King Edward's Hospital Fund, London

Kinnersly P 1973 The hazards of work: how to fight them. Pluto Press, London

Kirkham MJ 1983 Labouring in the dark: limitations on the giving of information to enable patients to orientate themselves to the likely events and timescale of labour. In: Wilson-Barnett J (ed) Nursing research: ten studies in patient care. John Wiley & Sons, Chichester, p 81–99

Klaus M, Kennell J 1976 Maternal infant bonding. Mooby, St. Louis

Klein R 1989 The politics of the NHS. 2nd edn. Longman, Harlow

Knaus W A, Draper E A, Wagner D P et al 1986 An evaluation of outcome from intensive care in major medical centers. Annals of Internal Medicine 194: 410–418

Knowelden J, Keeling J, Nicholl P 1985 Post neo-natal mortality. HMSO, London

Knox P L 1979 The accessibility of primary care to urban patients: a geographical analysis. Journal of the Royal College of General Practitioners 29: 160–168

Kobasa S C 1979 Stressful life events, personality and health. Journal of Personality and Social Psychology 37: 1–11

Kotarba J A 1983 Chronic pain, its social dimensions. Sage, Beverly Hills

Kramer M 1974 Reality shock: why nurses leave nursing. C V Mosby, New York

Kratz C R 1978 Care of the long-term sick in the community: particularly patients with stroke. Churchill Livingstone, Edinburgh

Kubler-Ross E 1970 On death and dying. Tavistock, London

Kuhn T S 1962 The structure of scientific revolutions. Chicago University Press, Chicago

Lachenmeyer C W 1971 The language of sociology. Columbia University Press, Columbia

Laing R D 1965 The divided self: an existential study in sanity and madness. Penguin, Harmondsworth

Laing R D 1967 Family and individual structure. In: Lomas P (ed) The predicament of the family. Hogarth Press, London, p 107–125

Laing W, Buisson 1992 Laing and Buisson review of private health care. Laing & Buisson, London

Lalonde M 1974 A new perspective on the health of the Canadians: a working document. Information Canada, Ottawa

Land H 1978 Who cares for the family? Journal of Social Policy 7: 257–284

Larkin G 1983 Occupational monopoly and modern medicine. Tavistock, London

Laryea MG 1984 Postnatal care – the midwives' role. Churchill Livingstone, Edinburgh

Laslett P 1965 The world we have lost. Methuen, London

Lawler J 1991 Behind the screens: nursing, somology, and the problem of the body. Churchill Livingstone, Edinburgh, p 1–247

Lazarus R S, Cohen J B 1977 Environmental stress. In: Altman I, Wohlwill J (eds) Human behaviour and environment: advances in theory and research. Plenum, New York, p 89–121

Leete R 1976 Marriage and divorce: trends and patterns. Population Trends 3: 3–8

Lefebvre H 1968 The Sociology of Marx. Pantheon, New York

Leininger M, Watson J 1990 The caring imperative in education. National League for Nursing, New York

Lemert E 1964 Social structure, social control and deviation. In: Clinard M,B. (ed) Anomie and deviant behaviour:a discussion and critique. Free Press, New York, p 57–97

Levin E, Sinclair I, Gorbach P 1989 Families, services and confusion in old age. Avebury, Aldershot

Levitt R, Wall A 1992 The reorganized National Health. 4th edn. Chapman & Hall, London

Lewis E 1976 Stillbirth: psychological consequences and strategies of management. In: Milunsky A (ed) Advances in perinatal medicine, Vol. 3. Plenum Press, New York, p 205–245

Lewis O 1964 The children of Sanchez. Penguin, Harmondsworth

Lindemann E 1944 Symptomatology and management of acute grief. American Journal of Psychiatry 101: 141–148

Lindesmith A R 1947 Opiate addiction. Principia Press, New York

Lindesmith A R 1968 Addiction and opiates. Aldine, Chicago

Litman T J 1974 The family as a basic unit in health and medical care: a social-behavioural overview. Social Science and Medicine 8: 495–519

Lloyd J, Laurence K M 1985 Sequale and support after termination of pregnancy for fetal malformation. British Medical Journal 290: 907–909

Locker D 1981 Symptoms and lless: the cognitive organisation of disorder. Tavistock, London

Lorber J 1975 Good patients and problem patients: conformity and deviance in a general hospital. Journal of Health and Social Behaviour 16: 213–225

Lovell A 1983 Some questions of identity: late miscarriage, stillbirth and perinatal loss. Social Science and Medicine 17: 755–761

Lyotard J 1984 The postmodern condition. Manchester University Press, Manchester

McCormick A, Rosenbaum M, Fleming D 1990 Socioeconomic characteristics of people who consult their general practitioner. Population Trends 59: 8–10

McDowell I, Newell C 1987 Measuring health: a guide to rating scales and questionnaires. Oxford University Press, New York

McEwen J, Finlayson A 1977 Coronary heart disease and patterns of living. Croom Helm, London

McFarlane J K 1976 A charter for caring. Journal of Advanced Nursing 1: 187–196

Macguire J 1969 Threshold to nursing: a review of the literature on recruitment to and withdrawal from nurse training programmes in the UK. Occasional Papers on Social Administration, No. 30. Bell, London

McHaffie H E 1990 Mothers of VLBW babies: How do they adjust? Journal of Advanced Nursing 15: 6–11

MacIlwaine H 1983 The communication patterns of female neurotic patients with nursing staff in psychiatric units of general hospitals. In: Wilson-Barnett J (ed) Nursing research: ten studies in patient care. John Wiley & Sons, Chichester, p 1–24

McIntosh J 1977 Communication and awareness in a cancer ward. Croom Helm, London

McIntosh J 1981 Communicating with patients in their own homes. In: Bridge W, Clark JM (eds) Communication in nursing care. HM + M, London, p 99–114

McIntosh J, Dingwall R 1978 Teamwork in theory and practice. In: Dingwall R, McIntosh J (eds) Readings in the Sociology of Nursing. Churchill Livingstone, Edinburgh, p 118–134

McIntyre S 1978 Obstetric routines in anatenatal care. In: Davis A (ed) Relationships between doctors and patients. Saxon House, London, p 76–105

McIntyre S 1980 Needs and expectations in obstetrics. Health Bulletin 38: 113–118

McIntyre S 1982 Communications between pregnant women and their medical and midwifery attendants. Midwives Chronicle and Nursing Notes 95: 387–394

Mackay L 1989 Nursing a problem. Open University Press, Milton Keynes

McKeganey N P 1990 Drug abuse in the community: needle-sharing and the risks of HIV infection. In: Cunningham-Burley S, McKeganey N P (eds) Readings in medical sociology. Routledge & Kegan Paul, London, p 113–137

McKennell A C, Thomas R K 1968 Adults' and adolescents' smoking habits and attitudes. Government Social Survey No. SS353/B. HMSO, London

McKeown T 1979 The role of medicine: dream, mirage or nemesis? Basil Blackwell, Oxford

McKinlay J B 1979 A case for refocusing upstream: the political economy of illness. In: Jaco E,G. (ed) Patients, physicians and illness. 3rd edn. The Free Press, New York, p 9–25

McKinlay J B 1984 Issues in the political economy of health care. Tavistock, New York

McKinlay J B, McKinlay S M 1972 Some social characteristics of lower working class utilisers and under utilisers of maternity care services. Journal of Health and Social Behaviour 13: 369–382

McKinlay J B, McKinlay S M 1979 The influence of a premarital conception and various obstetric complications on subsequent prenatal health behaviour. Epidemiology and Community Health 33: 84–90

Madge N, Fassam M 1982 Ask the children: experiences of physical disability in the school years. Batsford, London

Malinowski B 1922 Argonauts of the Western Pacific: an account of native enterprise and adventure in the archipelagoes of Malanesian New Guinea. Routledge & Kegan Paul, London

Maris R F W 1969 Social forces in urban suicide. Dorsey Press, Homewood, Illinois

Marris P 1958 Widows and their families. Routledge & Kegan Paul, London

Marris P 1986 Loss and change. 2nd edn. Routledge & Kegan Paul, London

Marsh G N, Channing D M 1986 Deprivation and health in one general practice. British Medical Journal 292: 1173–1176

Marshall G, Newby H, Rose D, Vogler C 1988 Social class in modern Britain. Hutchinson, London

Marshall G, Rose D, Vogler C, Newby H 1985 Class, citizenship and distributional conflict in modern Britain. British Journal of Sociology 36: 259–284

Martin J, Meltzer H, Elliot D 1988 Office of Population Censuses and Surveys Disability Surveys, Report 1: The prevalence of disability among adults. HMSO, London

May D, Kelly MP 1982 Chancers, pests and poor wee souls: problems of legitimation in psychiatric nursing. Sociology of Health and Illness 4: 279–301

Mayston Report 1969 Report of the UK working party on the management structure of local authority nursing services. HMSO, London

Mead G H 1934 Mind, self and society. The University of Chicago Press, Chicago

Mead G H 1964 On social psychology: selected papers. In: Strauss A (ed). University of Chicago Press, Chicago

Mechanic D 1962 The concept of illness behaviour. Journal of Chronic Diseases 15: 189–194

Mechanic D 1992 Medical sociology. 2nd edn. Free Press, New York

Melia K M 1987 Learning and working: the occupational socialization of nurses. Tavistock, London

Merton R 1967 On theoretical sociology. Free Press, New York

Merton R 1968 Social theory and social structure. Free Press, New York

Merton R K 1957 The role-set: problems in sociological theory. British Journal of Sociology 8: 106–120

Merton R K, Reader G, Kendall P 1957 The student physician: introductory studies in the sociology of medical education. Harvard University Press, Cambridge, Mass

Meyer E, Mendelson M 1961 Psychiatric consultations with patients on medical and surgical wards: patterns and processes. Psychiatry 24: 197–220

Miles A 1988 Women and mental Illness. Brighton, Wheatsheaf

Miles A 1991 Women, health and medicine. Open University Press, Milton Keynes

Miles I 1987 Some observations on unemployment and health research. Social Science and Medicine 25: 223–225

Miles R 1982 Racism and migrant labour. Routledge & Kegan Paul, London

Miller E J, Gwynne G V 1972 A life apart: a pilot study of residential institutions for the physically handicapped and the young chronic sick. Tavistock, London

Millman M 1976 The unkindest cut: life in the back rooms of medicine. Morrow, New York

Mills C W W 1970 The sociological imagination. Penguin, Harmondsworth

Ministry of Health 1966 Report of the committee on senior nursing staff structure (The Salmon Report). HMSO, London

Ministry of Health and Board of Education 1939 Interim report of the interdepartmental committee on nursing services (Chairman, The Earl of Athlone). HMSO, London

Ministry of Health and Department of Health for Scotland 1961 Medical staffing structure in the hospital service: report of the joint working party (Chairman, Sir Robert Platt). HMSO, London

Ministry of Health Department of Health for Scotland,and Ministry of Labour and National Service 1947 Report of the working party on the recruitment and training of nurses (Chairman, Sir Robert Wood). HMSO, London

Moos R H 1984 Context and coping: toward a unifying conceptual framework. American Journal of Community Psychology 12: 5–25

Mor V 1987 Hospice care systems: structure, process, costs and outcome. Springer, New York

Morris J N 1975 Uses of epidemiology. 3rd edn. Churchill Livingstone, Edinburgh

Moser C A, Kalton G 1971 Survey methods in social investigation. 2nd edn. Heinemann, London

Moser K A M, Fox A J, Jones D R, Goldblatt P O 1987 Unemployment and mortality: comparison of the 1971 and 1981 longitudinal study census samples. British Medical Journal 294: 86–90

Muetzel P A 1988 Therapeutic nursing. In: Pearson A (ed) Primary nursing. Croom Helm, London, p 89–116

Mulleady G 1987 A review of drug abuse and HIV infection. Psychology and Health 1: 149–163

Mullen K, Illsley R 1981 Unemployment and health: a review of findings and methodology. MRC Medical Sociology Unit, Institute for Medical Sociology, Aberdeen

Murcott A 1981 On the typification of 'bad' patients. In: Atkinson P, Heath C (eds) Medical work: realities and routines. Gower, Farnborough, p 128–140

Murcott A 1983 Introduction. In: Murcott A (ed) Sociology of food and eating. Gower, Aldershot, p 1–5

Murphy E 1982 Social origins of depression in old age. British Journal of Psychiatry 141: 135–142

Murphy J W 1988 Making sense of postmodern sociology. British Journal of Sociology XXXIX: 600–614

National Advisory Committee of Nutrition Education 1983 A discussion paper on proposals for nutritional guidelines for health education in Britain. The Health Education Council, London

Newsom J, Newsom E 1965 Patterns of infant care in an urban community. Penguin, Harmondsworth

NHS Management Executive 1990 Outpatients departments: changing the skill mix. HMSO, London

Nightingale F 1859 Notes on nursing: what it is, and what it is not. Reprinted (1980) Churchill Livingstone, Edinburgh

Nisbett R A 1967 The sociological tradition. Heinemann, London

Nursing Times 1987 Racism: the great divide. Nursing Times 83, 24: 24–31

Nutbeam D, Catford J 1987 Pulse of Wales social survey supplement. Heartbeat Report No. 7. Heartbeat Wales, Cardiff

Oakley A 1972 Sex, gender and society. Temple Smith, London

Oakley A 1976 The family, marriage, and its relationship to illness. In: Tuckett D (ed) An introduction to medical sociology. Tavistock, London, p 74–109

Oakley A, McPherson A, Roberts H 1990 Miscarriage. Penguin, Harmondsworth

Office of Population Censuses and Surveys 1982 General household survey 1980. HMSO, London

Office of Population Censuses and Surveys 1982 Studies in sudden infant death: studies on medical and population subjects No. 45. HMSO, London

Office of Population Censuses and Surveys 1986 Occupational mortality: the Registrar General's decennial supplement for Great Britain, 1979–80, 1982–83. Series DS No. 6. Part I: Commentary. HMSO, London

Office of Population Censuses and Surveys 1988 Occupational mortality, childhood supplement: the Registrar General's decennial supplement for England and Wales, 1979–80, 1982–83. Series DS No. 8. HMSO, London

Office of Population Censuses and Surveys 1990 Standard occupational classification. Volume 1. HMSO, London

Office of Population Censuses and Surveys 1991 Mortality statistics. Series DH2, No. 17. Table 2. HMSO, London

Office of Population Censuses and Surveys 1992 Mortality statistics. Perinatal and infant: social and biological factors. Review of the Registrar General on deaths in England and Wales, 1990. Series DH3 No. 24. HMSO, London

Office of Population Censuses and Surveys and General Register Office for Scotland 1992 1991 Census. Definitions Great Britain. HMSO, London

Office of Population Censuses and Surveys Medical Statistics Division 1978 Social and biological factors in infant mortality, 1975–76. Occasional Paper No. 12. OPCS, London

Olesen VL, Whittaker EW 1968 The silent dialogue: a study in the social psychology of professional socialization. Jossey- Bass, San Francisco

Oswin M 1991 Am I allowed to cry? Souvenir Press, London

Owens P, Glennerster H 1990 Nursing in conflict. Macmillan, London

Pamuk E R 1988 Social class inequality in infant mortality in England and Wales from 1921 to 1980. European Journal of Population 4: 1–21

Parkes C M 1965 Bereavement and mental illness. British Journal of Medical Psychology 38: 1–12

Parkes C M 1972 Accuracy of predictions of survival in later stages of cancer. British Medical Journal 2: 29–31

Parkes C M 1984 'Hospice' versus 'hospital' care: reevaluation after 10 years as seen by surviving spouses. Postgraduate Medical Journal 60: 120–124

Parkes C M 1985 Terminal care: home, hospital or hospice? The Lancet 155–157

Parkes C M 1986 Bereavement: studies of grief in adult life. 2nd edn. Penguin, Harmondsworth

Parkin F 1971 Class inequality and political order. McGibbon & Kee, London

Parkin F 1979 Marxism and class theory: a bourgeois critique. Tavistock, London

Parry N, Parry J 1976 The rise of the medical profession: a study of collective social mobility. Croom Helm, London

Parsons T 1937 The structure of social action: a study in social theory with special reference to a group of recent European writers. McGraw-Hill, New York

Parsons T 1951 The social system. Routledge & Kegan Paul, London

Parsons T 1954 Essays in sociological theory. The Free Press, New York

Parsons T 1964 Social structure and personality. Free Press, New York

Paxman J 1990 Friends in high places. Who runs Britain? Michael Joseph, London

Payne G 1987 Mobility and change in modern society. Macmillan, London

Payne G, Dingwall R, Payne J, Carter M 1981 Sociology and social research. Routledge & Kegan Paul, London

Pearson A 1988 Primary nursing. Croom Helm, London

Pearson A, Pontoon S, Durant I 1992 Nursing beds: an evaluation of the effect of therapeutic nursing. Scutari, London

Petrie AA 1967 Individuality in pain and suffering. University of Chicago Press, Chicago

Phillipson C 1990 The sociology of retirement. In: Bond J, Coleman P (eds) Ageing in society: an introduction to social gerontology. Sage, London

Phizacklea A, Miles R 1980 Labour and racism. Routledge & Kegan Paul, London

Pill R 1983 An apple a day ... some reflections on working class mothers' views on food and health. Gower, Aldershot

Pill R, Stott N C H 1982 Concepts of illness causation and responsibility: some preliminary data from a sample of working class mothers. Social Science and Medicine 16: 43–52

Platt S 1984 Unemployment and suicidal behaviour: a review of the literature. Social Science and Medicine 19: 93–115

Pocock S J, Shaper A G, Cook D G, Phillips A N, Walker M 1987 Social class differences in ischaemic heart disease in British men. The Lancet ii: 197–201

Popper K R 1961 The poverty of historicism. Routledge & Kegan Paul, London

Poulantzas N 1979 Classes in contemporary capitalism. 3rd edn. NLB, London

Pratt L 1973 The significance of the family in medication. Journal of Comparative Family Studies 4: 13–15

Prior L 1989 The social organisation of death. Macmillan, London

Psathas G 1968 The student nurse in the diploma school of nursing. Springer, New York

Quint J C 1967 The nurse and the dying patient. Macmillan, New York

Qureshi H, Walker A 1989 The caring relationship: elderly people and their families. Macmillan, London

Ramazanoglu C 1989 Improving on sociology: problems in taking a feminist standpoint. Sociology 23: 427–442

Ramazanoglu C 1992 On feminist methodology: male reason versus female empowerment. Sociology 26, 2: 207–212

Ransford H E, Smith M L 1991 Grief resolution among the bereaved in hospice and hospital wards. Social Science and Medicine 32: 295–304

Raphael B 1977 Preventive intervention with the recently bereaved. Archives of General Psychiatry 34: 1450–1454

Rapoport R N, Fogerty M P, Raporport R 1982 Families in Britain. Routledge & Kegan Paul, London

Rapoport R, Rapoport R N 1971 Dual-career families. Penguin, Harmondsworth

Rapoport R, Rapoport R N, Strelitz Z 1977 Fathers, mothers and others. Routledge & Kegan Paul, London

Raw M 1978 The treatment of cigarette dependence. In: Israel Y, Glaser F,B., Kalant H, Popham R,E., Schmidt W, Smart R,G. (eds) Research Advances in Alcohol and Drug Problems. 3rd edn. Plenum, New York, p 441–485

Reed J 1989 All dressed up and nowhere to go: nursing assessment in geriatric care. Unpublished PhD Thesis, Newcastle upon Tyne Polytechnic

Reed J, Bond S 1991 Nurses' assessment of elderly patients in hospital. International Journal of Nursing Studies 28, 1: 55–64

Reed M I 1992 The sociology of organisations: themes, perspectives and prospects. Harvester Wheatsheaf, London

Reedy B L E C. 1980 Teamwork in primary health care: a conspectus. In: Fry J (ed) Primary care. Heinemann, London, p 108–138

Registrar General for Scotland 1982 Annual report 1980. HMSO, Edinburgh

Registrar General Scotland 1992 Annual report 1991. HMSO, Edinburgh

Reid I 1989 Social class differences in Britain. 3rd edn. Fontana Press, Glasgow

Reiss D 1981 The family's construction of reality. Harvard University Press, Cambridge, Mass. Report of the Committee on Nursing 1972 (The Briggs Report), Cmnd. 5115. HMSO, London

Report of the Royal Commission on the National Health Service 1979 (The Merrison Report) Cmnd. 7615. HMSO, London

Rex J 1961 Key problems of sociological theory. Routledge & Kegan Paul, London

Reynolds M 1978 No news is bad news: patients' views about communication in hospital. British Medical Journal 1: 1673–1676

Richie J, Jacoby A, Bone M 1981 Access to primary health care. HMSO, London

Riley EMD 1977 What do women want? The question of choice in the conduct of labour. In: Chard T, Richards M (eds) Benefits and hazards of the new obstetrics. Spastics International Medical Publications, Heinemann, London, p 62–71

Roberts H 1981 Doing feminist research. Routledge & Kegan Paul, London

Robinson D 1973 Patients, practitioners and medical care: aspects of medical sociology. Heinemann, London

Robinson I 1988 Reconstructing lives: negotiating the meaning of multiple sclerosis. In: Anderson R, Bury M (eds) Living with chronic illness: the experience of patients and their families. Unwin Hyman, London, p 43–66

Robinson J 1991 Project 2000: the role of resistance in the process of professional growth. Journal of Advanced Nursing 16: 820–824

Robinson W S 1951 The logical structure of analytical induction. American Sociological Review 16: 812–818

Roemer J E 1982 A general theory of exploitation and class. Harvard University Press, Cambridge, Massachusetts

Rogers K B 1981 Face masks: which, when, where and why? Journal of Hospital Infection 2: 1–4

Roper N, Logan W W, Tierney A J 1990 Elements of nursing: a model for nursing based on a model for living. 3rd edn. Churchill Livingstone, Edinburgh

Rose D, Marshall G 1991 Constructing the (W)right classes. Sociology 20: 440–455

Rosenthal C J, Marshall V W, Macpherson A S, French S E 1980 Nurses, patients and families. Croom Helm, London

Roth J A 1963 Timetables: structuring the passage of time in hospital treatment and other careers. Bobs-Merrill, New York

Roth J A, Eddy E M 1967 Rehabilitation for the unwanted. Atherton, New York

Rowntree B S 1901 Poverty: a study of town life. Macmillan, London

Royal College of Physicians of London 1983 Obesity. Journal of the Royal College of Physicians of London 17: 5–65

Royal Commission on Marriage and Divorce 1956 Report 1951–1955, Cmnd 9678. HMSO, London

Royal Commission on the National Health Service 1979 (The Merrison Report) Cmnd 7615. HMSO, London

Runciman P 1982 Ward sisters: their problems at work – 2. Nursing Times Occasional Paper 78: 51: 145–147

Runciman P 1983 Ward sister at work. Churchill Livingstone, Edinburgh

Runciman W G 1966 Relative deprivation and social justice. Routledge & Kegan Paul, London

Russell M A H 1976 Tobacco smoking and nicotine dependence. In: Gibbins R J, Israel Y, Kalant H, Popham R E, Schmidt W, Smart R G (eds) Research advances in alcohol and drug problems. 3rd edn. John Wiley & Sons, New York, p 1–47

Rutter M 1972 Maternal deprivation reassessed. Penguin, Harmondsworth

Rutter M, Madge N 1976 Cycles of disadvantage: a review of research. Heinemann, London

Sainsbury P, Grad J 1970 The psychiatrist and the geriatric patient. Journal of Geriatric Psychiatry 4: 23–41

Salvage J 1992 The new nursing: empowering patients or empowering nurses? In: Policy issues in nursing. Open University Press, Milton Keynes, p 9–23

Sanson C D, Wakefield J, Yule R 1972 Cervical cytology in the Manchester area: changing patterns of response. In: Wakefield J (ed) Seek wisely to prevent. HMSO, London, p 151–159

Saunders C M, Baines M 1983 Living with the dying: the management of terminal disease. Oxford University Press, Oxford

Saussure F 1974 Course in general linguistics. 2nd edn. Peter Owen, London

Schachter S 1978 Pharmacological and psychological determinants of smoking. In: Thornton R E (ed) Smoking behaviour. Churchill Livingstone, Edinburgh

Scheff T J 1964 The societal reaction to deviance: ascriptive elements in the psychiatric screening of mental patients in a midwestern state. Social Problems 11: 401–413

Scheff T J 1966 Typification in the diagnostic practices of rehabilitation. In: Sussman M,B. (ed) Sociology and rehabilitation. American Sociological Association, Washington, p 139–144

Schott T, Badura B 1988 Wives of heart attack patients: the stress of caring. In: Anderson R, Bury M (eds) Living with chronic illness: the experience of patients and their families. Unwin Hyman, London, p 117–136

Schutz A 1972 The phenomenology of the social world. Heinemann, London

Schutz A, Luckmann T 1974 The structures of the life world. Heinemann, London

Seale C 1991a Death from cancer and death from other causes: the relevance of the hospice approach. Palliative Medicine 5: 12–19

Seale C 1991b Communication and awareness about death: a study of a random sample of dying people. Social Science and Medicine 32, 8: 943–952

Seale C 1991c A comparison of hospice and conventional care. Social Science and Medicine 32, 2: 147–152

Seale C 1992 Community nurses and the care of the dying. Social Science and Medicine 34: 375–382

Seale C F 1989 What happens in hospices: a review of research evidence. Social Science and Medicine 28: 551–559

Secretaries of State for Health Social Security, Wales and Scotland 1989 Caring for people: community care in the next decade and beyond. CM849 (White paper). HMSO, London

Secretary of State for Health 1991 The health of the nation: a consultative document for health in England. HMSO, London

Secretary of State for Health 1992 The health of the nation: a strategy for health in England. HMSO, London

Segal L 1983 What is to be done about the family? Penguin, Harmondsworth

Shaffir W B, Stebbins R A 1991 Experiencing fieldwork: an insider view of qualitative research. Sage, Beverly Hills

Shaw M, Heyman R, Harding J 1984 Competing ideologies: implications for nurse socialisation. Unpublished Mimeograph, Newcastle Polytechnic

Sheiham A 1983 Sugars and dental decay. The Lancet I: 282–284

Silverman D 1970 The theory of organisations. Heinemann, London

Silverman D 1987 Communication and medical practice. Sage, London

Simpson I H 1979 From student to nurse: a longitudinal study of socialisation. Cambridge University Press, New York

Sinclair H 1984 The career of nurse graduates. Nursing Times Occasional Paper 80: 56–59

Smith A, Jacobson B 1988 The nation's health: a strategy for the 1990s. King Edward's Hospital Fund for London, London

Smith D M 1977 Health care of people at work: agricultural workers. Journal of the Society of Occupational Medicine 27: 87–92

Smith H W 1975 Strategies of social research: the methodological imagination. Prentice-Hall, Englewood Cliffs, NJ

Smith P 1992 The emotional labour of nursing. Macmillan, London

Smith R 1987 Unemployment and health: a disaster and a challenge. Oxford University Press, Oxford

Sognnaes R F 1948 Analysis of war-time reduction of dental caries in European children. American Journal of Diseases of Children 75: 792–821

Solzhenitsyn A 1971 Cancer ward. Penguin, Harmondsworth

Sontag S 1983 Illness as metaphor. Penguin, Harmondsworth

Sontag S 1990 AIDS and its metaphors. Penguin, Harmondsworth

Sorokin P A 1959 Social and cultural mobility. The Free Press, Glencoe, Illinois

Spicer C C, Lipworth L 1966 Regional and social factors in infant mortality: studies on medical and population subjects No. 19. HMSO, Table 13, London

St. Christopher's Hospice Information Service 1992 Directory of Hospice Services. St Christopher's Hospice Information Service, London

Stacey M 1969 The myth of community studies. British Journal of Sociology 20: 134–147

Stacey M 1988 The sociology of health and healing: a textbook. Unwin Hyman, London

Stacey M, Dearden R, Pill R, Robinson D 1970 Hospitals, children and their families: the report of a pilot study. Routledge & Kegan Paul, London

Stacey M, Homans H 1978 The sociology of health and illness: its present state, future prospects and potential for health research. Sociology 12: 281–307

Stainton Rogers W 1991 Explaining health and illness. Harvester-Wheatsheaf, Hemel Hempstead

Stein L 1978 The doctor-nurse game. In: Dingwall R, McIntosh J (eds) Readings in the sociology of nursing. Churchill Livingstone, Edinburgh

Stein L, Watts D, Howell T 1990 The doctor-nurse game revisited. New England Journal of Medicine 322: 546–549

Stimson G, Webb B 1975 Going to see the doctor: the consultation process in general practice. Routledge & Kegan Paul, London

Stockwell F 1972 The unpopular patient. Royal College of Nursing, London

Strauss A 1987 Qualitative analysis for social scientists. Cambridge University Press, Cambridge

Strauss A N 1978 Negotiations. Jossey-Bass, San Francisco

Strauss A N, Corbin J 1990 Basics of qualitative research. Sage, Newbury Park

Strauss A, Fagerhaugh S, Suczek B, Wiener C 1985 The social organization of medical work. University of Chicago, Chicago

Strauss A, Schatzman L, Ehrlich D, Bucher R, Sabshin M 1963 The hospital and its negotiated order. In: Friedson E (ed) The hospital in modern society. Collier-Macmillan, London, p 147–169

Strong P M 1979a The ceremonial order of the clinic: parents, doctors, and medical bureaucracies. Routledge & Kegan Paul, London

Strong P 1979b Sociological imperialism and the profession of medicine: a critical examination of the thesis of medical imperialism. Social Science and Medicine 13A: 199–215

Strong P M 1988 Minor courtesies and macro structures. In: Drew P, Wootton A (eds) Erving Goffman: Exploring the interaction order. Polity Press, Cambridge

Strong P, Robinson J 1990 The NHS – under new management. Open University Press, Milton Keynes

Sudnow D 1967 Passing on: the social organisation of dying. Prentice-Hall, Englewood Cliffs, NJ

Szasz T S 1971 The manufacture of madness. Routledge & Kegan Paul, London

Tansey M J B, Opie L H, Kennelly B M 1977 High mortality in obese women diabetics with acute myocardial infarction. British Medical Journal 1: 1624–1626

Taylor Lord 1975 Poverty, wealth and health or getting the dosage right. British Medical Journal 4: 207–211

The Lancet 1977 Nitrate and human cancer. The Lancet II: 281–282

The Politics of Health Group 1980 Food and profit – it makes you sick, Pamphlet No.1. The Politics of Health Group, London

Thomas L H, Bond S 1991 Outcomes of nursing care: the case of primary nursing. International Journal of Nursing Studies 28, 4: 291–314

Thomas R, Elias P 1989 Development of the standard occupational classification. Population Trends 55: 16–21

Thomson A M, Black A E 1975 Nutritional aspects of human lactation. Bulletin of World Health Organisation 52: 163–177

Titmuss R 1968 Committment to welfare. Allen & Unwin, London

Todd J E, Dodd T 1985 Children's dental health in the UK, 1983. HMSO, London

Toffler A 1970 Future shock. Bodley Head, London

Towell D 1976 Understanding psychiatric nursing: a sociological study of modern psychiatric nursing practice. Royal College of Nursing, London

Townsend J, Frank A,O., Fermont D, Dyer S, Karran O, Walgrave A 1990 Terminal cancer care and patients' preference for place of death: a prospective study. British Medical Journal 301: 415–417

Townsend P 1962 The last refuge: a survey of residential institutions and homes for the aged in England and Wales. Routledge & Kegan Paul, London

Townsend P 1965 On the likelihood of admission to an institution. In: Shanas E, Streib G F (eds) Social structure and the family generational relations. Prentice-Hall, New York, p 163–187

Townsend P 1979 Poverty in the United Kingdom: a survey of household resources and standards of living. Penguin, Harmondsworth

Townsend P, Davidson N 1982 Inequalities in health (The Black Report). Penguin, Harmondsworth

Townsend P, Davidson N, Whitehead M 1988 Inequalities in health. Penguin, Harmondsworth

Townsend P, Phillimore P, Beattie A 1988 Health and deprivation: inequality and the north. Croom Helm, London

Turner R 1968 Talk and troubles: contact problems of former mental patients. Unpublished PhD dissertation. University of California, Berkeley

Turner R H 1962 Role-taking: process versus conformity. In: Rose A M (ed) Human behaviour and social processes. Routledge & Kegan Paul, London, p 20–40

Ujhely G B 1963 The nurse and her problem patients. Springer, New York

Ungerson C 1983 Women and caring: skills, tasks and taboos, the public and the private. Heinemann, London

Ungerson C 1987 Policy is personal: sex, gender and informal care. Tavistock, London

United Kingdom Central Council for Nursing Midwifery & Health Visiting 1986 Project 2000: a new preparation for practice. UKCC, London

Van Gennep A, Vizedom M B, Cassee G L 1960 The rites of passage. Routledge & Kegan Paul, London

Van Itallie T B 1978 Dietary fibre and obesity. American Journal of Clinical Nutrition 31: S43–S52

Venters M 1981 Familial coping with chronic and severe childhood illness: the case of cystic fibrosis. Social Science and Medicine 15A: 289–297

Vincent C E 1967 Mental health and the family. Journal of Marriage and the Family, February: 18–39

Vovelle M 1976 La redecoverte de la mort. Pensee 189: 3–18

Waddington I 1984 The medical profession in the industrial revolution. Gill & Macmillan, London

Waitzkin H, Stoeckle JD 1972 The communication of information about illness: clinical, sociological and methodological considerations. Advances in Psychomatic Medicine 8: 180–215

Walker A 1982 Community care: the family, the state and social policy. Basil Blackwell, Oxford

Wallace W L 1971 The logic of science in sociology. Aldine-Atherton, Chicago

Webb C 1984 Feminist methodology in nursing research. Journal of Advanced Nursing 9: 249–256

Weber M 1948 Science as a vocation. In: Gerth H, Wright Mills C (eds) From Max Weber: Essays in sociology. Routledge & Kegan Paul, London

Weber M 1948 The Protestant ethic and the spirit of capitalism. Unwin Hyman, London

Wells T J 1980 Problems in geriatric nursing care. Churchill Livingstone, Edinburgh

Werner E E, Smith R S 1982 Vulnerable but invincible: a study of resilient children. McGraw-Hill, New York

Westergard J H, Resler H 1976 Class in a capitalist society: a study of contemporary Britain. Penguin, Harmondsworth

Westermark E 1926 A short history of marriage. Macmillan, London

Whitehead M 1987 The health divide: inequalities in health in the 1980s. Health Education Council, London

Whitehouse C R 1985 Effect of distance from surgery on consultation rates in an urban practice. British Medical Journal 290: 359–362

Whorton D, Krauss R M, Marshall S, Milby T H 1977 Infertility in male pesticide workers. Lancet ii: 1259–1261

Wilkin D, Hallam L, Doggett A-M 1992 Measures of need and outcome for primary health care. Oxford University Press, Oxford

Wilkinson R G 1978 A classy way to die. Ecologist Quarterly Summer: 102–113

Wilkinson S 1991 Factors which influence how nurses communicate with cancer patients. Journal of Advanced Nursing 16: 677–688

Willcocks D, Peace S, Kellaher L 1987 Private lives in public places: a research-based critique of residential life in local authority old people's homes. Tavistock, London

Williams R 1983 Concepts of health: an analysis of lay logic. Sociology 17: 185–205

Williamson J, Stokoe I H, Gray S, Fisher M, Smith A, McGhee A, Stephenson E 1964 Old people at home: their unreported needs. Lancet II: 1117–1120

Wilson A, Startup R 1991 Nurse socialisation: issues and problems. Journal of Advanced Nursing 16: 1478–1486

Wilson E 1982 Women, the 'community' and the 'family'. In: Walker A (ed) Community care: the family, the state and social policy. Basil Blackwell & Martin Robertson, Oxford, p 40–55

Wolf Z R 1986 Nurses' work: the sacred and the profane. In: Behind the screens. Holistic Nursing Practice, p 29–35

World Health Organization 1971 Report on the statistical aspects of the family as a unit in health studies. December 14–20, DSI/72–6. WHO, Geneva

World Health Organization 1976 Nursing process workbook. WHO Regional Office for Europe, Copenhagen

World Health Organization 1983 Constitution of the World Health Organization, 33rd edn. World Health Organization, Geneva, p 1

Worsley P 1974 The state of theory and the status of theory. BSA presidential address 1973. Sociology 8: 1–17

Worsley P 1977 Introducing sociology. 2nd edn. Penguin, Harmondsworth

Wright E O 1979 Class, crisis and the state. 2nd edn. Verso, London

Wright E O 1985 Classes. Verso, London

Wright E O, Hachen D, Costello C, Sprague J 1982 The American class structure. American Sociological Review 47: 709–726

Wright M 1981 Coming to terms with death: patient care in a hospice for the terminally ill. In: Atkinson P, Heath C (eds) Medical work: realities and routines. Gower, Aldershot, p 141–151

Wright S G 1990 My patient – my nurse: a guide to primary nursing. Scutari, London

Yeandle S 1984 Women's working lives. Tavistock, London

Young K 1977 Values in the policy process. Policy and Politics 5: 1–22

Young M 1961 The rise of the meritocracy 1870–1933. Penguin, Harmondsworth

Young M, Benjamin B, Wallis C 1963 The mortality of widowers. The Lancet II: 454–456

Young M, Willmott P 1957 Family and kinship in East London. Routledge & Kegan Paul, London

Young M, Willmott P 1973 The symmetrical family: a study of work and leisure in the London region. Routledge & Kegan Paul, London

Zborowski M 1969 People in pain. Jossey-Bass, San Francisco

Znaniecki F 1934 The method of sociology. Farrar & Rinehart, New York

Index

SUBJECT INDEX

AUTHOR INDEX